THE DEVELOPMENTAL THERAPIST

A PROTOTYPE OF THE PEDIATRIC OCCUPATIONAL THERAPIST

BARBARA SHARPE BANUS

MAUREEN HAYES
CAROLYN ABBE KENT
M. PATRICIA KOMICK
DORIS A. SUKIENNICKI

Charles B. Slack, Inc.
Thorofare, New Jersey 08086

Acknowledgments

In order to write this book for you, we have sought help from many sources. We wish to thank you all. Carol Schad Bull and Shirley Perlmutter generated and nurtured the idea of the book several years ago. Wilma West generated action three years ago. Many other occupational therapists have helped make it a reality ever since by helping us clarify and critique our concepts and our writing: Martha Buskirk, Shirley Carr, Margaret Cooper, Claire Derry, Mary Fiorentino, Beverly Gladstein, Jerry Johnson and the faculty in the Division of Occupational Therapy at Boston University, Jim Oien, Judy Riesman, Ruth Wiemer and Betty Yerxa. All of my former occupational therapy students also must receive credit for regularly and emphatically complaining about the absence of one book which could replace the excessive number of hours spent in library research.

We also thank the nonoccupational therapists who were more than willing to help us understand and integrate material which is vital to our work with children, but less familiar to us as occupational therapists: Louise Bates Ames, Associate Director, Gesell Institute of Child Development; Amy Blackwell, Staff Psychologist, Children's Hospital Medical Center; Margaret Brewster, Education Director, Handicapped Children's Preschool; Ruth Butler, Harvard Research Associate and Consultant in Social Work in M & I and C & Y Projects in the Division of Family Health Services, Massachusetts Department of Public Health; William K. Frankenburg, Assistant Professor of Pediatrics, University of Colorado Medical Center; Andrew Sabersky, Research Division, Stanford Linear Accelerator Center; Bickley Simpson, Research Associate, New England Materials Instruction Center; Jerry Trimble, Professor of Child Psychology, Massachusetts Bay Community College; Irving Silverman, Assistant Professor of Pediatrics, Harvard Medical School.

The Boston University faculty who assisted us included Y.S. Chang, Professor, School of Business Administration; Frances K. Grossman, Associate Professor, Department of Psychology; Whitney Powers, Professor and Chairman, Department of Health Sciences; Don G. Sandy, Associate Professor, Director of Speech, Language and Hearing Pathology, School of Education; and Shirley Stockmeyer, Associate Professor of Physical Therapy, Sargent College of Allied Health Professions.

Finally, we say a special thank you to our husbands, families and friends, all of whom shared in the growth and development of this book: Mario Banus, Dave Kent, Bob Sukiennicki and Nick Haddad; Diane Kent, Ernie Way, Barbara Cohen and Beverly Green.

To all my students

who requested the book

and to Mario

whose love and encouragement

made it possible

Foreword

In beginning a course of study in development, we might well first reflect a bit on life as the student has experienced and observed it, and ask of the student, "What do you already know of growth and development?" The student may think she knows too little or too much — too little if she thinks she knows nothing, too much if she thinks she has understood it thoroughly. Can we in a foreword put *development* in perspective? I don't know. Perhaps the answer lies only in the student after she has read, reflected and discussed the textual material. A text can only illuminate what one already has experienced and can lead one further in pondering the experience of life. I would hope that a student would read the chapters that follow, bit by bit as I did, and think along the way of growing and developing things that she has encountered in her entire life experience, not just her clinical training. In this way, the student can multiply the examples available to her study, and can enrich her understanding of the world about her. This will lead her to becoming a wiser and more empathetic person, and inevitably a better professional, as she becomes more skilled technically.

What has fascinated me, as I have seen developmental therapy in practice, is that the developmental approach provides the link between the humane and the scientific in the understanding of the process of life. In the study of development, we begin to probe the mysteries and poetry of life. We ask what occurs in chemical or physical terms when change occurs in an organism. But to pretend that the scientific description of molecular processes is sufficient in understanding life is to ignore the tremendous gaps in our knowledge of the underlying principles of life and the unique characteristics of each individual. To look at human life as a developmental process, occurring in a predictable scientific sequence but in an unpredictable individual milieu, is the essence of the developmentalist's contribution.

The chapters that follow say much about development as a scientific discipline. They certainly do not say it all, nor do they say it the way every scientist would wish it put. But, in sum, this book only opens a door. Read on, dear student, after you finish this book, and continue to learn from other books. But, more important, learn from the world about you, about people and how they become what they are. If this book helps you do that, it will achieve its intention of helping you to help others better.

Dorothy J. Worth, M.D. Director
Division of Family Health Services Mass. Dept. of Public Health

Boston, Massachusetts   *July 26, 1971*

Preface

The reasons for this book are evident. You, the occupational therapy students, have been requesting a book on children, their development and disabilities for a long time. You and other students in the fields of health and education have spent too much time researching basic information about children that either was not available or not accessible in a single unit. When the material was found, it often seemed fragmented and only partially applicable to occupational therapy in pediatrics.

We, the authors, hope that *The Developmental Therapist — A Prototype of the Pediatric Occupational Therapist* will provide you with a framework which will motivate you to pursue your study of children. We will introduce you to basic knowledge, skills and attitudes which are necessary to successful work with children and we will only survey the highly theoretical and technical material which is used by experienced practitioners. Too often, practical basic information about children and their therapy is neglected by your professors and supervising clinical therapists. Because of this, you may not learn the answers to some fundamental questions such as: What are the theories of child development which can guide me in my day-to-day work with children? How do I plan a child's evaluation? How do I plan treatment? What tools can I use in treatment? What should I include in the child's treatment? When should I treat him? What are the common psychological problems of sick or disabled children? How can I work most effectively with other health care personnel? What are my responsibilities to the child? How can I help his parents? How can I describe my position as a pediatric occupational therapist to others?

Our objective is to provide you with a resource that will help answer some of these fundamental questions. We anticipate that you will be able to study and digest much of this material independently of classroom lectures. Your professors and clinical supervisors then will have the time to expand upon and integrate this material with the more complex and constantly changing material which is directly related to your developing competence in pediatric occupational therapy. With this combination, we hope that you will develop the ability to work with children, their parents and other health care personnel more rapidly and effectively than would otherwise be possible.

This text is based on the content and organization of the pediatric occupational therapy courses which I taught first at the University of Illinois and then at Boston University. In these courses, the students had lecture/discussion sessions adjacent to clinical experiences with handicapped children during which they applied their "book learning" to real children. Initially, the students asked, "Why do we have to study pediatric occupational therapy?" and "What is the purpose of the organization of this course?" We hope that you will answer the first question yourself after you become well acquainted with children through studying and playing with them.

The second question can be answered more easily. There are many ways to organize any course or any book. Consequently, my organization may or may not be the most meaningful for you. To help you understand my approach and to choose your own road through the contents, a brief description of each chapter and alternative approaches follows.

The Introduction very briefly defines my concept of pediatric occupational therapy which is expanded upon throughout the book. Chapter One, The Theoretical Basis for Development, reviews some of the common developmental concepts and terminology as well as developmental theories which are applicable to pediatric occupational therapy. Although it may be heavy reading because of its theoretical nature, Chapter One will help you to understand and use child development concepts and terminology more accurately. It will also facilitate your understanding of the following chapters and other related literature.

Chapters Two, Evaluation, and Three, Treatment, are two sections which students have found valuable because general information on the process of evaluating and treating children is almost nonexistent. You may want to scan these chapters and then refer to them when you undertake specific evaluation and treatment procedures such as setting up the evaluation room, sequencing the test items, interviewing parents or planning a child's daily treatment schedule. You can apply these practical ideas on evaluation and treatment to all work with children, irrespective of their abilities and disabilities. It is for this reason that the general description of evaluation and treatment precedes Chapters Four, Five and Six — Neuromotor Development; Psychosocial Development: Function and Dysfunction; and The Development of Visual-Perceptual-Motor Function.

In Chapters Four and Five, the contributing authors have prefaced their description of occupational therapy evaluation and treatment procedures with a review of the developmental sequences. Although this can be found in more detail in other literature, we have composited it for a readily available reference. Literature which contains more detailed developmental information can be obtained through the extensive bibliographies at the end of each of these chapters. I believe that the authors' introductions to the contemporary evaluation and treatment procedures used in pediatric occupational therapy will help you separate the psychiatric and physical disability theory and practice which is relevant to children from that which is useful only for adults.

Instead of identifying multiple approaches to visual-perceptual-motor evaluation and treatment, Chapter Six mainly offers one scheme for evaluation and treatment which is based on the work done at Meeting Street School in Providence, Rhode Island. This chapter offers less of the theoretical concepts of development, evaluation and treatment and more of the practical application than that suggested in Chapters Four and Five. Because of this and the fact that visual-perceptual-motor function has always been a basic component of treatment in both psychiatric and physical disabilities (derived from the occupational therapists' focus on eye-hand coordination), it might be helpful to study this chapter before those on neuromotor and psychosocial behavior.

Chapter Seven, The Development of Communication and Cognition, reviews these developmental processes and the ways in which the occupational therapist can stimulate them. Although these two areas are often not considered part of the occupational therapist's domain, it is essential that we understand them because of the complex interactions among all developmental processes. Also, we must be prepared to assess and stimulate the child's speech, language and thinking because our goal is to stimulate the child's total development.

Chapter Eight, The Integration of Development, focuses on the total child. It follows the chapters on specific areas of development because students have said that it is less confusing to look at the parts of a child before looking at the whole child and the complex interrelationships in his behavior. You may prefer to scan this chapter for an overview of the evaluation and treatment of the total child before delving into Chapters Four through Seven.

You will note that throughout all these chapters, specific diseases and disabilities are emphasized secondarily in the description of occupational therapy with children. We feel that because of your strong undergraduate education in pathology, you can study specific disease processes independently as questions arise. It is necessary that you understand a child's disease or disability before planning his evaluation or treatment. However, as occupational therapists, you will usually focus on the child's habilitation or rehabilitation within the limitations of the disease, rather than on the disease process itself.

Chapter Nine, Illness and Disability: Their Implications for the Child, focuses on the secondary affects of disease and disability, hospitalization and institutionalization, the parents and other health care personnel. More often than not, the occupational therapist is confronted with children who have difficulty in coping with at least one of these factors. Part of our responsibility is to help the child deal with any factors that inhibit his becoming a happy, healthy child. You may find some of the references at the end of the chapter particularly interesting in your study of the psychological affects of illness and disability.

The family and health care personnel are discussed in this chapter as well as in other chapters. The child and his family cannot be separated in our thinking, either in our planning for or execution of the therapeutic program. Therefore, the family and health community are integrated into discussions throughout the text to help you always think of them as an integral part of the child's life.

If you are interested in understanding occupational therapy and its relationship to the other child care and health care services and the roles that are emerging for the pediatric occupational therapist, Chapter Ten, Health Care for Children, may be most meaningful. We are trying to prepare you for today and tomorrow by exploring present and future health care concepts and practices. Some of the concepts are well-known and accepted by occupational therapists; others are just beginning to gain acceptance. This chapter is a plea to all of you to think of the nationwide health needs of children and to adapt yourselves and your professional roles to meet them.

Barbara S. Banus
July 1971

Introduction

Our main objective as pediatric occupational therapists is to provide children with opportunities to grow and develop to their potentials: to assist in the prevention of disease and disability which interferes with the child's development. Pediatric occupational therapists do not work alone to meet this objective. Child psychiatrists, child psychologists, early childhood educators, nutritionists, pediatricians, pediatric neurologists, pediatric nurses, physical therapists, social workers, special educators and speech clinicians are all proponents of health.

Confusion often exists, however, in understanding the role responsibilities of different health care groups because of the conflicts between traditional and contemporary definitions and individual and group definitions. We can alleviate some of this confusion by focusing on the *development of the child for whom the service is being performed.*

Development of the child, or *health* (which is synonomous with development), is our objective. In order to meet this objective we provide developmental evaluation, developmental stimulation and developmental therapy. *Developmental evaluation* is the process of determining the child's status in the neuromotor, psychosocial, visual-perceptual-motor, communicative and cognitive spheres of development, among others. *Developmental stimulation* is the provision of an environment through which all of the child's senses — visual, auditory, olfactory, gustatory, tactile and kinesthetic — are stimulated. Through experiences with his human and non-human environment, the child becomes aware of himself and his changing abilities, which, in turn, motivates him to pursue developmental tasks as they become increasingly more difficult.

Developmental therapy is an extension of developmental stimulation and is usually requisite to the handicapped child's development. Developmental therapy is planned specifically to meet the child's individual needs, while developmental stimulation meets the general developmental needs of all children. Because of his handicapping condition, the child may need guidance in choosing and assistance in using the appropriate stimuli. Most handicapped children are like other children — they want to use their minds and bodies as much as they can — but they need more help, or therapy, from knowledgeable adults in order to achieve their developmental potentials. In this context, the person who provides the help is the *developmental therapist.* When I introduced this term to some of the individuals who provide health or educational services to handicapped children, they spontaneously replied "That's what I am!" There was no longer a "communication gap" as we began to talk about the child, his developmental problems and each of our own specialties in developmental evaluation and treatment.

Occupational therapy historically provides the pediatric occupational therapist with a value system and corresponding ways to implement successful developmental evaluation and treatment. He values work or the meaningful activity which is known to the child as "play." He encourages and assists both children and adults in the mastery of the environment, development of independence and development of self-esteem. He frequently uses nonverbal communication as the link between therapist and client — its value with the child is evident.

My perception of the pediatric occupational therapist, who is a developmental therapist, enlarges upon the traditional values and techniques. The pediatric occupational therapist is a *generalist* whose breadth of knowledge in early child development might be compared with that of the general practitioner s breadth of knowledge in medicine. He has a knowledge based in human development which results from the combined physiological and psychological orientation to human development. He is acquainted with physiological and psychological diseases and disabilities and usually has a subspecialty in the area of disability, such as child psychiatry, physical dysfunction or retardation. Even with specialization, however, the term *generalist* applies to the pediatric occupational therapist. The therapist always looks at the child's disability in the context of his overall development. He evaluates the developmental delay or dysfunction and plans developmental treatment to meet the child's specific needs while planning developmental stimulation to meet his general needs.

I believe that our greatest strength lies in our knowledge of early neuromotor, psychosocial and visual-perceptual-motor development and dysfunction. With this background, we can work with children in terms of prevention, habilitation or rehabilitation. In the area of prevention, we can assist with the identification of potential developmental disabilities through routine developmental evaluations of children five years of age or less. Or we can work toward the habilitation or rehabilitation of children of any chronological age who show developmental delay or dysfunction which reflects early, detrimental sensorimotor patterns.

In a nutshell, this is my perception of pediatric occupational therapy which is relevant to the 1970s. Because the pediatric occupational therapist is a developmental therapist, much of the content that follows in this text is applicable to other health care workers. Its uniqueness for the occupational therapist is based on the traditional and potential strengths stated above, and on the therapist's individual integration of theory with practice in the developmental evaluation and treatment of children.

Barbara S. Banus
July 1971

Table of Contents

Chapter One

The Theoretical Basis for Development

Barbara Sharpe Banus, M.A., O.T.R.

(July 1970)

THE RELEVANCE OF THE DEVELOPMENTAL
CONCEPTS TO OCCUPATIONAL THERAPY

Developmental concepts provide the basis from which evaluation and treatment are formulated in occupational therapy and in some cases delineate the type, degree and direction of change which may be accomplished through treatment.

The occupational therapist is responsible for the child's total development — this statement does not mean that the therapist directly treats all aspects of the child's development. It means that he is aware of all aspects of development and makes significant contributions within the framework of his specific knowledge of development and its deviations.

Occupational therapy is the art and science of directing man's response to selected activity to promote and maintain health, to prevent disability, to evaluate behavior, and to treat or train patients with physical or psychosocial dysfunction.[1]

The pediatric occupational therapist or the occupational therapist who works with children has the same defined responsibilities as all other occupational therapists. However, the developmental model provides the foundation for evaluation and treatment of all pediatric patients. This model is essential to the identification of the goals for treatment. The term *developmental therapy* succinctly explains the process and goal of occupational therapy, particularly those aspects of occupational therapy which are concerned with children. The process of "habilitation" is one of developing individual skills and abilities: those which never

3

have been learned and developed; "rehabilitation" is the redevelopment or relearning of a lost skill or behavior. Habilitation is developmental, and directly or indirectly is always part of the rehabilitation process with children. For example, the child's manipulation of his below-elbow prosthesis in grasp and release patterns is not in itself a developmental process. The daily tasks such as eating, toileting, dressing and writing which require the manipulation of the prosthesis are developmental in character and indirectly become a part of the treatment process.

The child who is hospitalized for a long period (as with burns or an orthopedic handicap, for instance), receives developmental stimulation and treatment concurrently with medical treatment for his specific disability. In other words, developmental therapy must always be provided concurrently with any type of medical or surgical treatment.

In occupational therapy with children, all evaluation and treatment are coordinated with the child's developmental status. The child develops and changes more rapidly than the adult in all areas of behavior — physical, social, motor, and emotional. Thus, the statement "...directing man's response to selected activity to promote and maintain health..." implies that the therapist chooses and supervises the child's activity to encourage progressive, sequential development or to maintain the child's present developmental status. "Health" in terms of the child is translated into "continuous, progressive development." In maintaining health, therefore, the developmental therapist or occupational therapist assists in preventing developmental delay and the resulting additional disability.

DEVELOPMENT

Human development is the series of events which occur in the process of change from the fertilized egg at conception and continue through life until death.[2] The concept of recapitulation (ontogeny recapitulates phylogeny) further describes the process of human development. It states that the development of the human organism follows the pattern of the development of the phylum of animals, proceeding from a single cell organism to a highly complex multicell organism with an intricate nervous system which contains both intelligence and the ability to communicate through oral and written language. The human end product of recapitulation is composed of many behaviors. It is through these behaviors or actions that the development of an individual can be identified. The areas of development and behavior to be emphasized in this book are *neuromotor, psychosocial, visual-perceptual-motor, language and cognition.* There are many other facets of development not directly related to the work of the occupational therapist but which affect it, such as physical and moral development.

The understanding of normal patterns of development is requisite to the comprehension of their relation to pathology. Thus, these developmental concepts are emphasized before considering their application to the treatment of pathology. Pathology treated by the occupational therapist includes any psychosocial or physical dysfunction — or both — and may range from very mild to severe involvement with both overt and covert manifestations.

In this book the term *children* includes those human beings whose ages range from birth to thirteen years; from thirteen through nineteen years is the period of *adolescence*. We shall here focus upon developmental behavior which occurs within the first five years, since most basic patterns are established within this time and are only *refined* over the remaining years of life (except psychosocial development, which continues throughout the life cycle, and cognitive development). Early development must be studied in order to understand the presence of immature patterns in various disabilities, such as severe or profound developmental retardation, in which the child shows behavior of less than five years; and emotional disturbance, in which the child often shows regressed development of less than five years.

All the developmental units or areas are interdependent and must interact in order for integrated behavior to take place — even though they are separated superficially for the purpose of study (Chapters Four through Seven). For example, in order for a child to speak meaningfully or communicate coherently, he must have a language: he must intellectually recognize and understand words; he must have the vocal structure with the neuromotor function to permit the speaking of words; and he must be able to express his emotion through the tone, the loudness, softness, or harshness of his voice.

The "series of events" referred to in the definition of development are the processes or changes which occur during a lifetime. In order for the organism to function at its maximum potential, development of most behaviors must proceed sequentially and continuously; change must be in a positive direction and correlate with the increasing chronological age. Although development never totally ceases, one or more areas may show temporary regression, as in the case of the child who loses ambulatory skills due to bedrest or the child who shows neuromuscular deterioration due to a degenerative disease such as muscular dystrophy. Temporary regression is detrimental if it is extensive and if the child has no opportunity to regain function. Progressive regression is detrimental since it usually results in minimal function or death.

One area of development may show delay in the rate of its progression. This delay in one area usually affects the development of another area due to interdependence of behaviors. If the motor development of an eighteen-month-old child is delayed, social development may be affected because of the child's inability to move from one location to another. The normal child who sleeps in a crib learns to climb out of it after his nap, walk across the floor, open the door and go out to join his siblings or mother in social interaction. If the child is unable to move from his room for neuromotor reasons, his social development may be affected negatively or positively: he may withdraw and not attempt to develop social behavior — or his desire for socialization may stimulate verbal communication.

Development in one area of function can be terminated due to trauma. A child's neuromotor development in the trunk and lower extremities may be terminated in an automobile accident from which paraplegia results and prevents the child's learning to walk; or the child with the traumatic amputation of the hand no longer can use that hand. Although development of the traumatized part of the organism ceases, it is essential to maintain function and development in all other areas of behavior and, if necessary, to substitute mechanical devices to prevent regression of the *total* child.

The temporary or permanent leveling-off of the developmental process is described as *plateauing*. Temporary plateauing is the practice stage in development at which time the child remains at one level of function until he has mastered the behavior of that level. Plateauing is a normal part of the developmental and learning process. When a child plateaus he is therefore permitted practice time to solidify the behavior. At the same time, the therapist re-evaluates the child's progress and focuses on another developmental area. If the plateauing continues and change does not occur within a designated period of time, however, a decision must be made as to whether the plateauing is temporary or permanent. If permanent, treatment is discontinued in this area of behavior.

Each area or behavior *develops at different rates* for each individual. All behaviors of an individual do not — and need not — develop at the same rate on a parallel basis for the child to perform well in his environment. Although the greatest amount of energy may be expended in the area(s) which is foremost in the child's immediate developmental practice, other behaviors are not ignored. For example, the child who is learning to walk may focus on this area to the temporary exclusion of speaking. Once walking is mastered and becomes automatic, it is incorporated into the child's overall daily function. At this time the child progresses in the mastery of other behaviors, such as speech and language. While some development is always occurring in each area of behavior, it may be incipient learning in one and reinforcement practice in another.

A child develops or changes along two dimensions: the sequential and the cross-sectional. *Sequential* or *longitudinal development* refers to the ordered progression of a specific behavior. The behavior is studied in relation to its change over time without consideration for other behaviors present in the child's repertoire. Each of the child's behaviors can be analyzed in this way; however, qualitative and quantitative amounts of normative data on sequential behavior are limited; partly the result of limited studies on development and partly the problem of gathering developmental data longitudinally over an extended period of time. Sequential data provides guidelines for determining the progressive steps in developmental treatment. Although each individual develops at different rates and in different directions at any one time, there is a similarity in the sequencing of the mastery of skills. Most children recapitulate the same sequence, although some omit a few steps — and others take a long time to solidify the learning which occurs at each level.

The term *cross-sectional development* refers to the child's total development in *all* areas of behavior at one time. From this data a developmental profile which identifies present development in each of the areas is obtained. The therapist then determines the child's strong and weak developmental behaviors and plans treatment accordingly. The therapist's objective in planning treatment based on overall cross-sectional developmental patterns is to help the child attain his potential development in all areas of function. It is of limited value for the therapist to treat a dysfunction or developmental problem if other behaviors will interfere with the performance of the new behavior. For example, if the child who is severely disfigured by burns has regained the function of his hands and legs with which he now can participate in games with other children, it is of limited value if he has not been assisted in developing awareness of and a means of coping with the other children's social reactions toward him and his disfigurement. Without additional assistance, the child may withdraw and may not develop social competencies.

THE CRITICAL PERIOD AND THE CRITICAL EVENTS HYPOTHESES

Acceptance or rejection of the *critical period* or *critical events* hypothesis determines the type of pediatric problem in which the therapist will invest his effort. The *critical period hypothesis* is a construct which implies that there are outward limits for the timing of each developmental process beyond which a child is unable to develop a specific function. According to Caldwell,

> ...the critical period hypothesis seems to be used in two distinct ways: (a) a critical period *beyond* which a given phenomenon will not appear (i.e., a point in time which marks the onset of total indifference, or resistance, to certain patterns of stimulation); and (b) a critical period *during* which the organism is especially sensitive to various developmental modifiers, which, if introduced at a different time in the life cycle, would have little or no effect (i.e., a period of maximum susceptibility).[3]

For example, a rigid application of the critical period hypothesis to language development might imply that within a designated range of time (ten to eighteen months, for instance) the child develops his first words of language. The first definition of the critical period hypothesis, "a period beyond which a given phenomenon will not appear," suggests that the child who does not learn his first word by eighteen months will never learn verbal language. On the other hand, the second definition of a critical period is described as the "period during which the organism is especially sensitive to various developmental modifiers, which, if introduced at a different time in the life cycle, would have little or no effect." This statement indicates that the child learns the rudiments of language best before eighteen months — after this time, he might develop some language but never as proficiently.

Caldwell has identified literature from various sources in different contexts which substantiates each of these hypotheses. She suggests, however, that both interpretations of the critical period may be too rigid. It has been found that at the end of the critical period there is not an abrupt extinction of learning; there is, instead, a gradual decrease which terminates in the inability to develop further.

Most of the research which has been done on critical periods involves the use of animals. From this there is some question of the relevance of the theory for the human organism. It would be ideal if some of the research could be done on children, yet there are many problems in this area. Longitudinal studies are not complete because of the disappearance of children or families involved — when families move and leave no forwarding address, for example. Retrospective studies depend upon the family's memory or the child's memory of his past, which becomes fuzzy over a period of years and provides limited factual evidence of the early behavior. Cross-sectional studies provide a variety of information about different people at one time, but do not show the long range effects of certain behaviors, and therefore have limited use in the long term analysis of critical periods. There are many variables in the study of children in terms of home life, number of siblings, nutrition, breadth of experiences, degree of development and so forth. In addition, there are other variables correlated with illness which the child is unable to control (such as separation from family and its effect on the child, or medications which change behavioral responses).

In spite of all the complications in correlating animal and human research, let it be assumed for the purpose of discussion that there is some relevance between the patterns of animal and human development. And, assuming that critical periods do occur and affect the developmental process, it is essential that early diagnosis of developmental problems be made so that treatment will be able to utilize the period of maximum sensitivity within each phase of the child's development. This would be true of both congenital problems (which need to be diagnosed at birth) and traumatic events (which impose dysfunction and possible delay on the child at a later time in his development).

Caldwell also explores and compares the critical period hypothesis with the critical events theory. The *critical events theory,* according to Caldwell, suggests that the event is the most important factor in determining the development of a behavior — regardless of the time of occurrence, which may vary considerably among different children. In other words, if an event or behavior is inhibited or ignored during the child's development and if that event is critical to the child's full maturation as an adult, its omission will be detrimental to the child's development. For example, the critical events theory implies that the development of the first word can occur at any time in a person's life, but that it must occur if the child is to develop language — it may be possible, therefore, to stimulate the incipient language of a person five, ten, fifteen or more years of age. (Even if this is theoretically possible, it seems that the nonverbal behavior might be so well established through reinforcement that the child might be limited in the development of verbal communication.)

The time required for the stimulation of a behavior must be weighed against the realistic needs of the child and his society as a part of the application of the critical events hypothesis. Several questions arise immediately. How long can one or more basic skills — walking, talking or writing — be delayed without interfering with the development of other basic skills and the child's performance in his environment? How long can a therapist realistically work with an individual in order to attain development of a behavior? Or how many hours can a person realistically spend in stimulating a developmental process, such as walking?

If the assumption is made that the critical events theory is valid, the therapist treating the child is *obligated* to stimulate the desired behavior at whatever point in the child's (or adult's) life he is treated.

I do not accept the rigid limitation of the critical periods and events hypotheses; I do believe, however, that the longer development is delayed, the more difficult it is to stimulate. It seems highly unlikely that development is a random occurrence in terms of the timing and actualization of events. However, in accordance with the basic principles of development, the critical periods should vary with the individual; rates of development vary so much that the time at which critical periods occur must necessarily differ. Developmental schedules often incorporate a margin for delayed and advanced behavior. The critical period, therefore, focuses on the excessive delay, which reduces the possibility of total development within a behavioral area.

This concept has relevance to the physical and psychological care of the pediatric patient; the earlier a child's problem is recognized and treated, the more successful the treatment results will be in terms of maintaining continuity between the chronological and the functional developmental ages. With the implementation of this philosophy by early treatment, concern for critical periods is decreased in the care of handicapped children as the possibility of long term dysfunction and delay is reduced. The infant with visual problems, for example, may develop psychosocial problems in addition to faulty visual perception in his school years. Neither of these problems might have developed if he had been given appropriate treatment in the first years of life.

The concept also may be relevant when determining the appropriate time for initiating or discontinuing treatment. If the critical time has passed for the development of specific behaviors, continued treatment would not benefit the child.

Rejection of the critical period hypothesis in pediatrics might result in the attitude of "wait and see, the child will grow out of it." Perhaps this reflects the critical events hypothesis, since it essentially states that change occurs naturally, and that timing is not the important factor. However, this attitude may be appropriate only if the recommended treatment requires extreme and questionable measures such as experimental surgery or drugs. The wait-and-see approach may waste valuable time in the periods of sensitivity for development in the child's rehabilitation.

In occupational therapy, development and dysfunction can be evaluated, and treatment initiated within the first year. If, however, treatment does not result in developmental progress and function, it is not valid to say that the passing of the critical period or absence of the critical event is responsible for the lack of progress. It may be inhibited by the child's physiological makeup — his metabolic rate for instance — which is not dependent upon time or an event. The child's progress may also be affected by changes in his growth potential or by his maturation. When a permanent plateau in his development is reached, the child may have to compensate for the areas of dysfunction which cannot be changed in spite of appropriate treatment.

TWO THEORETICAL BASES FOR DEVELOPMENT

Before initiating any developmental therapy, the therapist must define the theoretical framework within which he chooses to function. This framework will determine his approach to evaluation and treatment; it may suggest the kinds of goals toward which he will aim, the degree of his involvement in the treatment process, the type of treatment media and, possibly, the outcome of the treatment. In making this choice, the therapist must ask several questions of himself: do I believe that the child has internal, intrinsic limits which automatically determine the degree to which he can develop? Do I believe that manipulation of the child's environment can elicit unlimited changes in the child? Or, do I believe that the child has intrinsic potential which can be achieved only with the addition of extrinsic stimulation? In relation to extrinsic stimulation, must it be imposed on the child or will he seek it out? Is one theoretical construct applicable to the development of all behaviors? Or, is a theoretical construct behavior specific? For example, can motor development be intrinsically stimulated while intellectual development is extrinsically motivated? Or, must one construct encompass all development?

In broad terms, it can be stated that the concept of development which is dependent upon *intrinsic,* internal elements of the organism primarily includes the concepts of growth and maturation of an organism and the cognitive, psychoanalytic, and self-actualizing theories of learning. The *extrinsic* developmental concepts look to reinforcement (stimulus-response) theories of learning as the basis for the development of the organism. These concepts infer that man is an organism which changes through his reaction to the environment.

Child controls.

Concepts of Intrinsic Motivation Toward Development

change of child comes from within (own self)

If motivation toward development is primarily intrinsic to an organism, the organism's interaction with its environment might be viewed as a supplementary function. This statement implies that the child is already programmed to follow certain developmental sequences — regardless of his environment. However, intrinsic programming is not an adequate explanation of motivation toward development, simply because the environment provides the framework in which the child progresses through the sequence. Therapy, according to this theory, is viewed as part of environmental stimulation and provides only the framework within which the child develops. It can give direction to the child's development, but it can only bring out that which is already present in the organism. Dr. Robert McCammon, a pediatrician, succinctly describes the limits of therapy, be it that of the physician or of the therapist:

> They (children) are changing rapidly so the things you saw at the beginning of your therapeutic experience certainly are not the things you're going to see at the termination of your therapeutic experience and remove the therapy and they still won't be. So don't kid yourselves (occupational therapists) anymore than I can as a physician and take credit for curing a child of any disease. Sometimes I can help a little, but most of the time what I do is stand by as a cheering section while he gets over it himself. This is true, I think, in all areas with children. We can help, but we're not doing it, the child is.

Among the intrinsic factors which determine the degree and direction of change in the child's development are growth and maturation. *Growth* will be defined as the "increase in size of the organism or its parts, measured as an increase in weight, volume, or linear dimensions."[5] In other words, it is a developmental increase in the mass of the organism as determined by the epithelial, connective, muscle, and nerve tissues. It is dependent upon the healthy internal environment of the organism and healthy external environment of air, water, food, and so forth.

Growth proceeds at different rates. Sometimes growth is slow, as seen in the child whose body is engaged in the process of regeneration after a period of deprivation or extended illness. At other times this process, as noted by Dr. McCammon, can be rapid because of changes within the child or the application of therapy, including food or medication.

The occupational therapist can alter the physiological systems, such as the cardiovascular or adrenal systems, by stimulating the child's physical activity or emotional responses. He can also alter the physiological growth negatively by inhibiting function, as occurs secondarily to the treatment of a dysfunction which requires minimum activity for the child.

The occupational therapist does not directly effect change on the basic anatomical structure — for example, he does not change the respiratory or skeletal structure. He does not physically add missing parts of the anatomy or replace dysfunctioning parts, as is performed in a heart or kidney transplant. He does, however, often add assistive devices such as prostheses, which are not true integral parts of the body.

The therapist may assist in the differential diagnosis of developmental problems which encompass problems of growth, as in the case of the child with retarded physical growth, called *failure to thrive,* evidenced in the retarded physical size of the child. If the retarded growth is internal, as in the heart or lungs, it may not be evident to the diagnostician without sophisticated instrumentation. The symptoms of the retardation may be visible, but the etiology of the retarded growth obscure. Failure to thrive is a problem to all health services because a tentative diagnosis is not adequate for the planning of any treatment. The etiology, be it physiological or psychological, must first be ascertained. The physiological components of failure to thrive are assessed by the physician; the evaluation of possible psychological problems in the dyadic relationship (in the feeding-eating process) may be provided by the therapist as he establishes rapport with the child, feeds him regularly, and stimulates his total development. If the problem is psychological, the therapist (who is essentially a parent surrogate) may elicit a positive response — and growth may occur, to be evidenced in the child's daily weight gain over a period of days. If such is the case, it becomes apparent that the source of the problem is probably in the home with the parents.

If, however, the problem is physiological, the relationship of the therapist to the child will not alter the child's physical growth and medical or surgical treatment will be necessary to elicit change. Once the problem is corrected medically or surgically, the therapist may train or retrain the child to use his body functionally. The therapist, therefore, *facilitates* maturation of the system, which reached its maximum growth at a given period of time for that child's age.

Maturation is the "process of coming to full development," [6] and occurs only if an organism continues to grow, since growth provides the foundation for maturation. Growth is initially requisite to the process of maturation; after which the organism functions in an alternate (but coordinate) manner. *Coming to full development* is defined as the child's maturity at different chronological ages: *the developmental age is equivalent to the chronological age.* The mature two-year-old, for example, is considerably different from the mature nineteen-year-old. At two years, walking, some language, and beginning skills in self care are mature behaviors for the chronological age of two, while a nineteen-year-old showing only the same behaviors would be considered immature for his chronological age.

The child's maturation is affected by the quantity and quality of stimuli available to him. He must be given the opportunity to use his developing body maximally, which requires a variety of stimuli to encourage maturation of all behaviors. Environmental, physical, or emotional factors may inhibit or delay maturation. These factors may be intrinsic (a physical handicap), or extrinsic (a deprived ghetto environment).

Immaturity may appear in one or more behaviors, depending upon the degree of stimulus deprivation and its effect on each area of behavior. An environmentally deprived child who has lacked qualitative and quantitative stimulation probably shows immaturity in several functions. The child may not have learned or been stimulated to use his neuromotor, perceptual or language abilities and may not have matured in some or all of these behavioral areas, although he may be *functionally* ready through the growth process. For example, the child may have all the components necessary for speech and language (he is functionally prepared), but he may have only a limited opportunity to practice these behaviors and, therefore, demonstrates immature speech and language.

The occupational therapist facilitates or inhibits maturation only within the limits of the growth potential. For example, the neuromuscular facilitation techniques stimulate the function of the receptors and effectors. This can occur only if the four basic tissues are normal and in harmony in the area of facilitation — and are available to the receptors and effectors which are to be facilitated. Because these tissues are the basis for growth, facilitation (which is a maturational process) is not possible without them.

When the basic tissues for growth are present but dysfunctioning and maturation are delayed, the goal of the therapist is to aid the child in the attainment of mature function within his

growth = increase
mature = come closer to
our age (*devel.*)

THEORETICAL BASIS FOR DEVELOPMENT 15

limitations. This process is accomplished through the evaluation of the child's physical and developmental status, from which treatment is planned which directly or indirectly incorporates the child's present abilities in the correction of the dysfunction. For example, if the blind infant does not use his tactile and auditory sensory mechanisms, he will not perceive the possibilities for locomotion and the exploration of his surroundings because of the absence of visual feedback. He will mature slowly in motor behavior because he cannot be stimulated visually and will not be tactilely or auditorily stimulated to explore his playpen or crib. He might not smile in response to the adult's smile because he could receive no cues which could be imitated. His intelligence might be masked; he might become handicapped in social behavior because of the reactions of others who believe that he is "stupid" or "dumb." In total, the blind infant may not mature in many areas of behavior because he is unable to learn or benefit from a normal child's environment and activities without assistance.

A theoretical question can be raised concerning the intrinsic and extrinsic properties of growth and maturation. It appears that growth and maturation have both intrinsic and extrinsic motivating properties. Is the child, therefore, internally motivated to interact with the environment, and does he seek out the stimuli or must the environment come to him and impose its stimuli on him? If the therapist accepts the hypothesis that the child seeks out the stimuli, he assumes that primary motivation for growth and maturation comes from within the child. Acceptance of the latter interpretation, which states that environment is the primary motivating force, emphasizes the extrinsic properties for motivation toward growth and maturation.

Environmt. Controls child!

Concepts of Extrinsic Motivation Toward Development

This second approach implies that man is a reactive organism whose development is dependent upon his environment. He learns from his environment through stimuli imposed upon him and to which he responds. The limits on potential development of an organism are minimal because of continuous interaction with and response to stimuli and reinforcement. According to this theory, the stimuli and the reinforcers (which strengthen an already present behavior or a developing behavior) are the therapeutic agents and can be human or nonhuman objects. Thus, depending upon the choice of media the therapist may be either the stimulus or reinforcer or neither within the extrinsic process of learning.

16

Learning is the process by which an activity originates or is changed through reacting to an encountered situation, provided that the characteristics of the change in activity cannot be explained on the basis of native response tendencies, maturation, or temporary states of the organism...[7]

Although this definition of learning is very broad and not entirely satisfactory, even to its author, it does acknowledge that change is not only a property of learning. In addition, it described learning in terms of development activity is referent to behavior and change is referent to the developmental process of the organism. The three properties which are not characteristic of learning are inherent to the organism and related to the intrinsic changes.

The difference between the intrinsic motivation theories of individuals such as Freud, Piaget, and Rogers and the extrinsic theories presented by Hilgard is in the placement of emphasis. The intrinsic theorists emphasize the organism's active role in its development within an environmental framework. The extrinsic theorists emphasize the environment as the organism reacts to it in the process of development. The latter theory suggests that the organism has little control over its development.

Hilgard describes each of the properties which are not environmentally controlled, and refers to his definition of native response tendencies: "activities as characteristic of various species and those more nearly idiosyncratic to one species specific."[8] These kinds of behaviors have formerly been called _innate_ or _instinctual_ behaviors. The one problem which arises is defining the point at which behavior changes from a native response to a learned response. Which elements are learned; which are innate to the individual species?

"If a behavior sequence matures through regular stages irrespective of intervening factors, the behavior is said to develop through maturation and not through learning. If training procedures do not speed up or modify the behavior, such procedures are not causally important and the changes do not classify as learning."[9] The complex interaction of behaviors within the developmental process makes it difficult to distinguish between a maturational and learning function. Maturation may be occurring but a known or unknown intervening variable may be affecting it. At what point does maturation cease and learning begin? At what point do they interact? Are they consistently concurrent? If so, can they be distinguished? How much learning can take place with limited maturation — and vice versa?

The third area which is distinct from learning — the *temporary state of the organism* — includes fatigue. It is commonly recognized that this factor negatively affects the performance of a person who is ill. If it is true fatigue, it cannot be controlled by external sources. Another temporary state is described as *habituation,* during which a person becomes accustomed to a stimuli that he ceases to respond to it. In other words, he *adapts* to the sensation. A patient might cease to listen to the constant chatter of the therapist or to hear the droning of the machine tool with which he is working. (The therapist does not notice the smells in a hospital after he has worked there for a while.) Again, the degree of learning which is involved in these processes is not known.

Using Hilgard's broad definition as a basis for all the theories of learning, two of the theories which may be most pertinent to developmental concepts and treatment of the child will be reviewed and compared: the first is the *stimulus-response* or *reinforcement* model; the second is the *cognitive* model for learning. There are differences and similarities in the models which cannot be completely clarified. Some of the distinctions may be a matter of the theorist's semantics; others may be implied differences in behavior. Because they are theoretical models, it is virtually impossible to "prove" that one is right and the other is wrong at this time given the available research. The developmental therapist, therefore, must make his own choice according to his knowledge, experience, and values.

One discrepancy between the theories is the method by which an individual connects each event with the next. The stimulus-response theorists believe that some kind of response or action is the connecting link or the integrating factor between behavior sequences which Hilgard describes as a "peripheral mechanism." The cognitive theorist, on the other hand, places the integrative mechanism within the "central brain processes." (This is a more abstract concept in that the processes such as memory, which connects past with present or anticipation of the future, are not visible.)

A second difference is in terms of what is actually learned. The stimulus-response theorist believes that habits (responses) are learned through continuous practice. An obvious question comes to mind: if a behavior is learned so that it becomes prominent in the habit hierarchy, how is this kind of behavior transferred to a new experience? Can this transference take place, or is all performance related to habit structure? If the latter is true, one wonders how far the individual can develop beyond a highly structured habit pattern through stimulus generalization. Perhaps this model is most relevant to the theory of operant conditioning (see Chapter Five), as in the case of severely retarded children who can function within a highly structured routine, but who cannot adapt to change.

The cognitive theorists believe that a cognitive structure is learned, not a habit hierarchy. This structure provides a means for approaching and handling new experiences, which implies a more complex (higher) thought process through which associations are made in learning. It is admittedly easier to visualize the retarded child in the previous example learning through habit formation using stimulus-response mechanisms than through the utilization of central brain processes. The implication is that the stimulus-response mechanism requires a lower level neuromotor response than the cognitive process, which functions at a higher level of integration.

The third difference described by Hilgard is *trial-and-error learning* versus *insight in problem solving.* The theorist who based his approach on the stimulus-response theory would apply the habits learned in the past to a new problem. The choice of habit hierarchy would depend upon the commonalities between the old previously learned situation and the new one (in terms of both the parts of the new situation *and* the whole). For example, a child may be able to learn about and relate to the hospital setting because some of its parts are similar to those at home, such as meals, the bed, and the toys. The situation in total, however, is very different in structure from home and would give him no cues as to which hierarchy of habits to use. If the individual has no habits upon which to base his choice, he resorts to a trial-and-error approach until he finds the correct solution — or until he gives up.

The insight in problem solving of cognitive theorists refers to the perceptual structuring which occurs in the central brain process, and which comes from learning and remembering. Insight may be used if the experience is old, new or if it is presented in a different context. If the situation is known and recognized, cognitive theorists accept the theories of stimulus-response; otherwise, they proceed beyond these theories to formulate new solutions. In the comparison of problem solving with trial-and-error learning, the stimulus-response theorist looks back into the past experience of the patient for the solution to a problem. The cognitive theorist looks into the past only for the structure from which a solution can be made based upon the immediate situation and the patient's ability to make use of the elements of the situation. Both theorists accept insight and skill learning as a result of experimentation, which has demonstrated both properties under separate circumstances. Although experimentation has not yet proven it, each may be useful in different kinds of learning situations.

From the general framework of the differences between the cognitive and the stimulus-response learning theories proposed by Hilgard, the theories can be explored in more depth. The elements of the stimulus-response theories will be discussed in this chapter. The theories of cognitive development (the formulation of a structure for learning) of Jean Piaget will be discussed in Chapter Seven.

A Concept of Motivation

In occupational therapy the patient's motivation to perform generally is focused on his health or illness: the person's desire to maximize his potential (which might be referred to as his desire to get better or to remain ill). The reason for and degree of motivation varies: it may be strong or weak; it may be in terms of an immediate goal in the rehabilitation process or the end goal of health and independence; the motivation may be intrinsic, extrinsic or both. If it is intrinsic, the drive may be based upon his desire to become healthy, to play outdoors, to earn a living, and so forth. The motives usually are interrelated and can seldom be separated completely.

If a person appears to have no internal motivation toward health, but instead has a drive toward illness, as in the case of the individual who gives up because he is no longer "like he used to be" and cannot perform "as he used to perform," extrinsic motivation is provided by the therapist.

Extrinsic motivation may be in the form of human relationships or objects. These motivators also might be reinforcers of the desired behavior. The person is motivated to perform to gain this behavior which then in turn becomes a reinforcer. Although it is most desirable for motivation to become internalized so that a person continues to be stimulated toward function, the process of maintaining or regaining health may be so extensive and complex or painful that the person may lose his internal motivation for health.

A Concept of Learning: Stimulus-Response and Reinforcement Theory

The *stimulus* or *cue* is that which leads a person into an overt or covert response — it can be human or nonhuman, and generally is external to the person. However, for a person to become aware of the stimulus in preparation for acting upon it, he must be motivated toward it. Motivation can be biological or environmental. If biological, it might be hunger, thirst, sex, elimination and so forth. The cookie may be a stimulus for a child, for example. If the child is not hungry and not motivated to eat for other reasons, the cookie stimulus will not be of value and will not encourage him to eat. Some stimuli, therefore, do not result in overt action. They may, however, elicit an internal change in attitudes — as in the positive change of attitude toward a previously disliked situation.

It is part of the therapist's responsibility to identify the stimuli which will elicit the desired response in the treatment process. Before this is possible, the therapist must first discover that which will motivate the individual to recognize and make use of the stimulus — it is possible that a stimulus will push the patient into action, but not automatically in the direction which the therapist wishes. For example, if the therapist wants to observe a child's hand function, he may give the child a number of objects, varied in size and shape, to determine the type and degree of manipulation he uses. The desire is that the child will respond to them appropriately according to their characteristics — building with blocks, cutting paper with scissors, drawing on a piece of paper with a pencil. However, the stimuli may elicit an entirely different response: the child may poke a hole in the table with the point of the scissors because the stimulus for him is the point, which makes a hole; he may throw the blocks if the stimulus is noise, and so forth.

Response is the act or thought made in reply to a stimulus. It may be active and overt to the observer or covert — a thought or intentional nonaction. A response is found in all behavioral areas; because activity is emphasized in occupational therapy, however, a motor response is usually expected. The motor response may be the objective (in the case of flexion and extension of the fingers) or it may be in conjunction with other behaviors (such as the child's talking). In order to encourage a particular child to talk, for example, he is actively involved in a gross motor activity through which he relaxes enough to talk. The motor response may be an immediate objective which will lead to long-range change or response in another behavioral area.

The nonaction response may be positive or negative. It may be important for the child not to respond to the stimulus if it will injure him — that he looks at the fire on the stove but that he does not respond to it with a touch. This is a positive, nonaction response. Nonaction in a negative sense may be seen in the child who is supposed to perform in a group activity but who instead withdraws and sits on the side, watching.

Reward or *reinforcement* is used in order to elicit the most desired response from the child. This is an implicit characteristic of occupational therapy. Reinforcement for children is usually derived from one of three sources in occupational therapy: (1) the child's own internal reinforcement or satisfaction from a job well done or the pleasure he receives through the performing of the task, (2) the social reinforcement of the therapist or parents who praise the child and encourage him to perform, or (3) the nonhuman or object elements — candy for the completion of a task, for instance.

The heirarchy of these rewards can be visualized in terms of the child's maturity: (1) the concrete object provides the most basic reward (for the infant, mother may be the human object); (2) the social extrinsic reward is more advanced; (3) the child's internalized satisfaction from his own performance is the highest level of reward. The latter is the level toward which the therapist is working in treating the child over an extended period of time.

As an adult, rewards are not always immediate or obvious; the individual must, therefore, receive internal satisfaction. Rewards are presented on different bases at different intervals. There is the reward which is given immediately for a first response. If the child has never performed before, has no desire to do so, and needs reinforcement to do the task, he will be rewarded immediately. As his performance improves, rewards are scheduled intermittently so that the child learns to perform without continuous rewards. Intermittent rewards based on short-term performance may be necessary initially to help the child maintain a basic level of work. As he becomes involved in the task and learns the procedure, random intermittent rewards are given to help the child maintain desired behavior and in order to assure the highest performance level. Another approach is based upon the child's output instead of upon time — instead of rewarding the child for the completion of a task, the required number of completed tasks or products is gradually increased before a reward is given. These rewards may be tangible (candy) or intangible (praise).

Rewards must be earned. If a poor performance is rewarded, it is the behavior which is reinforced and will be repeated. For example, the internal reward for the completion of the task of picking up a pencil with a new prosthesis may be the child's pride in his own performance. He will not be proud if he is unsuccessful and therefore will not feel rewarded. Praise from the therapist or family who is teaching the child is social reinforcement, and will encourage the child's continued performance if it is sincere and honest. (Social reinforcement of all behaviors may be given during testing to stimulate the child's performance. This is one exception to the child's earning of a reward.) The piece of candy or pencil are the materialistic rewards which may be most reinforcing.

If the child's response is not rewarded or is punished, the process of *extinction* occurs and the child's behavior ceases. For example, if the child has difficulty in manipulating the pencil with his prosthesis and receives no internal or social reward for his occasional success but continues to have difficulty with the task, the response of picking up the pencil may cease. As a result, the child will no longer practice the task and will not become proficient in it. The extinction process may be rapid or gradual, depending upon the strength of the reinforcement. For example, if the child hurts himself by poking the pencil into his hand, he may interpret the action as negative reinforcement and immediately discontinue the practice. If, on the other hand, the child has difficulty in performing and functions slowly he may become discouraged gradually and extinction will occur slowly.

Some behaviors are not desirable and are therefore intentionally extinguished by the omission of reinforcement. Unacceptable social behavior, such as the child's hitting the therapist when he (the child) doesn't get his own way or when he feels ignored by the therapist, is an example. The child may have learned this behavior because he found that such response achieved the attention he desired. To extinguish the behavior, the therapist may ignore the child as long as the behavior continues.

The stronger a behavior is, the higher it is on the hierarchy of responses, which means that it will appear more readily in the child's behavior repertoire. Because of the frequency with which it appears, a strong behavior habit is more difficult to extinguish, and consequently, requires a longer and more persistent extinction process and possibly a more potent extinction media than a behavioral habit which has not developed strongly. This is as true of motor behavior as it is of emotional, social or other responses.

The effectiveness and judiciousness of ignoring behavior in two situations must be seriously questioned. If the child's response is dangerous to himself and others, is ignoring the behavior realistic and effective? If the child has minimum energy and tolerance for frustration due to a severe illness, could he cope with being ignored as means of extinguishing undesirable behavior such as whimpering from loneliness and discomfort?

The process of generalization and discrimination also are very important concepts in the child's learning. *Generalization* is the process of associating and categorizing many things in relation to one thing that is known. The generalization may be appropriate or inappropriate, depending upon the knowledge and experience upon which the child's generalization is based. For example, at about two years of age, children are inclined to call all women "mommies" and all men "daddies."

Discrimination is the separation of two similar things into distinct categories. At this time the child realizes that Mommy is different from anyone else and that *only* Mommy is *called* "mommy" — other women are called ladies, grandmas, aunties, and so forth. Usually children discriminate ideas, meanings, or feelings before they can define the differences in words: the child may see, hear or feel the difference but may not be able to describe it verbally.

The *transfer of learning* seen in the processes of generalization and discrimination is an important concept to the occupational therapist. If the child cannot apply or associate his learning (as described in the stimulus-response model), from one situation to another, the implication is that only rote learning has occurred. (Rote learning is the learning of a single task without necessarily understanding it — and without applying the concepts learned in this task to another situation.) A single task which is learned but not applied to another situation is called a *splinter skill*. Thus, rote learning may conflict with the goals of occupational therapy, which generally are to encourage a child to apply his learning to a broad range of behavior in his daily tasks. In order to prevent the development of splinter skills, the child is given multiple tasks with the same or similar concepts, which encourage the recognition of similiarities and differences in a variety of objects or situations. This recognition, in turn, develops the child's ability to transfer his learning via the process of generalization.

When the child must develop a skill or habit which he can repeat automatically with little variation, rote learning is ideal — it requires no conscious thought beyond the initial stimulus-response process through which it becomes an automatic response. For example, the child who is learning to use his prosthetic hand needs to learn the process of opening and closing the hand by rote so that he can automatically approach an object, grasp it, and release it. This saves the child time and adds to a smooth performance. Other tasks, such as walking, self-feeding and hand washing, require limited variation and are also appropriately learned as mechanical tasks.

Suggested Application of the Stimulus-Response and Cognitive Theories to Occupational Therapy Hilgard has tentatively suggested that the following concepts may be pertinent to the application of theoretical concepts in realistic situations. As he has stated, it is very difficult to make the jump from theoretical research to the real world. He has categorized them according to the theory based upon their relevance to application, not on controversy.

Principles emphasized within the S-R theory:

1. The learner should be active, rather than a passive listener or viewer. The S-R theory emphasizes the significance of the learner's *responses,* and "learning by doing" is still an acceptable slogan.
2. *Frequency of repetition* is still important in acquiring skill, and in bringing enough overlearning to guarantee retention. One does not learn to type, or to play the piano, or to speak a foreign language, without some repetitive practice.
3. *Reinforcement* is important; that is, repetition should be under arrangements in which desirable or correct responses are rewarded. While there are some lingering questions over details, it is generally found that positive reinforcements (rewards, successes) are to be preferred to negative reinforcements (punishments, failures).
4. *Generalization* and *discrimination* suggest the importance of practice in varied contexts, so that learning will become (or remain) appropriate to a wider (or more restricted) range of stimuli.
5. *Novelty* in behavior can be enhanced through imitation of models, through cueing or through "shaping," and is not inconsistent with a liberalized S-R approach to learning.
6. *Drive conditions* are important in learning, but all personal-social motives do not conform to the drive-reduction principles based on food-deprivation experiments. Issues concerning drives exist with S-R theory; at a practical level it may be taken for granted that motivational conditions are important.
7. *Conflicts* and *frustrations* arise inevitably in the process of learning difficult discriminations and in social situations in which irrelevant motives may be aroused. Hence these have to be recognized and their resolution or accommodation provided for.

Principles emphasized within cognitive theory:

1. The *perceptual features* according to which the problem is displayed to the learner are important conditions of learning (figure-ground relations, directional signs, "what-leads-to-what," organic interrelatedness). Hence a learning problem should be so structured and presented that the essential features are open to the inspection of the learner.

2. The *organization of knowledge* should be an essential concern of the teacher or educational planner. Thus the direction from simple to complex is not from arbitrary, meaningless parts to meaningful wholes, but instead from *simplified wholes to more complex wholes.* The part-whole problem is therefore an organizational problem, and cannot be dealt with apart from a theory of how complexity is patterned.

3. *Learning with understanding* is more permanent and more transferable than rote learning or learning by formula. Expressed in this form the statement belongs in cognitive theory, but S-R theories make a related emphasis upon the importance of meaningfulness in learning and retention.

4. *Cognitive feedback* confirms correct knowledge and corrects faulty learning. The notion is that the learner tries something provisionally and then accepts or rejects what he does on the basis of its consequences. This is of course the cognitive equivalent of reinforcement in S-R theory but cognitive theory tends to place more emphasis upon a kind of hypothesis-testing through feedback.

5. *Goal-setting* by the learner is important as motivation for learning and his successes and failures are determiners of how he sets future goals.

6. *Divergent thinking,* which leads to inventive solutions of problems or to the creation of novel and valued products, is to be nurtured along with *convergent* thinking, which leads to logically correct answers. Such divergent thinking requires the subject to perceive himself as potentially creative through appropriate support (feedback) for his tentative efforts at originality.[10]

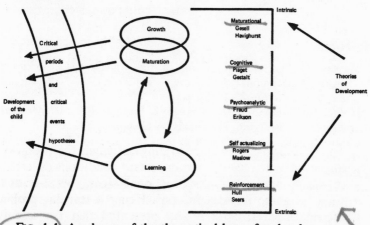

FIG. 1-1. A scheme of the theoretical bases for development.

SUMMARY

Figure 1-1 summarizes the interaction and relationships of the theoretical bases for development. Development of the child is the objective of therapy. To meet this end, the developmental therapist implements treatment according to his commitment to a theory or group of theories.

If the critical period or critical events hypothesis is accepted as crucial to development, it must be recognized as both a facilitator and obstructor of development — as indicated by the vertical divider between growth, maturation, learning and development. If it is not accepted as a theory, the divider is ignored and growth, maturation, and learning are not viewed as being impeded as indicated by the arrows.

Growth and maturation are parallel to learning; *both* constructs are essential to the understanding of development. The degree to which each of these factors influences development is the personal decision of the developmental therapist to be based upon his knowledge and experience. Belief in the growth and maturation theory of development and the intrinsic correlates of learning theory does not imply rejection of reinforcement theory. Nor does the belief in growth and maturation necessarily include acceptance of intrinsic learning theories. The theories of development are visualized on the continuum from emphasis on maturation through reinforcement theory. This, in itself, implies the gradual integration of theory between the extremes.

The complexity of each theory and its relationship to the others suggests the need for occasional review of the developmental concepts as the reader progresses through this text. These are the foundation for the developmental therapist.

References

1. Meyers, C. "Official Definition of the American Occupational Therapy Association." *Newsletter, The American Occupational Therapy Association* 22(1969), p.2.
2. Hoerr, N.L. and Osol, A. *Blakiston's Illustrated Pocket Medical Dictionary* (New York: The Blakiston Company, 1952).
3. Caldwell, B.M. 'The Usefulness of the Critical Period Hypothesis in the Study of Filiative Behavior." *Merrill-Palmer Quarterly* 8(1962), p.230.
4. McCammon, R.W. Proceedings of the Pediatric Occupational Therapy Meeting, American Occupational Therapy Association Conference. Denver, 1964.
5. Hoerr, N.L. and Osol, A., p.307.

6. Hoerr, N.L. and Osol, ., p.420.
7. Hilgard, E.R. and Bower, G.H. *Theories of Learning,* Third edition (New York: Appleton-Century-Crofts, 1966), p.2.
8. Hilgard, E.R.and Bower, G.H., pp.2-5.
9. Hilgard, E.R.and Bower, G.H., p.4.
10. Hilgard, E.R.and Bower, G.H., pp.562-564.

Bibliography

Ames, L.B. "Individuality of Motor Development." In Fehr, M.J. (ed.) *Normal Growth and Development with Deviations in the Perceptual Motor and Emotional Areas* (St. Louis: Washington University School of Medicine, 1966).

Bandura, A. and Walters, R.H. *Social Learning and Personality Development* (New York: Holt, Rinehart and Winston, 1963).

Bijou, S.W.and Baer, D.M. *Child Development, Volume I* (New York: Appleton-Century-Crofts, 1961).

Dollard, J. and Miller, N.E. *Personality and Psychotherapy* (New York: McGraw-Hill, 1950).

Erikson, E.H. *Childhood and Society* (New York: W.W. Norton, 1950).

Flavell, J.H. *The Developmental Psychology of Jean Piaget* (Princeton, New Jersey: D. VanNostrand, 1963).

Florey, L.L. "Intrinsic Motivation: The Dynamics of Occupational Therapy Theory." *American Journal of Occupational Therapy* 23(1969), pp. 319-322.

Gesell, A.L. *The First Five Years of Life* (New York: Harper and Row, 1940).

Gesell, A.L. and Amatruda, C.S. *Developmental Diagnosis,* Second edition (New York: Paul B. Hoeber, 1947).

Havighurst, R.J. *Developmental Tasks and Education,* Second edition (New York: David McKay, 1952).

Llorens, L.A. "Facilitating Growth and Development: The Promise of Occupational Therapy." *American Journal of Occupational Therapy* 24(1970), pp. 93-101.

Mosey, A.C. "Recapitulation of Ontogenesis: Theory for Practice of Occupational Therapy." *American Journal of Occupational Therapy* 22(1968), pp. 426-438.

Rogers, C.R. *On Becoming a Person* (Boston: Houghton Mifflin, 1961).

Staats, A.W. and Staats, C.K. *Complex Human Behavior* (New York: Holt, Rinehart and Winston, 1963).

Valentine, C.W. *The Normal Child* (Baltimore: Penguin Books, 1956).

NOTES

Chapter Two
Evaluation

Barbara Sharpe Banus, M.A., O.T.R.

(July 1970)

DEFINITION OF EVALUATION

The occupational therapist's evaluation of a child is the critical observation and analysis of behavior from which the treatment needs are determined and the procedure and goals are established. The choice of evaluation method is determined by the therapist (evaluator), based on his assessment of the child's needs and problems, the materials and space which are available, and his experience with and knowledge of testing. There are three types of evaluation: informal, formal, and standardized — any of which may be specified for group or individual testing.

The *informal evaluation* provides a general overview of a child's performance. It may cover a broad area of behavior or a more limited area. The evaluation tools may be selected by the therapist, the child, or both; or they may be used at random with no preselected sequence of presentation and with no time limits on performance. This method of evaluation has both assets and liabilities. It can be used at any time with a minimum of preparation — or even no preparation at all — at almost any location. It has no specific criteria for testing and is, therefore, adaptable to any child. These attributes lend to its serving as a precursor to formal or standardized testing by providing the therapist with general information from which further discriminative tests are chosen. Informal tests are too general, however, to allow the statement of definitive judgments about a child and his performance.

The *formal evaluation* usually evolves from informal observations and subtests (from standardized testing), which are combined formally to permit repetition. The method of formal evaluation is determined by the institution and is specific to one place with one particular patient population. It is seldom totally usable by another therapist within another institution because of the variables within the patient populations. The evaluation contains specific objectives: it defines a limited area of behavior to be observed and it is organized for a structured presentation to the child. Specific tools for the evaluation are chosen by the therapist for the purpose of eliciting specific, identifiable behavior.

The *standardized test* or evaluation, which is constructed from the testing of a sample of children, provides normative data on specific behavior of a specific population. To obtain meaningful and valid results from the testing of a child, specific procedures must be followed in presenting the test to a child (for example, the sequence for testing, the time limits if any, and the test instructions). Standardized tests have a narrow range for adaptation if standardized normative data are to be the baseline from which the child's performance is evaluated.

Individual and group evaluations have specific advantages for different types of children and problems. Individual evaluations may be appropriate for the neuromuscularly involved child or the infant, while a group structure might be vital to the diagnostic evaluation of the emotionally disturbed child with social problems or of the child who must be treated within a group because of space and staff limitations within an institution. It is ideal for the child to be evaluated in both situations.

Individual evaluation sessions permit an uninterrupted, close observation of the child by the therapist. Instead of observing several children superficially, the therapist can concentrate on the behavior of one. On the other hand, society dictates that children and adults interact with their contemporaries as well as with the "other generation," and group function is a natural and functional practice for children five years and older. Because of this practice, the school-age child may be more relaxed and natural in his behavior when with peers than if isolated with an adult. However, a child's behavior can readily be influenced by other children in the group. It may be difficult to distinguish his personal abilities from those of other group members whom he imitates or copies.

THE PURPOSE OF EVALUATION
IN OCCUPATIONAL THERAPY

The purposes of an evaluation are (1) to define or diagnose a problem or its attributes in one or more areas of behavior, such as a deficit, developmental delay or dysfunction in psychosocial, neuromotor, or perceptual-motor behavior, and (2) to establish the baseline of a child's performance from which his treatment program is to be developed. The evaluation of a child and his problem is primary to the success of treatment in occupational therapy.

The occupational therapist has several sources from which to gather information about the child. He performs the specific evaluation of the child for treatment of the problem within the occupational therapy department. This evaluation may include those developed by other professions, which have been legitimately adapted for occupational therapy (units from the Gesell Developmental Appraisal or the Stanford-Binet, for instance), as well as units devised specifically for occupational therapy.

The therapist also may use evaluation results of the psychologist, physical therapist, or other professionals to supplement or corroborate his own findings. If the results do not agree, as occasionally occurs when one evaluator repeats the evaluation at two different times or when two different professionals test the same child using identical or overlapping tests, the evaluator must decide which test results provide the most accurate assessment of the child's behavior. This is done in collaboration with the other evaluators. Even then, only through several treatment sessions can the validity of the evaluation be confirmed or rejected. If the assessment is incorrect or inadequate, revisions in programming are made to insure effective treatment.

The evaluation procedure introduces and familiarizes the child with the occupational therapist and, possibly, the treatment facilities and the type of therapy which he will encounter. The evaluation gives the therapist an opportunity to observe and evaluate the child's problem directly; to establish an initial relationship with the child; and to explore a variety of therapeutic behaviors and attitudes such as firmness or supportiveness, which will help determine the most effective approach with each child. If the occupational therapist who will treat the child does not perform the formal or standardized evaluation (not recommended), it is important that another occupational therapist do it and present his observations and treatment recommendations to the therapist who will treat the child. The therapist doing the treatment inevitably must then supplement the reported evaluations with his informal observations of the child during the initial treatment sessions.

The occupational therapist formally re-evaluates each child while he is being treated in occupational therapy. The frequency of the evaluation depends upon the changes which were anticipated in the child's behavior and the changes which have actually occurred. Evaluation for the child making rapid progress is more frequent than for the retarded child, whose changes are slow and require only periodic evaluation, whenever change becomes apparent.

Each treatment session is an informal and ongoing evaluation of the child's behavior: the therapist is always seeking cues which indicate needed change in the treatment process or in treatment goals. These changes are then implemented in successive treatment sessions. There may be a general increase or decrease in the rate of treatment because of growth spurts or plateauing; or trauma may have affected the child's health and required a change. A series of seizures which result in brain damage will, for instance, decrease the child's potential for learning specific behaviors.

There are both positive and negative factors which influence the therapist's decision to perform his own evaluations. Because the therapist knows his patient better than his associates, he can elicit a better performance, both quantitatively and qualitatively, than the others. In conjunction with this fact, the child may desire to perform his best for his own therapist.

On the other hand, an evaluator unknown to the child can put pressure on a child to perform beyond his apparent abilities and know that it will not jeopardize his own future treatment sessions. Information from the child's response is then relayed to the child's therapist, who decides what information and how to incorporate it into the treatment program. If a child is difficult to evaluate — or if the therapist has strong positive or negative feelings about him — it may be essential to use another evaluator. The therapist's subjectivity can invalidate the results if he sees only what he wants to see.

The registered occupational therapist (OTR) administers the complex formal evaluations or those standardized tests which require a high degree of examiner skill. Through these evaluations and re-evaluations, he determines the needed changes in treatment and recommends changes in procedures to his associates, who include the certified occupational therapy assistant (COTA) and the occupational therapy student (OTS). The evaluations and their recording may be done by a qualified person on the occupational therapy staff (as designated by the OTR), and, if appropriate, they are performed under his direct or indirect supervision.

The informal evaluation is performed by all occupational therapy personnel. Its value is in the degree to which the evaluator can observe and assess both the overt and subtle behaviors: the greater the professional skills, the more thorough the evaluation. However, all levels of observation are important in the analysis of a child's problem. By combining and evaluating all observations under the guidance of the qualified OTR, decisions about the child's program can be made.

The final evaluation precedes discharge from treatment and commonly is called the *final progress report.* This report provides a complete outline of the child's status at discharge for the health care professional who may treat the child as an outpatient (or as an inpatient) in the future. It may include a report and recommendations for professionals who work with the child outside the health care services, such as the educator or others within the child care services.

PREPARATION FOR THE EVALUATION

Preparing for an evaluation is standard procedure for every evaluator or examiner. This preparation includes the reading of reports written by other professional personnel; the interviewing of people who know the child, such as the parents and the nurses; the preparing of the child for the evaluation prior to the evaluation; the preparing of the testing room and testing materials for the evaluations; and the study of the examination procedure. With thorough preparation in all of these areas, the evaluation can proceed more smoothly than is otherwise possible and more complete evaluation results can be expected than if the preparation were incomplete or careless.

Pre-Evaluation Information Gathering

The gathering of information about the child from charts or records and interviews with parents and staff prior to the evaluation of the child has both advantages and disadvantages. Under most circumstances, however, the advantages are greater than the disadvantages. The evaluator can gain a perspective of the child's problem and obtain specific information about the behavioral area which is to be evaluated, and about the developmental range within which the child is performing. This information simplifies the therapist's preparation for the evaluation, since it decreases extraneous (but sometimes necessary) preparation for unexpected situations. For example, the therapist knows a child developmentally performs tasks within the two- to three-year-old range, although the child is chronologically six years. An evaluation, therefore, is chosen which incorporates the two- to three-year-old range of behavioral tasks — with a few additional tasks at both extremes to assimilate behavior not noted in the reports or interviews.

Precautions and restrictions noted on a chart give the evaluator cues for the handling of the child's medical or behavioral problems. This information prevents injury to the child through ignorance and provides the evaluator with constructive suggestions for the handling of problems that may occur. In addition, the therapist can "expect the unexpected," be comfortable with his knowledge and be able to function in a more confident and more responsible manner than would be possible if he were not mentally prepared.

Through the use of charts or interviews, the therapist seeks information necessary to the timing of the evaluation. Young children may have naps daily, and physically ill children may have naps at irregular hours daily. It is important to choose the child's best and most alert time during the day for his evaluation or treatment — after his nap, for instance, or after his breakfast. This reduces the possibility of one negative variable affecting the evaluation, and may eliminate the need to repeat an evaluation.

Interviews with the parents or family prior to the child's evaluation provide useful information about the child's behavior within the home and surrounding environment which can be compared with his behavior in the institution. There may be a marked behavioral change in the child because of the changes in his physical and social environment; the physical facilities and the people within an institution usually differ considerably from those within a child's home. The parents can give the staff information about the child's daily routine, his interests, his fears, the family complex and so forth which may facilitate the development of rapport between the therapist and the child. It also may be used in evaluating the child's knowledge about himself and his family in terms of names and ages of siblings, his school and his own diagnosis. By presenting the familiar material to the child, the evaluator can explore the child's ability to communicate both receptively and expressively — what he understands of questions and what he can communicate in return. The parents' communication is useful in itself; both the content and the attitude with which it is expressed indicate some of the positive and negative elements within the home environment. This information helps the evaluator to understand the family problems with which the child must cope during his treatment, and, later, upon his return home.

The major disadvantage in reading charts and interviewing families prior to interviewing and evaluating the child is the possible development of "tunnel vision" by the therapist. The evaluator may look only for those behaviors which he *expects* from the child as a result of the reports and interviews. He may not be alert to unreported and consequently unexpected behavior. For example, if it is known that a child is three years and five months old and has begun nursery school, it is expected that this child will demonstrate behavior within the normal range for the three-year-old. Although the child may be within the normal range of expectation, he also may show some advanced or regressive behaviors which may affect the progress he will make in nursery school.

Reports also may be inaccurate from the standpoint of emphasis upon unimportant or incorrect information. Reports of other professionals may emphasize factors which are irrelevant to the child in treatment in occupational therapy, facts which are no longer true of the child, possibly due to developmental changes which have occurred since previous evaluations. If the therapist is an acute observer who separates report information from direct observation, there is no problem; if he is careless, however, his observations may substantiate the previous irrelevant or incorrect information.

The Parent Interview

To procure maximum information from the interview, skill in interview techniques is required. The following guidelines for the interview process are adapted by each therapist to match his personality, his abilities, his situation, and to meet the needs of his client.

At the beginning of the interview, the therapist introduces himself to the parents and tells them the purpose of the interview, the purpose of occupational therapy, and, possibly, the purpose of occupational therapy for their child. The therapist then focuses on the parents and his immediate objective — which is to help the parents to feel comfortable with him. The parents may be made comfortable through the therapist's showing an interest in them and their child as a professional who has specific skills with which to help the child — and as a human with genuine concern for and sensitivity toward other humans.

It is important that the parents feel the therapist's interest in their problem and his willingness to listen to their discussion. The tone expressed by the therapist to the parents is, "I care about you and your child and want to help you." The therapist gives his complete attention to the parents during the interview, which is preferably held in a quiet place with a minimum of interruption from people or the telephone. Once the parents recognize the therapist's concern and begin to trust his interest in them and their child, they may become immersed in the interview and react adversely to any interruption in the conversation. An external interruption may create internal interruptions in thoughts and feelings for both therapist and parents. The parents may be unable to reorganize their thoughts or feelings — or may begin to feel that the therapist does not really care about them because he permits other factors to interfere with the interview.

P →

Parents have many feelings (some of which are ambivalent) about the child and his illness or injury which may be difficult to discuss easily. They may deny the child's problem or the extent of the problem — for once they do recognize it, they may begin to feel guilty. They may feel responsible for the child's illness or injury; they may feel anxious or frightened about the outcome of treatment; they may feel that their child will not perform well in the evaluation, which may reflect on their handling or raising of the child; or they may feel incapable of helping the child in his rehabilitation. The parents may want the therapist to see and hear only about the positive qualities of the child. On the other hand, the parents may have only negative comments about the child if they reject him — as in the case of the child who is the result of an unwanted pregnancy, or the child who does not meet their expectations because he is not perfect.

O.T. →

The parents must feel that the therapist accepts them as they are and does not condemn them for their behavior; that he accepts their feelings and their actions toward the child. The therapist refrains from projecting his personal values upon the child's family. Instead, the interviewer is an active listener who gathers information. To show the parents that he is actively listening, the therapist replies both verbally and nonverbally. He may restate or rephrase the parents' comments, which both clarifies his understanding of the communication and reinforces it in his thinking and also helps the parents to be accurate in their statements. The evaluator shows a listening attitude by visually and nonverbally attending to the interviewees, nodding his head and smiling at the appropriate times, and avoids extraneous interruptive behavior of manipulating papers, cleaning fingernails, and so forth.

The therapist gives no advice and demands no changes in the parents' behavior at the initial interview. Only by demonstrating the attitude of acceptance and openness are parents able to explore and discuss their child's problem in an initial interview. Later, during treatment, it may be appropriate to advise parents on the care of their child or to instigate change in one of their value systems which is detrimental to their child's health. At the time of the initial interview, however, the therapist does not have enough knowledge about the problems and should seldom offer suggestions or attempt to initiate change.

Too often, relatives, friends, and specialists in the health-care fields give advice to the parents concerning the management of their child. If these suggestions are contradictory, the parents become confused and may be inhibited in making any decision about the care of their child and his handicap. For example, one individual may tell the parents that "There is nothing wrong with your child"; others may say "Your child should be in an institution."

Having prepared the interview situation to maximize the parents' physical and emotional comfort, the interviewer is ready to proceed to the central issues. The question is "How do I elicit from the parents — without antagonizing them — accurate and useful information which is relevant to the evaluation and treatment?"

The natural response is to begin asking the parents semi-significant, basic questions, such as the name and age of the child, the problem and the past treatment. Usually, the parents already have been asked these same questions by other staff. The parents legitimately may be angry that they must repeat the information again; their question is "Don't you know this already? Can't you get these answers and leave us alone? We've already talked to the doctor, the nurse, and the social worker."

To decrease the parents' stress, rather than increase it through repetitious questioning, the therapist learns the basic facts prior to the interview through his communication with other staff. Facts include information about the etiology, diagnosis, prognosis, medical care, past treatment in occupational therapy, or other health services involved in the child's care, parental attitudes toward the child, the evaluations to be made, and the treatment procedures. With this background, the therapist then interviews the parents asking for clarification of confusing, nebulous or incomplete facts. He may state some of the known information, crosscheck it for accuracy, and ask the parents to add important points, such as, "Your child had been treated in occupational therapy for six months? Where? By whom? What was the treatment?" With this information, the therapist can contact the previous department for progress reports on the child and thus develop an appropriate treatment plan. In addition, any discrepancies between the therapist's and the parents' information can be clarified before they grow into a problem.

Questions are asked in a manner which elicits open and honest answers. The therapist avoids putting the parents on the spot or on the defensive. It is the interviewer's responsibility to raise important issues in a way which encourages the parents (1) to talk and (2) to give as complete answers as they are capable of giving at that time. The parents' answers are based on *what* the interviewer says and *how* he says it. If the interviewer formulates a question correctly but shows an attitude of condemning the parent when he states it, the parent may be afraid to answer and may remain quiet, and no information is gained. If, on the other hand, the interviewer formulates the question poorly but shows an accepting attitude toward the parents, he may receive a response. The answer may be incomplete or inaccurate, however, and therefore actually useless.

Open-ended questions, such as "Tell me about your child's play habits" are presented in order to avoid yes or no answers, and to encourage the parents to answer within their own frame of reference. If a parent replies, "What do you want to know about my child's play?," the interviewer explains more specifically and may say, "With whom does your child play? With what kinds of toys does he play? What hours of the day does he play?" This type of question has two functions. It prevents the yes and no answers (which seldom are informative) and it prevents the interviewer's projection of his own thoughts and values onto the parents. If the therapist asks, "Does your child play with his brothers or his sisters?" the parents might say yes or no and may not think beyond the obvious limits of the question — beyond the scope of the family group to the child's peers. If the interviewer reports only this information to other personnel, it may be assumed that the child does not play with his peers and that this is one of his problems. In reality, the child may play more with his peers than with his siblings. But, due to *specific* rather than *open-ended* questioning (which can be followed by specifics in order to locate missing material), the accurate facts do not appear in the interview.

The interviewer must be aware of the parents' changing reactions during the interview and be ready to clarify misunderstandings as they occur so that they do not multiply and affect the total interview. The parents may interpret the question, "Does the child play with his brother or sisters?" in a different way than that intended by the interviewer — the child *should* play with his brothers and sisters. Although the interviewer has not placed a value judgment on the question, the parents may think that this is the case. They may assume responsibility for the lack of interaction among their children and feel defensive of their own behavior because they do not want the therapist to think they are poor parents. Concern for this one situation may then dominate the remainder of the interview as the parents amplify its importance into a primary issue.

Some parents answer questions succinctly, others answer them expansively. The reasons for these differences are many. The parents whose child recently had a traumatic injury differ from the parents whose child has a chronic or congenital condition which has been recognized and accepted for a long time. The energy and concern of the first parents are focused upon their child as they deal with the immediate problem. Due to their inability to think clearly about the questions concerning the child's past or future, the interviewer must take the initiative to reschedule the interview for a later date.

The questions asked of parents vary considerably according to the purpose of the parent interview and the evaluation of the child. If it is anticipated that the child will be evaluated, institutionalized and treated within the institution over a period of time, questions asked of the parents by the occupational therapist, nurse, or social worker might focus on the child's daily routine at home. The objective is to gather information relevant to the child's specific treatment and his general developmental needs. This information is applied to the daily care of the child to make his institutionalization beneficial by maintaining the child's present developmental patterns and by encouraging further development. For example, the parent of a two-year-old may be asked to describe the child's words for needed items, such as "water," "mommy," "toilet," "get out of bed," "something hurts." Once the staff knows what the child is communicating, they can respond appropriately to his needs and decrease stress for the child. In addition, through the staff's using words which are familiar to the child, such as "potty" instead of "urinate," the child can understand the communication to him and can respond appropriately.

If the child is an outpatient and the parents are to carry out treatment in the home, the interviewer and the parents may discuss the family's daily routine and may tentatively plan a daily treatment schedule convenient to the family. The parents help choose the room in the home which provides the needed space. The parents and therapist discuss the treatment media and its availability in the home. If it is not available, the therapist suggests how and where it can be procured, how much it costs or how materials within the home can be adapted to meet the treatment needs.

This communication between parents and interviewer has two purposes. First, it provides the factual information necessary for effective treatment planning. Second, it considers the parents' need to assume responsibility for their child's rehabilitation; the parents need not abdicate their positions as the primary caretakers of the child. They become necessary members of the treatment team; they are decision makers who participate in the planning and initiation of the rehabilitation program, rather than technicians who only carry out the plans once they are made.

Because the parents are team members, the parent-interviewer roles are switched at some time during the interview: the parents become interviewers and the therapist the interviewee. The parents have an obligation to ask questions about the services to be provided by all the team members. They are, in effect, the consumers of the product which occupational therapy is selling. Although they may be naive about the new product they should explore its value for themselves and for their child.

Parents often ask questions of the person with whom they feel most comfortable. These may extend beyond the knowledge of the individual from whom they are seeking help. The occupational therapist, for example, might be questioned about other therapies, medical treatment, drugs and surgery for the child. Depending upon his knowledge of the questions and answers, the individual asking them, and the parents' communication with other staff, the therapist may give some information but *must* use his discretion in answering questions and offering suggestions. For example, parents might ask the therapist to explain the surgical procedure their son will receive. An appropriate response would be, "What do you know and understand about the procedure?" From the parents' reply, the therapist has several options: (1) to state openly that he is not qualified to give that information, (2) to confirm the answer and suggest that the parents seek further information from the surgeon or the pediatrician, (3) to state honestly that he does not know the answer, or (4) to supplement their information. In most cases, the first answer is the most appropriate and honest.

In addition, the parents may ask several staff members the same questions, hoping to get the answer they want to hear. Once they obtain the desired answer, they may use the information to manipulate the staff's handling of the child. For example, the parents may want to keep the child home because the child "doesn't seem too bad" and the hospital is expensive. They talk with the staff until finding one member who agrees that the child can stay at home. This comment is then used to confront the head of the treatment team with the demand that the child remain at home.

It is the responsibility of every member of the health-care team, including the therapist, to help the parent communicate with the appropriate personnel. The therapist contacts the appropriate individual to make an appointment for the parents to talk with him. This part of the procedure includes the referral of medical questions to the physician, referral of the family problems to the case worker in the social service department and so forth. This is realistic; the occupational therapist is not a psychiatrist, a pediatrician, or a social worker, and consequently cannot presume to know or to interpret the full responsibilities and knowledge of these individuals.

The Parent Interview in the Home

The interview process which has been discussed focused on the parents who seek help from the institution and are interviewed within the institution — the therapist's own territory. However, more health care is being provided in the home and community now than in the past and it may be desirable to interview the parents in their own home under certain circumstances.

The interviewer's attitude and the statement of the question is basically the same, but the physical environment in which it occurs is very different. The therapist may or may not be welcome in the home. The parents may feel embarrassed about their home if it is in a poor neighborhood, or if it lacks the material goods they assume are important for their child and they may be concerned about the advantages they cannot afford for their child, particularly if the child is handicapped.

The parents may not want help and may not have sought it — a neighbor or friend may have referred the health care center to the family. A health-care team or one of its members then may be sent to the home to evaluate the total situation. Under these circumstances, the parents may be angry at the intrusion into their private lives and reject the therapist's offer of assistance. To decrease the possibility of rejection, the therapist prepares the family for the interview by making an appointment for the interview via telephone or a brief visit before interviewing at the home. This gives the parents an opportunity to prepare themselves — both emotionally and socially — for the interview by thinking about the problems and needs, dusting the floor and so forth. Once at the home (as in any social situation) the therapist again introduces himself by stating who he is, where he is from and the purpose of the interview. This will be brief but will review the objectives of the visit for the family.

The therapist's behavior and personal appearance may be more critical in a home than in an institution. It may be the therapist's responsibility to help the parents become comfortable in their own home by showing them that he accepts them and their home and is comfortable in it, though sitting at the kitchen table with a cup of coffee or on an old sofa. The therapist's personal appearance should be congruent with his behavior, for it visually conveys a message to the family. The therapist avoids embarrassing the family by dressing comfortably, not exotically and not sloppily. The actual and real differences between the therapist and parents as people may be few, but extremes in dress can exaggerate the differences between two socioeconomic groups and can elicit antagonism. There is, however, no one mode of behavior or physical appearance for all communities.

To gather all information necessary for the planning of evaluation and treatment and to answer the parents' questions adequately, several interviews may be necessary. These may extend over a short or long period, during which time the parents are developing a sense of trust in the therapist as a person who can and will help them. The parents may feel that the therapist is assuming responsibility which belongs to them and may not trust the therapist's dominance in the situation. The therapist, in turn, must always remember that the child belongs to the parents.

If the therapist alienates the parents through his attitude or behavior, the parents may be reticent to accept him, his evaluation of their child, and his recommendations for treatment. If this occurs and the parents are responsible for the daily treatment of their child, the child's treatment may be neglected and he may suffer because of the parents' anger and disagreement. Generally, however, most parents want their children to improve and, when given the opportunity, will work with the therapist to meet the goal.

The Initial Interview with the Child

The therapist introduces himself to the child prior to a formal or standardized evaluation. The resulting interaction might be described as an informal evaluation for both the therapist and the child. The therapist previews the child's behavior and then plans the testing accordingly. Interactional play with the toddler and informal discussion with the teenager help the evaluator to determine the therapeutic approach to the child. The therapist may find that a particularly quiet and dependent child will need frequent reinforcement from the therapist and that a hyperactive child will need firm limits to maintain his performance during the evaluation.

In addition, the therapist briefly informs the child about the evaluation procedure and answers questions about it to prepare the child for evaluation. By making him comfortable, evaluation helps the child become more relaxed when taking the test and improves his performance. If the child shows a high degree of anxiety, such as physical tension or crying, it may be useful to show him the evaluation room. The very anxious child may be visualizing a hurtful room like the doctor's office rather than a playroom type of atmosphere. If the interview cannot be made prior to the evaluation, it is included in the evaluation at the child's room, on the way to the evaluation room or at the beginning of the evaluation.

The descriptive explanation of the evaluation given varies according to the age of the child. It is brief — with a goal of alleviating the child's anxiety — it is not an in-depth discussion. The child is given only basic information which clarifies facts for him, rather than extensive data which confuse him. Throughout the interaction, the therapist watches for cues which indicate concern or questions about the new information. He attempts to clarify the problems immediately before the evaluation session.

The explanation needs to be appropriate to the cognitive development of the child: factual information and details are increased with the age of the child. The explanation for a toddler is very simple, "I'm going to play with you after your nap. We have toys like blocks, story books..."A direct explanation may be given to the adolescent:"According to Dr. Smith, you have a perceptual problem in what we call basic motor planning. I will evaluate this problem tomorrow at ten o'clock, at which time I will tell you more about the testing. Any questions about it for now?"

The Physical Preparations for the Evaluation

The physical arrangement of the evaluation room is critical to the success of the formal or standardized evaluation. (During the *informal* evaluation, it may be desirable to make cabinets, closets, etc. accessible to the child so that he will be able to demonstrate his varied interests.) Prior to the child's arrival in the evaluation room, a table and chair appropriate to the size of the child are procured — there is nothing more uncomfortable than dangling feet in combination with a table upon which one rests his chin! The work area for the child is cleared of extraneous materials that can or may distract him. This includes the table, shelves, cupboards, and floor: the table top is cleared except for the examination material in use. All other examination materials are removed from the child's reach and, if possible, from his sight, perhaps in a box. Cupboard doors are closed. Shelves which have materials on them are emptied or arranged neatly. The floor is cleared of dangerous articles in order to prevent the child's hurting himself when engaged in gross motor tasks. These precautions are not necessary for all children; however, the precautions may eliminate much wasted time and frustration for the evaluator and the child if he should be more distractable and active than anticipated. This preparation prior to the evaluation may actually be "preventive chaos."

The evaluation materials, which are out of sight in a box, are kept in easy reach and arranged in order of presentation to the child. This prevents the child's attention from being lost while he waits for the evaluator to find the missing materials. Also, the child may become tired or wiggly if the evaluation is unnecessarily extended. All evaluation media must be in good working condition. A broken toy or test object can frustrate a child, in addition to invalidating formal or standardized test results.

In addition to gathering and ordering the appropriate evaluative tools, it is essential that the examiner study the test, the test order, and the materials before the evaluation. If using a standardized test, the tester or evaluator must practice administering the test to become familiar with it so the test administration proceeds smoothly. The evaluator's objective is to focus on the child's performance rather than on the test materials. When compiling the results of the evaluation later, the evaluator mentally reviews specific tasks which demonstrate the behavior; consequently, he must have closely and accurately observed the child. In the formal or informal evaluation, the therapist is also concerned with the timing of the evaluation and the ordering of the tasks. In order to do this effectively, the therapist must be familiar with the evaluation tools, their purpose, the behaviors they demonstrate and the way in which the child must use them.

THE PROCESS OF EVALUATION

The evaluation process incorporates all the dynamics of the child-adult, child-media, and adult-media relationships which occur from the time the child enters the evaluation setting until the time he leaves. It includes behavior observed in standardized or formal testing, as well as in the informal or supplementary observations. The _evaluation_ is the specific content or material through which the observations are made; the _process_ is the total procedure of functional evaluation. The child and the evaluator show many subtle behaviors throughout the evaluation, both in relation to objects and to one another. If ignored, they can affect the evaluation process and, consequently, the results. The evaluator demonstrates behaviors, such as a well modulated voice, a quick but easy presentation of test materials, which subtly enhance the evaluation procedure by influencing the child's behavior.

The therapist introduces observers or therapists external to the evaluation to the child before embarking on the test procedure. The child then does not wonder about the identity of the observers throughout the evaluation; otherwise, he may be anxious about them and their possible relationship to him. Once he knows them, he is free to ignore them or to incorporate them into his play. It is the therapist's responsibility to determine the role of the observers and to tell them and the child.

The Presentation of Directions and Media

Once the evaluation begins, the evaluator must concentrate on several aspects of his own performance. One of the most important is the manner in which he gives directions. The therapist-evaluator differentiates between *types of cues* he gives to the child when giving directions for a task. He avoids giving the child inappropriate cues for his performance. These may be conflicting cues, nondiscriminatory cues, or cues which interfere with the behavior being tested. For example, if the therapist says, "Give me the red block," and at the same time points to the red block with his finger, the child may respond correctly and give him the red block. However, the therapist does not know whether the child understood (1) the direction, "Give me the red block," (2) the word "red," from which he took his cue and, therefore, picked up the object which was red, or (3) the visual cue only, with no comprehension of the verbal command.

To determine the child's ability to understand *directions* and to learn from them, the evaluator systematically presents directions in a progressively more complex sequence. If the child's level of comprehension is unknown, the therapist begins at the lowest level for giving directions. He provides maximum stimulation if he is demonstrating the use of a tool at the lowest level. He may use tactile stimulation initially to reinforce verbal and visual stimulation; he may hold the child's hand on the object and go through the motions for the child. The therapist may, for example, hold the child's hand on a paint brush and move it across the paper in order to stimulate the child's tactile, visual, and kinesthetic senses (the touch of the brush against the paper, the sight of the results of the painting, and the feel of the gross arm movement). As the child begins to perform this task by himself, the therapist gradually reduces his assistance — the amount of stimulation from the pressure of his hand — until the child performs independently.

The next level is the giving of verbal directions in combination with visual demonstration: the task is described verbally while the action is demonstrated in order to help the child learn the words and associate them with the action. In the example described above, the words might be, "Hold the paint brush," "Dip the paint brush into the paint can." A complex task may require this level of directions at any age. A child learning to lace shoes may watch the therapist's demonstration on his own shoe, listen to the verbal directions, and then initiate the same process on his shoe. (This task is considerably more difficult than learning to manipulate a paint brush.)

The visual demonstration may be used alone for the child who does not understand words (a Spanish-speaking child in an English-speaking community) or for the child who cannot hear the words. The demonstration must be made carefully in order to avoid blocking the child's view with the therapist's hands or the materials. It must be made slowly and precisely in order to show the specific movements in the correct sequence.

Verbal directions are next in the hierarchy. In this case the therapist describes the task and, perhaps, gives the child a written description of the process to be followed. Verbal directions can be given independently of other directions *if* the child has some comprehension of the task required of him.

Written directions may be the most difficult to understand because such directions cannot respond to the child's questions — they provide no feedback. If the directions are poorly formulated or complicated, the therapist may need to interpret them for the child.

The words used in giving directions must be in the child's terminology rather than the professional's. The therapist changes and increases the complexity of the directions with the increased development of the child. At all times the therapist avoids the unnatural falsetto, frequently described as "baby talk." Young children imitate speech as they learn it and may develop undesirable speech patterns if given poor models.

As a secondary evaluation, the therapist may present the child with a task sequence which demonstrates his level of understanding directions. Suggestions for the use of directions in the child's treatment can then be based on specific observation rather than on guesswork.

The evaluator not only differentiates between the type of cues he gives to the child, but also between evaluation tasks and teaching tasks, which he presents within the evaluation. When giving a standardized test, the therapist must follow the structure of the formal test. If the structure is not followed, the evaluator cannot analyze the results according to the standardization and cannot therefore legitimately accept the test results as valid in comparison with the normative data. (The therapist cannot compare the child's performance with the normative data because the test has not been presented to the child in the same manner as it was presented to the sample populations on which it was standardized.) There is very seldom opportunity to teach the child a task during standardized testing. However, in the informal evaluation — or at the end of a formal evaluation — a short-term task can be taught to help determine the child's level of comprehension and his ability to learn progressively more difficult tasks, such as sequenced puzzles.

In addition to demonstrating the child's comprehension of directions, the task shows the child's approach to problem solving — his use of trial-and-error learning, for example, as opposed to action preceded by cognition — the speed with which he learns a specific task, and his response to frustration when the task becomes too difficult. Teaching is useful in both evaluation and treatment sessions, since it identifies the child's level of comprehension, his response to various teaching techniques and his approach to problem solving.

The choice of *media* for the informal and formal evaluation is critical. Before it is determined, however, the behaviors which are to be observed and evaluated must be identified. Then the media or material that will elicit the desired behavior is chosen. (See Chapter Three for a complete discussion of activity analysis.) Several factors are considered for each media chosen: these include the number of materials to be used and the discriminatory characteristics of each. One material cannot be used to test a variety of behaviors within the same task if these behaviors are overlapping or contradictory. In order to determine the child's ability to discriminate form, a formboard with matching blocks is used. The board must illustrate form only; the formboard and the forms must be one color only, or the board one color and the forms another color. If each form is a different color, and the hole into which it fits is the identical color, the evaluator cannot judge the child's ability to match forms according to the shape of the hole. He may be matching the color of the form to the color of the board. If the child is to match colors, the forms on the board should be identical so that only the colors are being matched (Figure 2-1).

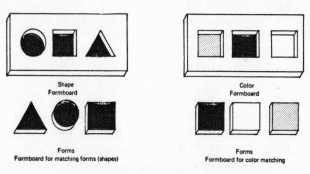

Shape
Formboard

Color
Formboard

Forms
Formboard for matching forms (shapes)

Forms
Formboard for color matching

FIG. 2-1. Discriminating formboards.

A single media can elicit several different responses in different areas of behavior (perceptual, social, and motor, for instance). From the analysis of the responses, it is possible to determine the child's developmental level in each area. For example, a child who holds a pencil demonstrates his hand coordination by the way he holds the pencil; his conceptual abilities by the kind of picture he draws; his receptive language by the way in which he follows directions; his expressive language by the manner in which he takes directions; his expressive language by the manner in which he talks about the picture; his perceptual-motor abilities by his manipulation of the pencil, and possibly his self-image by a drawing of a human figure. Although the pencil is used to demonstrate each of these behaviors, each is distinctly separate from the others and can be identified specifically within the total task.

In most situations, the fewer the test materials used for an evaluation the better. The child can focus on one task without constant change, for he has fewer distractions, and fewer media require less testing time. In most tasks more than one behavior is evident. Therefore, there is repetition of performance which can confirm or reject the integration of the behavior in the child's repertoire. A second media which demonstrates similar or identical behavior to that elicited through the primary media may be chosen for emergencies. It may be necessary if the first breaks or the child refuses to perform with the original material. For example, if the child refuses to use the crayon while testing his ability to draw form, a pencil or felt-tip pen may be used as a substitute. The child may have learned to use a pencil recently, or he may have learned that a felt-tip pen is special, while thinking that crayons are babyish and appropriate only for coloring pictures. Sometimes the child gives the evaluator reasons for his actions; at other times he simply refuses to perform.

Multiple media can be effective when used in quick succession either to maintain the child's attention or to determine the child's discriminatory abilities. When similar items are applied quickly, the child's level of task integration also can be assessed. If he knows the concepts of the media well, he can apply them readily to a variety of tasks; otherwise, trial-and-error learning may be evidenced.

All evaluation or standardized test media do not have substitutes. One or more variables of the material may be changed if the behavior being tested will not be affected. In standardized tests, particularly, it is essential that identical or equivalent materials be used. For example, two-inch blocks are not equivalent to one-inch blocks in tests of hand function based on motor coordination and range of motion. The two-inch blocks are more easily manipulated than one-inch blocks and balance better when stacked. Therefore, the child's hand and finger function need not be as refined for manipulating two-inch blocks as one-inch blocks. One-inch blue blocks, however, are equivalent to one-inch red blocks in the same tests simply because color does not influence hand function. If the child's behavior is being compared with standardized norms, there is no substitute for a specific media in testing a specific skill. If the child's concept of building in a vertical plane is being tested and not the motor skill, the size of the blocks is irrelevant and does not effect the test. It is the evaluator's directions that are crucial.

The therapist creates his own specification or *procedure for testing* if he is devising a formal test or presenting an informal evaluation. These specifications include the objectives of the test, its content and the procedure for presentation to the child. The first two factors are test dependent, the third is test independent and can apply to standardized, formal, and informal tests. Generally, however, directions for standardized tests accompany the test and describe the testing procedure in adequate detail.

The following procedures are recommended for all testing. Directions for a task are repeated a specified number of times (usually three or four), and they are repeated by the evaluator in the same manner with the same words. By observing the child repeating a task, the examiner can discriminate between a chance response and an intentional response. If the child understands the task and has the developmental abilities to perform the task, such as a motor or verbal task, he will repeat it in the same way; however, if the behavior is new to his repertoire, the response may not be consistent. The inconsistency also may indicate other problems: that the child is bored with the task and is being creative in order to alleviate that boredom or that he does not understand the task.

A child may refuse to perform a task upon request rather than to risk failure — he may suspect or know the response but may lack the self-confidence to experiment. Later, the same child may respond in the evaluation. He may develop trust in the evaluator and be willing to show his inadequacies; he may consider the problem and figure out the answer; or he may choose to be independent in determining the time at which he will answer.

One factor may invalidate the delayed response: standardized test items are sequenced to eliminate responses influenced by immediate previous learning. For example, the Gesell *Incomplete Man* and *Draw a Man* tests (1940) have different objectives. The former can interfere with the latter if it is presented first, because the *Draw a Man* test is a spontaneous drawing preceded by only the verbal directions of, "Draw a man." A developmental level can be established based on the child's awareness of people and his ability to draw a man prior to the testing. The *Incomplete Man* is presented after the spontaneous drawing to avoid giving the child cues about the parts and their relationships which can improve his independent drawing of a man. If the *Draw a Man* test follows the *Incomplete Man,* the results may indicate only immediate recall and short-term learning rather than long-term and visual memory (Figure 2-2).

The Sequencing of a Test

The sequencing of test items has relevance to other aspects of testing and can help or hinder the total evaluation. The evaluator considers the developmental range of the child, the behavioral characteristics and then sequences the test items appropriately for that child. He chooses an introductory media which initially motivates the child to perform, the materials for the body of the evaluation from which most of the specific behavioral data is obtained, and the final media to give the child a feeling of completion and satisfaction at the end of the evaluation.

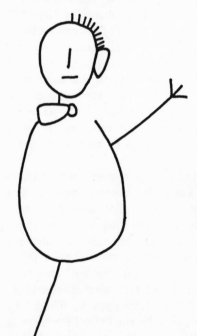

FIG. 2-2. Incomplete man by Gesell, Arnold, et al., from Part One of the *First Five Years of Life* by Gesell, Arnold, et al. Copyright, 1940 by Gesell, Arnold. Reprinted by permission of Harper & Row, Publishers, Inc.

To *introduce a test,* free play materials may be presented to motivate the child's interest and participation in an informal or nonstructured setting: the child is permitted to choose the toy or object he wants to use and to decide how he wants to use it —with no direction from the evaluator. In the formal or standardized test situation, a semistructured task may be presented to the child to help acclimate him: blocks may be presented with only the directions, "Make something with these blocks." This provides the child with both a structure for his work and some freedom within the structure. The freedom from direction may encourage the child to talk with the evaluator and thus begin to develop rapport. The nonstructured or semistructured tasks may frustrate the child who lacks creativity and spontaneity; it may distract the hyperkinetic child from further performance; and it may excite and involve the child who thrives on building and making things.

In both the free play and semistructured introduction, these behaviors may be demonstrated and must therefore be evaluated by the therapist for their effect on future treatment. If the child is given complete freedom in his choice of an activity, he may choose the activity which he enjoys or which he can most efficiently manipulate. Then he may refuse to continue the test with another task! If the child's favorite activity or toy is known, it may be saved and used as a reward at the end of the evaluation. The use of the toy at the end may permit the completion of the evaluation and leave the child with positive feelings toward both the evaluator and the evaluation — which may facilitate the initial treatment sessions.

Specific objectives for the *body of the evaluation* are established, and the session is organized accordingly. A limited and carefully preselected group of materials is provided for the child. The materials are specific to the range of the developmental abilities and interests of the child being tested, which insures some success and reinforcement for each task. The child will not be overwhelmed with a large variety of materials which may only confuse him — he may want to try everything! Most of the materials will be used at some time during the evaluation; the child need not feel unnecessarily restrained from the "things" he wants to try.

The sequence of the tasks presented within the body of the evaluation is determined by the behavior to be evaluated and by the developmental age of the child. The body of the evaluation is divided into primary behaviors within the developmental range of the child, such as activities of daily living (ADL), neuromotor and perceptual-motor. Each of these areas is then subdivided into its specific elements and the media or tasks are chosen to test the behavior. Each task presentation within the unit is then ordered according to the developmental sequence within the child's developmental range.

The evaluator begins testing at or below the baseline of the child's developmental ability and progressively increases the difficulty of the task until the child is unable to continue further. The baseline is defined as "the level at which the child can perform all the behaviors in the required tasks." It can be established for the total test or units within the test, such as a baseline for neuromotor, perceptual-motor or emotional behavior. (It may be known from previous reports or contacts with the child or it may be unknown, the only information available being the child's chronological age.)

If there is no baseline known, the evaluator prepares a broader sequence of presentation of increasingly and decreasingly difficult tasks from the child's chronological age. If there is any question, it is preferable to begin below the child's baseline in order to provide him with a successful experience before he begins to make mistakes and become discouraged. If one task is the building of block structures from which the child's conceptual and neuromotor abilities will be evaluated, the evaluator reviews the total sequence of the developmental process in block construction (which is as follows if the Gesell schedules are to be the guideline). The building of two or more structures occurs within the same developmental period. A child may solidify his knowledge and skill at a lower level of competence — building a horizontal structure, for instance — while experimenting and developing incipient skills at the higher level by combining vertical and horizontal patterns. Another child may omit one step in the sequence by combining two steps or may learn the advanced behavior before practicing a lower level behavior. Generally, however, the development is orderly as the child gains skill in many areas of behavior which are interdependent (Figures 2-3 through 2-8).

At the lowest level of learning, the child *imitates* the evaluator's building of a structure: the child watches the evaluator build the structure and imitates his actions step by step to complete the task. Next the child *copies* the already complete structure of the evaluator: the evaluator builds the structure without the child observing his building and the child copies the final product. Third, the evaluator gives only *verbal directions,* such as "Build the blocks as high as you can," with no visual cues for the child. The evaluator presents concrete directions to the preschool child and gradually increases the conceptual elements of the directions as the child's cognitive skills develop.

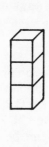

FIG. 2-3. Tower building. The structure incorporates only the vertical dimension. (Figs. 2-3 through 2-8 by Gesell, Arnold, et al., from Part One of the *First Five Years of Life* by Gesell, Arnold, et al. Copyright, 1940 by Gesell, Arnold. Reprinted by permission of Harper & Row, Publishers, Inc.)

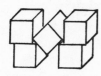

FIG. 2-4. Train. Simple two-dimensional vertical and horizontal structure.

FIG. 2-5. Bridge. Two-dimensional structure with spatial considerations which require balance.

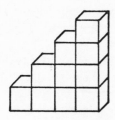

FIG. 2-6. Gate. Two-dimensional structure with spatial considerations and angulation of block which requires increasingly refined manipulation.

FIG. 2-7. Steps. Two-dimensional structure with increased quantity of blocks which increases complexity of visual-motor task.

FIG. 2-8. House. Three-dimensional structure.

A diagram of the process of single-task evaluation appears in Figure 2-9. It begins at or below the child's baseline performance and ends with the child's best performance.

The last step of the single-task evaluation example is identified with a broken arrow indicating the continuation of the process until the child shows his most advanced performance. The column on the left shows the sequential decrease in task difficulty for the child who is unsuccessful. The column on the right shows the sequential increase in task difficulty. It can be noted that the evaluator omitted one step in the sequence of the child's learning ability on the last task: imitation of the structure with the angulated block. If this is included, the more advanced task of copying is invalidated due to immediate previous learning. However, if the child is unsuccessful in copying, the evaluator can

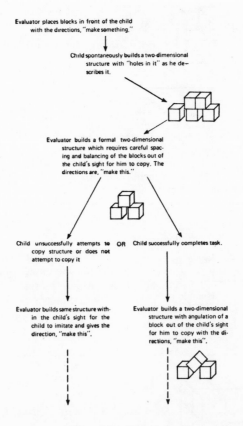

FIG. 2-9. Single-task evaluation process.

revert to imitating with no side effects. The evaluator also can advance the task if the child can copy, for it is then known that he can imitate the task which is on a lower level.

Primary behavior tasks, such as neuromotor, perceptual-motor, and ADL, can be sequenced in many ways. The most successful evaluation sequence is that which is most logical to the child and that which matches his immediate needs and desires.

The first sequence in Figure 2-10 shows no awareness of a child's habits and his inability to comprehend the reasons for doing a task strictly for the test, such as putting on a coat at the end of the evaluation prior to demonstrating that he can take it off! It shows a lack of knowledge about three-year-olds, who need gross activity after sitting still — and frequent toileting.

In formal, informal, or standardized tests, fine motor tasks generally are presented early in the evaluation of the child who is developmentally five years or less. He is often familiar with the test objects and can be readily involved in the tasks. Also, he is most alert and least desirous of gross activity at this time. This sequence may not be as important to the school-age child or adolescent who does not get as restless and who understands the purpose of testing.

Verbal response test items — the naming of specific objects, talking about the child's family and himself — may be answered most completely and easily when the questions are presented midway in the evaluation. Children communicate more freely after they become acquainted with an individual — they do not have the

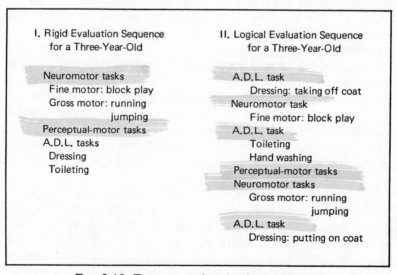

I. Rigid Evaluation Sequence for a Three-Year-Old	II. Logical Evaluation Sequence for a Three-Year-Old
Neuromotor tasks	A.D.L. task
Fine motor: block play	Dressing: taking off coat
Gross motor: running	Neuromotor task
jumping	Fine motor: block play
Perceptual-motor tasks	A.D.L. task
A.D.L. tasks	Toileting
Dressing	Hand washing
Toileting	Perceptual-motor tasks
	Neuromotor tasks
	Gross motor: running
	jumping
	A.D.L. task
	Dressing: putting on coat

FIG. 2-10. Two types of evaluation sequences.

social amenities which lead to conversation as a polite gesture. And, once children become restless, they focus less on verbal communication and more on motor tasks. Talking also decreases when a young child is under stress. Although the child of five years or less may not intellectually understand the meaning of testing, he feels the pressure or insecurity of the new situation and becomes nonverbal. Emotionally charged content in a discussion also may elicit a negative reaction which can be nonverbal, or verbally disorganized. If a subject of great concern is raised, the child may become very tense and react in his normal pattern for stress.

Speech increases as the child becomes comfortable — as he is led into conversation, not forced into conversation. Initially, no demands are placed on the child and no questions asked of him. "Hi! You are Johnny Jones. I'm glad to see you again...We're going to play... Here is the table and chair for you... Look at the red block. It's bright..." General comments from the evaluator give the child cues about the adult who is evaluating him through the voice, his smile and his movements. The silent therapist gives the child no cues about his thoughts or actions or reasons for them and unintentionally may frighten the child. Once verbal communication is established, the evaluator proceeds to this aspect of the evaluation.

Activity of daily living behaviors may be observed at appropriate times during the evaluation such as removing sweaters at the beginning of the evaluation and putting them on again at the end; opening and closing doors; recalling the location of the evaluation room after toileting. A child may refuse to perform these tasks if they are imposed on him at an illogical time in his frame of reference. Through these tasks, the evaluator can make an initial assessment of the child's social behavior and his short-term memory in practical situations.

Peer interaction may be observed at the time of evaluation. If a single observation is made in a setting unfamiliar to the child such as a children's hospital ward or institution waiting room, the accuracy of the observation is questionable when compared with the child's behavior with his friends. The judgment resulting from a single observation may be inaccurate and later detrimental to the child unless this behavior is found to have a high positive correlation with his behavior with friends.

It is advisable to present active tasks at the *conclusion of the evaluation.* Some tests or evaluations specify that gross motor activities be done at the end of the test or at the point at which the child becomes restless. Although some children are able to return to quiet activities once they have been physically active, others become excited and cannot return to the testing.

The Therapist-Child Interaction

Interpersonal or social behavior between the child and the evaluator is evident throughout the evaluation, particularly with the child who is not knowledgeable about testing and reacts spontaneously. Once this child begins to talk and is encouraged to continue, he may be quite verbal. Some school-age children, however, have learned to focus their full attention on the test and show little personal interaction unless it is built into the evaluation and elicited by the evaluator.

One of the evaluation objectives is to determine the child's reaction toward the therapist. Because the child responds to the evaluator, the evaluation, the materials which the evaluator presents, and the way in which he presents them, the child's response usually indicates his perception of an authority figure who is unknown to him, makes demands of him and sets limits on him. It is the therapist's responsibility to be consistent and honest in his behavior, make realistic demands, follow up the demands and set realistic limits. An evaluator probably will not elicit the child's best behavior if he does not provide a good model of behavior.

A consistent and honest evaluator is careful and consistent in all aspects of his communication; he asks or states what he wants to say, and shows it in his face, his body and his voice; he makes a single request and accepts the child's response. The therapist asks the child to demonstrate the desired behavior in a specific way and accepts the child's action. If the therapist says, "Would you like to sit down?" actually meaning, "Sit down," but feeling that the former is the polite or nice way to present the command, the child may not sit down. The child is correct because he has interpreted the question literally. If the therapist pursues the topic and demands that the child sit down, the child may reject, accept or ignore the evaluator. He does not trust the evaluator or his statements because of the incongruence of the initial statement and the final demand. As a result of the confusion, the child may begin to question or doubt the evaluator's following statements or questions. This leads to poor development of rapport and, consequently, a poor response to verbal test items.

Requests in the form of a question can be made only if the evaluator intends to accept the response given by the child. The child will respond appropriately only if the demand is reasonable according to his frame of reference. If the therapist wants a specific response, but also wants the child to have some control of the situation, the question must be self-limiting, "Would you like to sit down on this chair, at this table, or on the floor?" The therapist's question is reasonable and the child makes the choice. If the evaluator does make the demand, "Sit down," it is important that he means it and follows it up; that he does not permit the child to control him and the evaluation. The child may know that the limits are reasonable and seek the therapist's control by testing him. To know which child needs limits and which limits are appropriate for him, it is useful to have reports preceding the child's evaluation.

The child's emotional response to frustration also is observed by the evaluator: it sometimes is called *frustration tolerance.* In this text it refers to the child's perseverance in working on a difficult task before or while showing a negative emotional reaction. Maximum inability to tolerate frustration is demonstrated by the child's quitting the task.

Before frustration is elicited for evaluation, the evaluator assesses the child's physical and emotional condition. The physically ill child may have a very limited tolerance for any difficult situation. He may lack the physical or emotional resources to cope with problems other than his illness; he may tire very rapidly or may focus only on the constant pain. Other children, who have learned to work with problems until a solution is reached or several alternatives attempted, may have very high tolerance for frustration — it is possible for the child to control this situation, while it is not possible for him to control pain.

After the assessment of the child's general condition, he is involved in the test situation and rapport is established between him and the evaluator. Otherwise, the evaluator may be unable to reinvolve or redirect the child's attention once frustration is elicited and the session may end. It is preferable to frustrate the child toward the end of the evaluation to prevent this occurrence.

Frustration can be elicited in several ways. The examiner may demand that the child continue to work on a difficult task: "Try again," until the child reacts negatively; the child may be refused a desired toy; or the evaluator may remove a material which he is enjoying and using successfully from the child. Generally, one or more of these situations occur naturally or the child becomes frustrated spontaneously due to the difficulty of the tasks in the evaluation.

Once frustration is elicited, it is the evaluator's responsibility to set limits on the child's emotional expression and to redirect the child's attention to the task. Limiting the emotional expression of frustration may be relatively easy or difficult depending upon the degree of the child's reaction as seen in the comparison of anger expressed by "No!" and refusal to continue the task with a temper tantrum. The child is not pushed into explosive behavior beyond which he has no control of himself and becomes incapable of functioning. The objective is only to determine the point at which he becomes frustrated and begins to have difficulty in performing for the purpose of planning his treatment: to determine the amount of pressure the child can tolerate, his reaction to stress, and the most effective method for handling the reaction of that particular child should it occur spontaneously. Once in the treatment setting, the child's tolerance for frustration usually increases because he knows the therapist and the treatment routine.

A basic problem which leads to a child's upset and frustration in both evaluation and treatment is "time." Preschool children have very little concept of time as identified by the clock and, like other children and adults, they do not like to be interrupted in their "work." It is only fair to give children a warning before a task must be completed and then give them time to complete the task. For a preschool child, the statement may be "When you have finished drawing the house, the crayons must be put away so you can do something else." The statement for a school age child might be "When the clock over the door says 11 o'clock, all toys must be put away on their shelves and you must return to the ward with the other children." Reassuring statements, such as "You have lots of time before lunch," decrease stress created by time pressures and also are helpful to the child.

Some evaluations or standardized tests are timed so a warning is unrealistic and unnecessary, as seen in the test in which each subtest is very short. However, in the semistructured or free play section of an evaluation, time warnings help the evaluation proceed smoothly and comfortably for the child. He is already functioning under stress and to demand an unnecessary abrupt change may increase his anxiety.

Frustration tolerance decreases as a child begins to tire. Thus, it is important to stop the evaluation at the first indication of real fatigue, as differentiated from the "I'm tired" avoidance type of fatigue, and continue again when the child is alert. Symptoms of real fatigue include the rubbing or closing of eyes, thumb-sucking, increased sitting and decreased gross motor activity and talking, slouching and whimpering or crying. The results of the evaluation cease being an accurate indicator of the child's potential once fatigue develops. Also, the child may develop negative feelings toward the evaluation which he may project into the treatment setting at a later date.

There are a few attitudes and behaviors which all evaluators and therapists need to respect when working with children over fifteen months of age. Some are mechanical reactions which automatically demonstrate basic good manners. For example, interruptions are not permitted during an evaluation. A sign may be posted on the door that evaluation or treatment is in progress. Telephone conversations are very brief and held only if absolutely necessary; these interruptions break the continuity of the evaluation session and may interfere with the child's ability to concentrate on the task or the sequence of tasks before him.

Commitments to children are kept and are kept on time. If changes are to be made in the child's schedule, he is notified directly and as soon as possible. If the child is not notified of the changes, he may become anxious and wonder what to expect. He may have been anxious about the evaluation and rather than alleviating the anxiety by ignoring the change, the evaluator may increase it. Careless behavior indicates that the evaluation is unimportant to the child and that the initial preparations were irrelevant to the child's welfare!

The therapist is a model of responsible adult behavior for a child. He demonstrates the behaviors which the child may imitate in interacting with his peers or other adults. The evaluator's behavior shows his respect for the child by recognizing that the child's time is valuable to him, that he wants to complete the necessary tasks and return to his play. In turn, the child learns to respect the importance of the therapist's work and interrupts him less frequently.

The response of the adult to the child in the evaluation relates directly to the adult behavior described in the adult-child relationship. Some examiners maintain both a physical and emotional distance from the child. They do not smile; they show no physical attention to the child and do not put a needed hand on the shoulder of a tense child to help him relax; they may give directions and physically remove themselves from the child. It seems, instead, that human warmth — the sincere smile or the pleasant comment or genuine pleasure in the child's success — usually motivates a child to perform his best without detracting from the reliability of his test behavior in the informal evaluation. Insincere "gushing" by the evaluator, however, may be questioned by a child and may elicit as poor a response as total indifference or negativism. Children usually discriminate between honest, real reactions and those that are false and superficial.

Evaluator behavior is not the same for every child in the informal evaluation, since his behavior is not interpreted in the same way by every child. However, in the formal or standardized testing, the examiner may have specific directions for his response to the child when the child gives a right or wrong answer. Sometimes the examiner is required to reply only in a positive manner — "Good" — in all situations, so that the child does not become discouraged but continues to perform until stopped by the examiner. Some children need feedback about their performance and constantly glance at the evaluator for his approval; others focus intently on the task and seldom acknowledge the evaluator's presence.

Note-taking by the evaluator during the evaluation may elicit a reaction or questions from the child being evaluated. Depending upon the criteria for the evaluation, an explanation may be given to the child about the note-taking, "I want to remember what you did today so I can help you the next time you come to see me." A school-age child and adolescent may request to see the notes. In this case, it is suggested that instead of showing him the notes, the evaluator offer to discuss his findings with the child at a later date, once the information is compiled. The raw data which the evaluator notes is of little actual value to the child, may have little meaning for him, and only may confuse him at this time. Once the evaluation is completed and the child is reinvolved in his daily routine, he may or may not forget his request. If he is in occupational therapy it will be logical and appropriate to discuss the problems found in the evaluation and the treatment which will be used to correct them.

The process of note-taking by the examiner during the evaluation is an acceptable and often necessary procedure. In standardized or formal testing it may be required and is usually necessary; and in the informal evaluation notes are taken depending upon the evaluator's ability to recall the details of a child's performance. The evaluator cannot risk forgetting or misrepresenting details of the child's performance.

Interaction with the child, and close and accurate observation of the child's performance is primary in evaluation; note-taking is secondary and therefore kept to a minimum. It is difficult, if not impossible, to observe a child, to present the test materials orderly and quickly, and to make extensive notes at one time. Sometimes it is useful to have an "open" outline (Figure 2-11) which helps to order the presentation of the evaluation and to organize the compilation of the results. In this type of outline the evaluator can make comments about the child's behavior, which may or may not be relevant to the final evaluation report when the outline is reviewed after the evaluation session.

```
Upper Extremity Function

      Strength                    of shoulder
      Range of motion             of elbow
      Coordination                of wrist
                                  of fingers


      Function: pronation
                supination
                reach
                grasp
                release
                transfer
                bilateral function:  dominant hand
                                     supporting hand
```

FIG. 2-11. Sample of an open outline for organizing evaluation observations and compilation in one area of behavior.

THE COMPILATION AND ASSESSMENT
OF THE EVALUATION RESULTS

The compilation and assessment of evaluation information is equal in importance to the process of evaluation. Inaccurate oral and written reporting of the evaluation can lead to inappropriate treatment or recommendation for treatment. Detailed notes on all relevant behavior are written up immediately following the evaluation session from the notes taken during the evaluation or information recalled from the evaluation. (See the informal developmental evaluation in Chapter Eight.)

Because there are many different ways to organize evaluation reports, the following example primarily identifies the factors which are pertinent to most reporting, suggesting ways of including the information into the report and means of organizing it and compiling it. This information is included in most reports. although the different sections may be emphasized or omitted. The general information included below is not necessarily in order of importance:

1. Name, age, and diagnosis of the child.
   Name of the evaluation.
   Name of the evaluator.
   Date of the evaluation.

2. The area(s) of behavior for which the evaluation is performed, and possibly the materials used to elicit the behaviors which explicitly identify and describe the behavior.
3. Assets and liabilities — primary and secondary.
4. Treatment precautions and restrictions.
5. Information from records, parents and other sources which is pertinent to the evaluation.
6. Summary of the evaluation.
7. Recommendations for treatment.

The child's neuromotor, perceptual-motor, or psychosocial behavior is the focus of the report, not the activities or media used to elicit the performance. Emphasis is on the behavior the child demonstrates when he performs with an object, and not on the object itself. For example, to describe a child's hand function, the following information might be included.

The child has bilateral hand and arm function (he throws and catches an eight-inch ball); he transfers objects easily; he shows consistent unilateral dominance of the right hand and uses the left hand for support (drawing); he has a smooth, direct reach from the shoulder using the total arm, wrists and hand. He demonstrates opposition of the fingers and thumb; he shows a mature pattern of release with no hyper-extension of the fingers.

The description of the media used to elicit the behavior singularly clarifies a concept or further verifies the child's performance. "The child has opposition of index finger and thumb. He can pick up a one-inch block, but not a 3/8-inch pencil." This gives the reader a clear visual image of the tasks. This specific identification may be important in planning treatment or in giving factual evidence of the behavior for other staff who read and use information from the report. Identification of a specific task eliminates incorrect or inappropriate assumptions, particularly in the area of psychosocial behavior. For example, to say that a child: "behaved well during a test," means nothing to the reader of the report because the words are vague and invite multiple interpretations. A meaningful description might be:

The child cooperated with the examiner by performing all the tasks upon request and by answering questions. The child, however, did not initiate any task or questions. He was very restless and wiggled in his chair — it was difficult to determine the degree of his concentration.

In comparison with the many uncooperative children the evaluator had tested, he thought this child "behaved well." However, from reading the details of his behavior, the staff member might question the broad statement which described the child as behaving well. In addition to clarifying the demonstrated behavior, the extended comments give other staff members information about the child and his behavior which can be valuable in their future contacts with him — this is not true of the first statement.

A standard for comparison of the child being tested must be identified prior to an attempt to describe the child's behavior. It may be valid to examine the child in the light of the standards for healthy children and of those for other children with his dysfunction. If behavioral standards for the healthy population of children are ignored, the therapist may develop a distorted view; he may begin to compare the handicapped child only with others who are handicapped and, consequently, lose sight of the overall degree of healthiness of his patient. It is essential that the therapist maintain feedback from normal children in order to keep a realistic perspective of the abilities and limits of his patients.

Having identified all relevant behavior and having compiled and organized it in the format acceptable to the institution, the problem behavior or the area of the child's specific problem is identified. At this time, the child's primary and secondary assets and liabilities are defined on the developmental or dysfunctional profile. The *primary assets* and *liabilities* are those factors directly related to the injury or dysfunction. For example, a child with a below-elbow prosthesis of the right arm has both assets and liabilities directly related to the prosthesis and its functional use. The child's primary liability is that his right side is his dominant side. His primary asset, directly related to the dysfunction, is the use of his own elbow for flexion and extension of the forearm and the full use of his shoulder. In addition, he has full use of his left arm.

The healthy or positive elements of the child's total behavior, apart from the handicap, are his *secondary assets* and are identified for use in the correction of the dysfunction and for supportive measures during the rehabilitation process. These assets indirectly and positively influence the rehabilitation. For example, a six-year-old child has poor perceptual-motor skills in the advanced visual motor behavior, but he has a strong desire to print his name on his drawings "...like the other kids," as he told the evaluator during the evaluation. One of the secondary goals for his treatment which will motivate him to work is the printing of his name legibly. This is a very real goal to the child, not a manufactured goal. The child's secondary asset in this situation is his recognition of the problem and his desire to be like his peers.

A *secondary liability* can be a disabling factor beyond the original disability — as can be seen in the case of a twelve-year-old girl who has been burned and is receiving treatments of splinting and exercise for the prevention of contractures and further dysfunction. The primary liability is the actual burn and the physical dysfunction it has imposed on the preadolescent. The girl, however, is very conscious of her appearance and has withdrawn from her peers as a result of the disfiguration. The scarring and consequent distorted physical appearance is the secondary liability. It does not hinder her function directly, but it strongly and negatively influences her self-image — and thus her emotional behavior. Over a period of time, this influence may become the primary liability and require direct treatment.

Secondary assets and liabilities are identified in the evaluation report to insure awareness of and the need for continuous treatment in areas other than the overt dysfunction. Socialization becomes an important goal in the treatment of the twelve-year-old burned girl as she gradually learns to deal with her disfigurement in public. The gradual introduction into printing prior to completion of treatment will be an asset and motivator for the boy with the advanced visual motor deficit. In both cases, the therapist and all other personnel treating the child are aware of these problems and the assets so that treatment will be effective from the beginning.

Treatment precautions and restrictions are also identified to prevent any further injury to the child. Precautions are those measures which are taken by the therapist and the child in order to prevent further injury or dysfunction and to prepare for emergency situations in the event of illness. Specific precautions are taken for the child with seizures and for the child who is taking special medication which has side effects. In addition to knowing the preventive measures to be taken in order to avoid injury, the therapist also is aware of the treatment precautions and first aid relevant to possible problems.

Treatment restrictions include the motor or social limitations or both which are imposed on the child to prevent injury or illness. The child with rheumatic fever may need bedrest and quiet activity; the child in a lower extremity traction unit may need physical restraint; the child with temper tantrums may be restricted from social interaction for behavioral management.

Being aware of and knowing precautions and restrictions, the therapist can plan the appropriate treatment program which will incorporate all the specific needs of the child. Without considering these aspects the treatment might be unrealistic and even dangerous to the child.

The source of information not observed directly by the evaluator must be noted in the report. The person reporting may be subjective in his feelings because of strong positive or negative reactions toward the child — or he may not have observed the child's performance closely. If this is a possibility, the evaluator must crosscheck the reference's reports with his own observations. observations.

If treatment is to be focused on problems reported by others, it is particularly important for the therapist himself to observe the child's behavior. A parent may report, for example, that he must feed his two-year-old child. Upon direct observation by the therapist, it is found that the child can feed himself. Through further questioning of the parent, it is found that the parent dislikes the messiness of self-feeding, so does not permit the child to feed himself. If only the parent's information on the child's self-feeding is included on a developmental evaluation, an inaccurate picture of the child's immediate developmental skill and potential development is presented. As a result, valuable time may be lost in planning and in executing the appropriate treatment.

A summary is included at the end of an evaluation. This is a definitive compilation of the primary and secondary assets and liabilities of the child which broadly define the problem in relation to occupational therapy. The summary does not repeat the report in detail, but only highlights important behavior. In one sense, the summary can be compared with the introduction of a book: it succinctly explains the contents of the report to the reader. The reader then can determine the applicability of the report for himself as a staff member and decide whether or not to study it further. An example of a meaningless versus a meaningful summary statement is:

1. The child's social behavior is good for his age.

2. The child socially is at the stage of gang play which is appropriate for his age.

Recommendations for treatment may or may not be included in an evaluation report. If the individuals who will receive the report are to use it directly in their treatment or handling of the child, it may be useful to make appropriate and easily understood suggestions. If the report is to be used by teachers, the terminology should be familiar to them and the medical and occupational therapy jargon should be omitted. Recommendations for occupational therapy aides or COTAs are written in detail — as a prescription is written for a technician who performs a given task. For another OTR, ideas and theoretical questions may be posed concerning treatment rather than detailed instructions for treatment.

If the evaluation is performed completely and written skillfully, with treatment recommendations included, the task of planning treatment is greatly simplified. The basic information in the evaluation serves as a guide for the initial treatment session. If the evaluation is not completed due to a limited or poor performance by the child, the evaluator can continue or repeat the evaluation during the first treatment session.

Each treatment session is an evaluation of a child's behavior on a specific day and the treatment plan is revised daily if the child's behavior indicates this need. The child may progress beyond the expected point, regress or, maybe, show no change in behavior. Because each evaluation shows only what the child does on that day and at that hour when the evaluation is done, evaluations are ongoing and an integral part of the treatment process.

Bibliography

Arbuckle, D. S. *Counseling Philosophy, Theory and Practice,* Revised edition (Boston: Allyn and Bacon, 1965).

Arbuckle, D. S. *Counseling and Psychotherapy* (New York: McGraw-Hill, 1967).

Cohen, D. H. & Stern, V. *Observing and Recording the Behavior of Young Children* (New York: Teachers College Press, 1958).

Gesell, A. L. *The First Five Years of Life* (New York: Harper & Row, 1940).

Rogers, C. R. *Client-centered Therapy* (Boston: Houghton Mifflin, 1951).

Spock, B. M. *Problems of Parents* (Boston: Houghton Mifflin, 1962).

Takata, N. "The Play History," *American Journal of Occupational Therapy* 23 (1969), pp. 314-318.

Terman, L. M. & Merrill, M. A. *Stanford-Binet Intelligence Scale: Manual for the Third Revision, Form L-M* (Boston: Houghton-Mifflin, 1960).

Wechsler, D. *Wechsler Intelligence Scale for Children* (New York: The Psychological Corporation, 1949).

NOTES

Chapter Three
Treatment

Barbara Sharpe Banus, M.A., O.T.R.

(July 1971)

DEFINITION OF TREATMENT IN OCCUPATIONAL THERAPY

Treatment in occupational therapy consists of tasks or actions which an individual performs — passively or actively — under the supervision of the therapist, in order to gain or to improve his function or performance. (*To perform a task* implies interaction between the human and a nonhuman object or environment. *To act and change function* means to use oneself and to make a change in oneself.) The patient is an active participant in the treatment process and, if possible, helps to determine the treatment objectives, adjust them, and to carry out the treatment process — with the assistance of the therapist.

The treatment process is cyclical and continuous from its inception to its completion. It is composed of four units: (1) the setting of treatment objectives, (2) the formulation and analysis of the means of attaining the objectives, (3) the implementation and process of treatment, and (4) the evaluation of the success in meeting the treatment goals.

THE APPLICABILITY OF THE SYSTEMS ANALYSIS PROCESS TO THE TREATMENT PROCESS

There are organizational models in industry, education, and government which can be adapted for use in the analysis of treatment objectives and the formulation of treatment programs. The educational model analyzes the cyclical process described above in three steps: objectives, learning experiences, and evaluation.[1] The model is very general and must be further analyzed by the therapist who uses it; its primary emphasis is on the clear statement of objectives succeeded by the implementation.

The models used in industry and government have been derived from an approach which emphasizes economic output: in industry they are titled *management science* or *operations research;* in government and defense programs they are a form of *systems analysis.* Systems analysis was developed for use in the United States Department of Defense, in order that it could utilize its income, resources, and services to their maximum effectiveness. The basic concept of systems analysis can be defined as: "a systematic approach to helping a decision-maker choose a course of action by investigating his full problem, searching out objectives and alternatives, and comparing them in light of their consequences, using an appropriate framework — insofar as possible analytic — to bring expert judgment and intuition to bear on the problem." [2]

An adaptation of this model, the "scientific decision-making process in occupational therapy," provides a logical, systematic framework for determining a treatment program. In the application of the model of systems analysis to occupational therapy, two important modifications are necessary: (1) the emphasis on noneconomic objectives must be increased in occupational therapy and (2) variations in human behavior must be taken into account. The first modification refers to the equating of the cost-benefit concept, with all the positive and negative aspects of treatment — including financial and nonfinancial factors. The second modification refers to the inclusion of a unit (*Implementing Treatment*) to the cyclical process of iteration (Figure 3-1).

A modification of Quade's definition for occupational therapy reads: a systematic approach made by a trained individual (an *occupational therapist*) as he chooses and implements a course of treatment by investigating the patient's problem and the institution's responsibilities, searching out treatment objectives and alternatives and implementing them in the light of their consequences and the subtleties affecting them, and using an analytic framework in order to bring expert judgment and skilled intuition to bear on the problem.

This systematic approach can be used to organize a broad program within an occupational therapy department or a narrow program for the treatment of one patient. It illustrates and suggests a systematic approach to planning treatment for children in occupational therapy and will, therefore, be applied in the narrower context. The total process of setting treatment

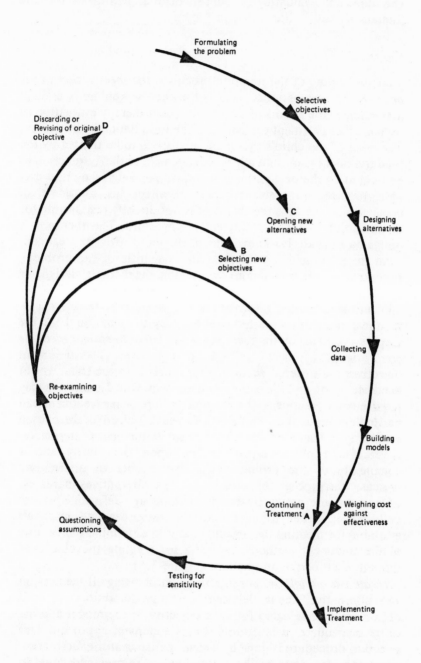

Formulating
the problem

Selective
objectives

Discarding or
Revising of original **D**
objective

C
Opening new
alternatives

Designing
alternatives

B
Selecting new
objectives

Collecting
data

Re-examining
objectives

Building
models

Continuing
Treatment **A**

Weighing cost
against
effectiveness

Questioning
assumptions

Testing for
sensitivity

Implementing
Treatment

FIG. 3-1. Adaptation of the iteration process of systems analysis to occupational therapy.

objectives, systematically analyzing and implementing treatment activities, and evaluating the success of treatment is described as "iteration" and is illustrated in Figure 3-1.

Iteration

The beginning of the iteration process is the *formulation of the problem*. In occupational therapy the child's problem is defined according to the results of the occupational therapy evaluation as well as other pertinent evaluations. The formulation is the general statement of the child's dysfunction which is to be treated by the total treatment team, and a specific statement of the dysfunction to be treated by the occupational therapist. Although the child may have multiple problems which will affect his treatment in occupational therapy, the therapist is not directly responsible for their resolution in his treatment of the child. The therapist is obligated to share his knowledge of the child with the treatment team in order to help complete the diagnosis of the problem. From this information and his own testing, the therapist designates the problems with which he will be concerned.

From the compiled information, the *objectives are selected* — for the treatment of the total problem by the team, and for the specific problems by the therapist. *Alternative treatment methods are designed* to meet each of the objectives. The treatment objectives are ordered according to priorities in the treatment of the dysfunction and the child's development. One dysfunction may require some treatment, for example, before other treatment can be implemented; the alternatives for each objective are chosen accordingly. There may be a large or small number of alternatives to meet the objectives, depending upon the clarity and/or complexity of the problems. As the number of alternatives increase, the problem of selecting the best alternatives increases.

Once the alternative treatment methods are defined, *data are collected* in order to determine the resources and materials available for meeting the objectives and to determine the validity of the treatment methods or media for meeting the objectives through each of the alternatives (Figure 3-5).

Treatment models are constructed incorporating all the data on each alternative. The models must meet a predetermined standard of performance selected for each objective; if the model appears to be inadequate, it is dismissed as a treatment approach. This selection procedure is done by *weighing cost against effectiveness,* commonly described as the evaluation of the pros and cons. In occupational therapy, "cost" may be defined in terms of money received for treatment; the child's energy expenditure; the quantity of time required for treatment; and the number of personnel required to perform the specific method of treatment. These costs are then weighed against the degree of effectiveness or the value of the specific treatment. The goal is to obtain the most effective treatment for the most reasonable cost. In rehabilitation, it may be necessary to increase the cost if a minimum standard of effectiveness in treatment is to be met. If the cost is very low, the effectiveness may be low. The cost, however, can be very low but effectiveness high. When neuromuscular facilitation techniques are applied to the appropriate dysfunction, for example, the cost in terms of the child's energy expenditure is very low but the effectiveness or benefits are high — an ideal situation.

The alternative treatment method which appears to be most effective is chosen and *treatment is implemented.* Treatment elicits practical considerations, as opposed to the theoretical ones which have been considered to this point. All people involved in treatment have different responsibilities which effect the fulfillment of the objectives. In *testing for sensitivity,* both the theoretical and the practical factors are evaluated in the initial phase of treatment — which is a period of time specified for experimentation to determine the effectiveness of the model chosen by the decision-maker.

The expert, professional judgment of the therapist or decision-maker is the key to the successful planning of treatment: the greater the knowledge of the decision-maker, the greater the possibility of accurate and objective decisions. This reduces subjective interpretation and inaccurate judgment based on incomplete facts. Treatment within the first cycle of iteration can be called "short term" and thus might be considered experimental because of the alterations which are usually necessary because of development or changes in the child's dysfunction.

The last three steps in the iteration process form the monitoring (or evaluation) system. Through this system the treatment model, which has been implemented in the occupational therapy model, is scrutinized to determine its success or failure in total or in part and thus determine the need for change. First, the *assumptions are questioned.* The treatment model originally chosen, which was developed from the decision-maker's knowledge and expertise, is analyzed as treatment proceeds and success or failure in meeting the treatment objectives becomes apparent.

If upon *re-examination of the objectives,* gains are being made by the child at a consistent pace, treatment is continued (*arrow A in Figure 3-1*). If progress is slow or nonexistent, it is evident that a problem exists somewhere in the cycle of iteration. If the objective has been met, treatment toward this objective is discontinued and the process of planning, analysis, implementation and evaluation for other objectives is begun (*arrow B*). If the original alternatives to the treatment are inadequate or inappropriate, or if new alternatives appear (*arrow C*), the first two steps in iteration are omitted as the iteration process continues. Another possible problem (*arrow D*), is that the original objective was poor and needs to be revised or discarded.

The assumptions of the decision-maker in building the original models may have been influenced by unexpected factors or unplanned situations, which appear upon implementation. It may have been assumed, for example, that X hours would be available weekly to treat a child. If the time cannot be available, the objectives must be re-examined in line with the new information and the child's progress to date. *New objectives are written, new alternatives are explored, data collected* and so forth through the cycle.

Iteration continues until treatment is completed. The more often the process is repeated, the less useful it becomes unless new material appears (for example, negative changes in the child's progress due to a setback from his illness or positive changes from the administration of a new and effective drug). All normal and handicapped children eventually develop to a point after which their conditions cannot be changed or improved despite the cost expended and the effectiveness of the treatment methods.

FORMULATION OF THE PROBLEM

Factors Which Indirectly Affect the Formulation of the Problem

Treatment is affected by the total institution and by the specific department in which the occupational therapist functions. The function of the occupational therapy department is contingent upon the institution and its philosophy, goals, and financial status. The type of treatment provided is contingent upon the policies and practices of the occupational therapy department.

The institution's policies and procedures determine the treatment programs throughout the institution. They define the type of evaluation and treatment programs for which the institution provides service, as seen in the titles *Child Psychiatry Clinic, Outpatient Medical Service,* and *Amputee Clinic.* The institution is established in order to render specific services and may, therefore, restrict the type of patient problems it accepts, based on its physical facilities, the qualifications of personnel, budgets and so forth. For this reason, it may not be possible for the therapist to treat a child with one kind of problem, although he may be qualified to do so. For example, a medical ward in a general hospital does not have the staff, physical facilities or personnel training to care for a severely emotionally disturbed child. Although the therapist may have the training to treat the child as well as some of the necessary tools, the child must be sent to another institution which is fully equipped to handle him.

In addition, the policies of the institution directly or indirectly define the way in which treatment is given. They may encourage experimental procedures — or they may require the use of conventional techniques. This policy is determined by the philosophy of the administrators, the type of physical facilities, the space available for treatment, and the equipment, and the number and types of ancillary services available (psychology, occupational therapy, physical therapy). A private hospital may give stipends to its staff for specialized study; money for the purchase of special equipment; and support and encouragement in experimental research on its patient population. A state hospital may lack money for anything other than the continuing of conventional, well established programs: it may be unable to supply new personnel, extra training or new materials.

Permanent and expendable budgets, research grants, fellowships and so forth determine the growth of an institution and its departments. Without financial backing, the quantity and quality of materials available to the therapist for evaluation and treatment are limited. It may be impossible to purchase up-to-date testing and treatment materials, which, in turn, affects the total quality of treatment available to the patients.

A second factor which directly affects treatment is the list of policies and procedures of the occupational therapy department (which are based primarily on those of the institution). In addition, the occupational therapy department develops policies and procedures for its own specific function within the institution. These can differ but must be complementary: the objectives of one department should not conflict with those of the other departments because of the cooperation necessary for a patient's rehabilitation. In order to maintain consistency, the individual department may be prevented from employing new evaluation or treatment methods; if this situation occurs, the therapist makes the decision about staying or leaving the institution.

Factors Which Directly Affect the Formulation of the Problem

The *child's problem is defined or formulated* from the evaluations of the total treatment team. With this information, the staff decides whether or not it can treat the child in accordance with the institution and department policies. If the decision is negative, the child is referred to the appropriate institution; if positive, broad treatment goals are defined and treatment tentatively considered. From this information, each team member identifies the problems which can be treated by his service: the occupational therapist formulates specific problems to be treated in occupational therapy .

After the specific problems which can be treated in therapy are determined, the factors which will influence their treatment are identified. These may or may not be "problems," but are presented at this point because they can create varying degrees of difficulty in treatment. Questions raised about the following factors may be evaluated quickly and dismissed — or may require further investigation. In other words, all information possibly relevant to the setting of objectives and the choosing of alternatives for treatment is noted.

Precautions and restrictions (identified in Chapter Two) may be a problem to the child if they contradict one set of his needs to meet another, as in the case of the nine-year-old boy who needs bed rest prior to open-heart surgery, but who desires activity. *Medical treatment* may actively interfere with treatment by the ancillary services when it affects the child's behavior — as, for instance, in the case of the drugs which have a secondary, sedative effect on the child.

The *developmental level or range* of the child is identified in each area of behavior. The child's development always influences treatment and is considered in planning treatment whether it is primary or secondary to the dysfunction. The following areas of development are considered when formulating the child's problem to be treated in occupational therapy:

Ego development: the child's sense of identity or self image, his personality dynamics and modes of emotional expression

Social development: his social conscience or superego — as seen in his group and individual behavior; his need for and reaction to adult and peer relationships

Neuromotor development: the degree of skill and coordination in gross and fine motor behavior, balance, and posture

Perceptual-motor development: his sensory-perceptual-motor performances in relation to vision, audition, kinesthesia, touch

Cognitive development: his ability to use his intelligence and adapt to his environment with its changes

Speech and language development: his receptive-expressive language, verbal and nonverbal expression of it and comprehension

The members of the *family complex* and their concern for the child are assessed in order to determine their ability to assist in the child's treatment and their positive or negative influence on the child's treatment.

Information about the *child's past experience* is useful for several reasons. First, the kind and degree of competencies of the child prior to his illness indicate his original potential in several areas — motor, social, intellectual and others. If there is a gross discrepancy between the child's former and present function — and if the child is aware of it, there is a problem. The positive elements of knowing breadth and depth of the child's living experience, such as his education, hobbies, travels, and contacts with peers, gives the therapist cues about the type of interaction the child may need and will indicate the level of his communication to the therapist.

The *child's daily schedule,* which includes hours for treatment, may create conflicts between services. Priorities for treatment must be chosen when there is a time conflict which indicates, subtly, the importance of the different services in the institution. It is a problem to schedule occupational therapy, physical therapy, and school when all three must occur within the same overlapping three hours. Which has priority?

Figure 3-2 is an example of the formulation of the problem of Susan Barkley. Susan's case will be used to demonstrate the application of the iteration process to occupational therapy. The planning of her treatment is much simpler than that of the usual handicapped child and is described strictly to illustrate iteration in a simplified manner.

SELECTING OBJECTIVES

Each of the factors stated above is pertinent to the selection of treatment objectives. The limited problem of Susan permits explicit objectives. If the diagnosis indicates multiple developmental or dysfunctional problems, however, treatment may be very complex. The family and its relationship to the child affect the number of objectives which the occupational therapist can meet. If the

Name: Susan Barkley

Date of report: Dec. 6, 1969

Sex: female

Birth date: Dec. 5, 1966

Age: 3 years

Diagnosis: traumatic below-elbow amputation of the right forearm, which is the dominant side

Diagnostic problems to be treated in occupational therapy:
1. training of the right prosthetic hand in ADL (eating, dressing, toileting) bilateral functions; transferring; and unilateral, supporting functions.
2. training of the left hand in dominant hand functions.

Precautions and restrictions: Stump is slightly tender.

Medical treatment: None presently.

Developmental ranges:
social behavior—2 to 2½ years. Susan clings to adults, watches but does not interact with peers. (Regressive behavior as a result of trauma and hospitalization?)
Emotional expression—2½ to 3 years. Cries when stump is hit or rubbed against. Says "no" emphatically when angry. Shows problems of separation: needs attention of adult to involve self in play and cries for mother at bedtime.
Neuromotor behavior—range of 3 years plus or minus a month. Right upper extremity function is poor to nonexistent.
Perceptual-motor behavior—adequate for age 3 except as affected by hand function.
Language abilities—2½ to 3 years. Problem seems to be shyness rather than inability to speak. Receptive language is good.

Family complex: Parents, no siblings. The parents are helpful to the child by requiring her independence. The home is 300 miles away and parents visit only on weekends during the training session period of hospitalization.

Child's past experience: Susan had limited contacts with other children in her first three years. Prior to the injury, she was a talkative, active, independent child who played well alone when in the same room with a parent (report of mother).

Child's present daily schedule from which to plan occupational therapy: Physical therapy for whirlpool treatment of the stump: 9-9:30 A.M. and 3-3:30 P.M.; Playroom group: 10-12 Noon and 4-5 P.M. (Susan can be taken out for treatment.); Rest hour: 1-3 P.M.

FIG. 3-2. Formulation of the problem.

family is cooperative and can supplement the treatment hours provided by the therapist, the objectives may be expanded. However, if the therapist must do all treatment, the range and quantity of treatment is necessarily smaller.

The selection of objectives may be easy or it may be complex. If the initial evaluation defines the problems of the child clearly and if there are a limited number of problems, the objectives for treatment can be stated clearly and concisely. Once chosen, the objectives are arranged according to priority in treatment. They are sequenced on the basis of the child's immediate needs and ability to function. Only the obvious objectives may be apparent immediately following evaluation — others may appear as the child performs in treatment. These then will be incorporated into the treatment program.

Secondary objectives are those which are not directly related to the dysfunction, but are important to the child's development and rehabilitation. They are analyzed according to the same format as the primary objectives, and implemented on a parallel basis at the appropriate treatment stage (Figure 3-3).

The secondary objectives may appear to be primary, as in Susan's case. Treatment of the dysfunction may be simplified once the child's problems of separation and peer interaction are resolved. Thus, they may have priority in treatment over the primary dysfunction. This is one of the situations in which the decision-maker's professional judgment is critical in cost-effectiveness analysis.

Primary objectives:
1. Develop dominance in left hand for unilateral function.
2. Develop right hand (prosthesis) in reach, grasp, and release for assistive functions.
3. Develop transfer between left and right hand.
4. Develop bilateral hand function.
5. Develop functional independence in ADL skills appropriate to Susan's developmental level.

Secondary objectives:
6. Develop self-confidence during mother's absence.
7. Develop peer relationships.

FIG. 3-3. Selection of objectives in order of priority.

DESIGNING ALTERNATIVES

Designing the alternatives is the name given to the process of choosing a variety of possible media and methods to meet each objective. This process is based upon the correlation of the compiled information from the evaluation with the activities or treatment media available within occupational therapy. The method of obtaining and compiling the basic information from the evaluations has already been discussed. The focus is now on the correlation of activity with objectives and analysis.

Media in occupational therapy may be defined as the stimuli which elicit specific goal-directed behaviors or responses. They range from static nonhuman objects to the dynamic human object of the child's self and others within the child's environment. The degree of the child's involvement with human or nonhuman media varies: the child may perform with the media for an indeterminate time and expend minimum to maximum physical or emotional energy. The modality may have practical application to the child's immediate situation, or long-range value, as seen in the learning of a task which later evolves as a hobby. The child may use the media as either the means to the end or as the end result itself, or both.

Activity can be analyzed from two perspectives: *cross-sectional* and *sequential* or *longitudinal*. These perspectives parallel those for the human developmental patterns — in other words, media or nonhuman objects follow a developmental sequence which makes correlation of media with the child's treatment possible. Data collected from the observation of the children's use of materials show that materials are used in the same sequence by all children, with only limited variation.

The cross-sectional analysis of media is the comparison of one media with others at the *same* developmental stage — the comparison of drawing, blocks, puzzles, ball, and utensils as used by a five-year-old, twenty-four-month-old, or a twelve-month-old child. With cross-sectional knowledge of media, the therapist can observe a child's use of a variety of media and determine the child's developmental and functional profile (evaluation). In planning treatment, the former pattern is followed in order to provide the child with a broad and appropriate range of media.

The sequential analysis is the study of the same material over a period of time, for example, the block structures built sequentially by a child from age nine months through five years. This shows the changes in the child's ability to use materials as he progressed developmentally. Media are analyzed from the longitudinal perspective in order to determine their sequential use in treatment.

Change in the way the child uses the media or the kind of media demonstrates his development. It is therefore essential to know the child's progressive use of media.

Media also are analyzed for their practical use in the treatment of specific dysfunctions. A medium which offers the greatest overall use is favored over that which is appropriate occasionally. The material most easily handled is introduced at the beginning of treatment, while complex media are reserved until the child indicates readiness for challenge.

There are several possible classifications of the broad variety of media available to occupational therapy. The following classification has been chosen because of its adaptability. The list is not all-inclusive, but it does show some of the possibilities for treatment media in pediatric occupational therapy.

Use of self is a term that refers to the therapist's use of his own personality and body in the interaction between child and adult during treatment. This is emphasized particularly at the beginning of treatment when the child may be anxious about the treatment, the strange room or the unknown adult. The therapist may need to actively involve himself in the relationship in order to reduce the child's concern, or he may interact minimally as the child uses the media, rather than the therapist, as he adapts to the new situation.

The therapist is himself an essential medium: all treatment is dependent upon some interaction and direct supervision (except in specialized cases which use behavior modification techniques). Small children, in particular, need mechanical assistance and emotional support in learning the required task because of their limited cognitive, language, and emotional development. Adolescents may require less direct assistance. For example, the treatment objective may be to shift the responsibility for the adolescent's treatment from the therapist to the adolescent himself as he gradually internalizes the need to perform and provides his own reward through the results of this performance. Even then, the therapist uses himself as motivation for the adolescent to perform the desired task independently.

The therapist also serves as a model for the child. His behavior, which includes the helpful behavior and the idiosyncrasies, is observed and may be imitated. These behaviors may be intentionally or unintentionally passed on to the child, although they may not be the primary objectives of the child's treatment. The therapist is consciously honest and open with the child; unconsciously, he speaks with an accent and has the mannerism of scratching his ear.

The *child's body* may itself be a treatment media directly (physically) or (psychologically) indirectly. His total self-image — which includes the social, emotional, and physical self and his body image — is based upon the perceived self and may or may not be realistic; upon the actual self, which is seen in his performance; and upon the view of himself by others. The handicapped child's reaction to his own physical body is dependent upon the real or imagined degree of disfigurement, distortion, or dysfunction.

When the child's body is used as a treatment medium to elicit a change or response, the body itself may be the only medium through which and for which the treatment is done, or an external media may be used in addition. For example, some neuromuscular facilitation techniques require only the child's body in order to change the neuromotor function of the child. With other neuromuscular facilitation techniques, tools external to the child are applied in order to change the neuromotor function The child may use other materials on himself to create visible change which affects his psychological perception of his body; or he may perform behaviors which change him, although the change may not be obvious to others. The uncoordinated child who does not respect his own performance may exercise to improve his poise and motor performance by improving muscle tone and coordination.

In spite of physical change, the child's attitude toward himself may remain the same; he will need to work on understanding and accepting his own body and its changes. Teenagers, particularly, are very aware of the changes occurring in their bodies. Exercising, grooming, dressing and so forth become important media for eliciting healthy responses to the changes that naturally occur. In addition, the adolescent's posture and poise improve. It is easy to understand the frustration of the handicapped teenager whose problems with his self-image may multiply his problems resulting from dysfunction.

Manipulative materials are developmental toys which are used to meet the manual manipulative needs of the child. The child learns his abilities by using a variety of materials. These "toys" include the preschool learning, put-together type of toys and the advanced manipulative materials such as construction sets, blocks, and so forth. The materials stimulate the development of refined motor skills in coordination with tactile, auditory, visual, and kinesthetic function. Perceptual-motor behaviors are developed. These materials can be varied to be appropriate at many developmental stages.

Gross motor media are those materials which develop the child's kinesthetic and postural behavior. They are used to stimulate total body posture and gross motor movements of the lower extremities or the large muscle movements of the upper extremities. These include games of running, jumping, hopping, and so forth; and swimming and activity with objects such as bicycles, tricycles, wagons, large balls, swings, climbing apparatus. Gross motor media meet the need for total body expression and total body stimulation.

Symbolic-creative materials are used by the child to express his feelings and talents without the imposition of a predetermined end product — the process and goal are chosen by the child. The materials include painting, drawing, freeform claywork, etc. They may be made into a useful or decorative end product; they may be permanent (loom-woven cloth mat) or temporary (woven paper mat). Additional tools may be used as an advanced means for the child who wishes to produce a refined piece of work his hands cannot perform alone.

Symbolic materials help the child to express nonverbally the feelings and thoughts which he is unable to describe verbally; he may feel restricted socially and fear repercussion, or he may not be consciously aware of his behavior and feelings. The materials provide him with a means of expression which needs no explanation but which does provide him with a release. However, the freedom which accompanies the release can elicit anxiety. If the child is rigid in his behavior, the permission to be explosive, in even a minimally contained manner, can frighten the child — the child who never has fingerpainted because it was "messy" may be quite fearful of expressing himself this way. But, with the use of a piece of paper (the edge provides natural boundaries) and a tool which serves as an extension of himself (the child will not become a part of the mess), the child gradually may become free in his behavior. The same procedure also restricts the child whose expansive behavior needs limits.

The symbolic work of children, such as painting, sometimes is used by the therapist to interpret the child's feelings and behavior. There are some common interpretations of children's artwork; however, interpretation of work done by children must be specific to the child and his problems; interpretation of art is speculative and subjective. The therapist's comments and interpretations to the child about his work may be more detrimental to the child than the therapist's general acceptance and encouragement for continued performance. As the child becomes more comfortable with his feelings, or cognizant of their meaning and begins to verbalize them, the therapist may make comments or question him tactfully.

Sometimes comments made to the child about his artwork can be both realistic and symbolic. The therapist combines his hypothesis about the meaning of a piece of artwork with the child's own comments, attitudes and behavior regarding his work.

When this hypothetical material is combined with the realities of the child's life, it may be appropriate to present the child — directly or indirectly — with an interpretation. For example, it may be hypothesized from a child's drawing, attitudinal comments, and behavior that he interprets his traumatic injury as proof of his worthlessness. Perhaps the child is making a figure of clay during the treatment session and he is distressed over the fact that it breaks: "It is no good," and must be thrown away. Perhaps the therapist already has a strong hunch that the child thinks *he* is himself no good and should be discarded. The therapist can say, "It can be fixed," because, in reality, clay figures can be put back together, and so the therapist's remark points out reality. In addition it can be interpreted symbolically by the child to mean that he, too, can be fixed. If and when appropriate, the therapist can escalate and be more direct: "The figure of clay can be fixed and people can be fixed." The therapist must be sure that his realistic-symbolic comments have the same meaning for the child. The therapist must not imply, even symbolically, that a body part, such as an amputated arm, can be replaced by a live body part.[3]

Structured activities require a certain procedure for the production of the end result or specific tools to produce the results. Their characteristics provide a sense of predictability and security; they tend to reduce anxiety and to organize thoughts and actions in this way. The activity may be self-limiting because of the kind or number of its parts, or because of the types of tools available. The tasks may be repetitive or varied; each task may be singular and repetitive or it may contain many steps, each of which is different.

The repetitive or singular task may be used for rote training; for example, in the teaching of grasp and release for a prosthetic hand. This situation is one in which it is important that the child perform repetitively in order to make the opening and closing of the prosthetic hand an automatic behavior. The process then is broadened and a variety of tasks such as self-feeding, dressing, and developmental play are added. This type of behavior requires a variety of motions which must be repeated — it gives the child with the prosthetic hand a variety of positions at which the hand can be opened and closed.

Structured activities organize or specify the range of the child's behavior rather than enlarge and expand upon it as symbolic-creative media usually do. However, creative materials (such as clay) can be structured in order to stimulate a specific behavior — if it is desirable to combine structure and creativity. If, for example, a specific hand function is desired, such as the stretching of the palm and finger flexors, clay coils can be rolled. In this step of the project, there is little freedom for the child to be creative; creativity would appear only in the size of the coil and the shape of the final object.

Prevocational tasks are those tasks that help to develop behaviors important to work or that prepare the child for future vocational tasks. Prevocational tasks in the widest sense are the functional work-oriented behaviors taught from the toddler years through the adult years. This training and exploration begins in the toddler years[4] and frequently is more meaningful to the young child than a play activity.

The prevocational task may be indirectly and unobtrusively used to train a child in specific developmental behaviors without developing useless splinter skills. An example of this is seen in "stacking," which is an important concept and function in both the child and adult worlds. The child can implement this concept by the time he is two years old: he can help mommy stack towels from the laundry for the bathroom; he can stack the magazines on the living room table; he can pile the cake and pie pans on the bottom kitchen shelf; and he can pile his own clothes in his own dresser drawer. These are practical applications from both points of view. Education and possibly treatment can occur without expending extra time or energy.

The narrow and more common use of the term *prevocational tasks* or *training* includes training in all areas of development which are essential to work. A specific area may be focused upon: for example, the training of a basic skill such as color-sorting and the matching of objects. Or, a more specific work-oriented situation is created (an assembly line for building hobby horses in quantity, for example), in order to encourage correct work habits, such as punctuality and acceptance of supervision.

Prevocational training is among the most important areas of treatment in occupational therapy with children. The therapist reasons: "This child is learning this particular behavior at this particular time because it is leading him through a specific progression which will be useful to him throughout his life."

Sexual identification tasks are those tasks which symbolize the male and female roles according to the rules of a specific society: homemaking tasks of sewing, cooking, child care for the girl; outdoor and indoor work and simple repairing tasks with basic mechanical tools for the boys. Although some distinction is made between male and female roles, suggested materials are appropriate for both boys and girls — chef's clubs for boys, for instance. The sex roles and responsibilities in society are changing; it is now acceptable for males and females to exchange some responsibilities; this circumstance need not decrease a healthy individual's ability to identify with his own sex. In spite of the exchange taking place, male and female types of play begin to differentiate at three to four years of age — boys begin to imitate daddy and the girls begin to imitate mommy.

Materials used to reinforce sexual characteristics are closely related to those used to enhance body image. The girl who has the body build of a boy may have more desires to play with boy-types of materials and vice versa. Depending upon the degree to which the girl identifies with the male role, specific male behaviors may be discouraged and female behaviors encouraged — the teenage girl may be encouraged to use make-up, wear dresses, dance instead of playing baseball, and grow long hair. Rigid demands need not be made of the child unless the behavior is pathological and is interfering with his development and function.

Imitative and imaginative play are related to sexual identification play when the child's primary objective is to learn about his role in society. In its narrowest form, imitative play refers to the mimicking of a very specific action from watching someone perform. Imaginative play expands upon imitation and implies the application of real behavioral situations to make-believe ones for further understanding of another person's behavior.

The child projects many of his own feelings into imaginative play. The projection is generally derived from his wishes, fantasies or real situations with which he has dealt in the past (similar to the use of symbolic creative media). In this play, he can express his real feelings in an acceptable way as seen in the case of the child who paddles his doll and says, "Bad baby, bad baby!"

Imitative play also demonstrates the child's use of models in learning new modes of behavior. The models may be other children or adults — and may be negative or positive in helping the child develop acceptable behavior.

Activities of daily living (ADL) are the basic self-help behaviors essential to everyday living, including dressing, eating, toileting, and grooming. The objective of ADL training is to help each child to care for himself. He never may have learned the skills due to some congenital dysfunction or early trauma; he may be relearning skills he lost because of dysfunction; or he may be learning them within the context of normal development, such as the three-year-old who is learning how to dress himself. The adolescent with a traumatic injury must relearn the tasks which he once had mastered — he may relearn the behavior or he may have to learn a behavioral adaptation for a task. The problem of relearning is discouraging because of his memory of previous "normal" behavior which was easy and automatic, the change in his body image and so forth.

Children who are learning to perform normally within the context of a single, specific handicap (a prosthesis, for example) receive ADL training. Children who are learning to use adaptive techniques and equipment also receive ADL training.

It is important that adaptive equipment be used in activities of daily living only when essential. The more equipment that an individual needs to function independently, the greater his social and functional handicap will be. For example, if the cerebral palsied child can use a regular spoon with difficulty in grasping, it is still preferable to his using a built-up spoon — even though the training which is required so that he can use his own body may not be traditional and may take longer. Otherwise, he will have to carry the special spoon with him every time he goes out to eat.

In summary, the designing of alternative treatment media is done after the correlation of the child's development with his handicapping condition and the activities which have been analyzed for the particular child. Media are not diagnosis-specific — they can be used interchangeably with a variety of treatment problems. For example, all children must develop self-images and handicapped children have more difficulty in doing so. Emotionally disturbed children have self-image problems which are different from those of congential amputees — and these amputees have problems different from traumatic amputees.

Although similar media may be used with a variety of handicapped children, different objectives may be established and different treatment methods developed for each child. In addition, there may be some different materials used for each specific condition in conjunction with the parallel media (Figure 3-4).

Objective 1
    Develop dominance in left hand for unilateral function.
Alternatives
    1. coloring
    2. eating with a spoon
    3. block building
    4. ball throwing
    5. holding things for mother when helping in the kitchen
    6. feeding doll from a toy bottle

FIG. 3-4. Designing alternatives to meet the first treatment objective. Alternatives are designed in the same manner for each of the other six objectives.

COLLECTING DATA

The following data are now collected on each of the media (alternatives) to determine the reality of employing it in treatment. The data usually include the availability of the material, the analysis of the components of the media in relation to the child's development and his handicap — the characteristics which permit varied use of adaptation. Additional general data are collected on services other than occupational therapy which are treating the same problem, to avoid duplication of services and conflicting services; the available location and time for treatment; the personnel and staff requirements; and on the child's individual schedule and personal preferences.

Components of the Media

The *neuromotor requirements* of a media determine the type and degree of function necessary for the child to manipulate the media motorically. The type of function includes the quantitative requirements of the upper and lower extremity and postural involvement. The degree of function consists of the requirements in strength, range of motion, and coordination. Resistiveness and malleableness determine muscle strength; size and purpose of the media determine the range of motion and coordination. Some media require minimal quantitative motor involvement (sewing), others require maximum involvement (swimming). Qualitatively, however, sewing may be a more difficult task than swimming because of the degree of fine motor skill involved.

The *emotional elements* of media are those which can elicit an emotional response in the child. Although media have characteristics which commonly elicit identifiable reactions, responses are specific to the individual and may be positive for one and negative for another; some children enjoy the coolness and smoothness of Plasticene; others detest the stickiness.

Structured activity and creative activity elicit different kinds of emotional behavior — the former encourages specific organization of behavior; the latter provides latitude and encourages a variety of behaviors. Structure may be essential to one child's successful performance; for another, creativity may be important to self-expression and successful performance.

The degree of neatness and cleanliness is considered both in the choice of activity and in the planning of the total atmosphere of the treatment setting. Some children can focus on a specified task only if the room is neat and tidy and may become upset or distracted by sloppiness. Others function readily in messiness.

Both aggressive and passive elements of an activity must be considered for each child. Aggressive behavior may be triggered by activities which require considerable muscle strength because of resistivity, size, degree of energy expenditure. One child may become frustrated with resistive materials, feel unable to compete with them and quit; another child may need and enjoy the resistive qualities which assist him in expending energy for an emotional release. Passivity generally results from activities which require minimum motor involvement. These are necessary to the child — the post-surgical patient, for example — who needs quiet rather than the excitement which may be aroused from a stimulating material.

Familiar materials elicit behaviors different from unfamiliar materials; familiar media generally make the child feel more comfortable when he is in an unfamiliar setting. These media include objects from the child's home or objects similar to those from his home which can be used in a way that is familiar to him. Emotionally, these objects associate the institution with his home in a positive way, serving as a positive introduction to treatment. (If the familiar has previously been used inappropriately by the child, or has raised negative connotations for him, however, problems may be created rather than alleviated by the association.) The unfamiliar or semifamiliar, though sometimes unpopular, is necessary in order to expand the experience and learning of the child. The therapist continuously watches for anxiety provoked by the media which can hinder performance — if it increases beyond the level of stress with which the child can cope.

A combination of *sensory-perceptual elements* are found in all media — tactile, visual, auditory, kinesthetic, olfactory, gustatory. In occupational therapy, the tactile, visual, auditory and kinesthetic are most often considered. The tactile elements include size, shape, and texture, which the child can determine when manipulating the material. Shape and size can also be identified visually, but color is specific to visual perception. Each medium is analyzed according to its sensory-perceptual elements to determine which of the child's senses can and should be stimulated and the degree of comprehension or integration necessary for output or response. For instance, if the child has no vision, but in all other areas functions adequately, the other senses are stimulated excessively to balance the absence of one sensory mechanism.

Social elements of the material are explored in order to determine its requirements for individual or group function. These are then correlated with the child's ability to interact with peers and adults — his ability to cooperate and compete, to lead and follow, to learn and teach. This information reveals the child's developmental level of socialization; it is necessary to determine the social competencies of the child before the media are chosen because some media require participation by others and cannot be used independently.

The type of therapist-child relationship which the child can tolerate also affects the choice of media. (Does the child require help; can he accept and handle help; or must he function independently from the therapist?) If the child cannot interact with the therapist initially, a familiar material is chosen which requires little supervision or immediate interaction. Gradually media are introduced which necessitate involvement with others. It is important that the child function in a group setting (from the practical standpoint of cost in terms of time and money and from the reality standpoint in that children function in a multiperson society from infancy through adulthood). This may be a secondary objective which is met through a source other than occupational therapy if his particular behavior requires individual treatment.

The *cognitive-language elements* of a media are of primary importance and include input-integration-output as correlated with the child's ability to hear, interpret directions, and use the information as it is required for completion of the task. First, the quantity and quality of sound production within the media are explored by the therapist. The medium is then evaluated for its complexity in terms of the necessary directions — for which the child must have some degree of receptive language as well as problem-solving ability. The quantity of information which the child can retain, use correctly and in sequence, determines the number of directions given at one time and, therefore, the degree to which he can work independently. The third cognitive-language element of the media is the verbal and expressive language requirement: the degree and quality of the child's vocalization and the complexity or sophistication of the content. For example, the infant's expressive language is nonverbal and generalized behavior; the adolescent may have excellent diction and an extensive vocabulary.

The choice of media is based partly upon the child's need for parallel traits in his behavior; for example, if the primary treatment objective is to change the child's constrained neuromotor behavior into active behavior, the neuromotor (and possibly the social) elements of the media will be considered first. More active motor behavior can be encouraged through gross motor activity or resistive media such as clay throwing or hammering. Other elements and other media will be considered as the child is ready for the development of other behaviors. Language will become important to the child's verbal expression of his independence and aggression, as opposed to his present physical expression. And the social elements become much more important for the practice of his newly learned behaviors.

The Analysis of Data According to the Handicapping Condition

In the process of analyzing media developmentally, questions are raised which concern the effect of the child's dysfunction on his ability to use the media. How does his handicap affect the physical, emotional, social skills required by the media? In what ways does his handicap inhibit the use of media? How does his own healthy function assist? Which of his needs can best be met by a particular medium? Which variables of the media are particularly important to consider because of the child's handicap (color, if the child has some visual loss)?

The child's overall developmental level is compared with his performance level in the area of the handicap. It is possible that the child's performance in the area of his handicap may be much lower or earlier than the child's developmental levels in other areas of performance. For example, a child with a new prosthetic hand may be able to grasp and release a single two-inch block by opening and closing a hook, but he may not be able to grasp and stack one-inch blocks at the beginning of treatment. This may create a problem for the child if he is intellectually, socially, motorially, verbally and so forth at the level of a twelve-year-old child. He may consider the task of stacking, grasping, and releasing "infantile," since a twelve-month-old does this as part of his play. In planning for the child's treatment, therefore, tasks given to the child are appropriate for his other areas of development even though the actual process of grasping and releasing is an immature pattern for him. (This conception is not accurate because of the addition of the mechanical device, but the child may interpret it this way.) A twelve-year-old child may enjoy the competition of checkers, which requires grasping, stacking, and releasing.

One medium may have many components, all or part of which are therapeutic for a child: another medium may have a combination of therapeutic and nontherapeutic elements. If the latter medium is chosen over the former, the nontherapeutic elements may cancel out whatever beneficial results would have occurred. For example, the child who is receiving tactile perceptual-motor training is given tasks which require maximum tactile sensation.

The value of pasting and fingerpainting is diminished if a paste stick or a paint brush is used in place of the child's hand. The variety and quantity of tactile stimulation is decreased.

Some activities can be adapted in order to meet the treatment objectives. Before adapting the media, however, a theoretical analysis of the elements of the product is made in relation to the dysfunction. Its utility is correlated with the problems it can create via its adaptation. If the media has to be adapted grossly so the child only can function with that specific media, he will have a difficult time functioning in the every day world outside the treatment setting, as noted in the example of the adapted spoon.

Finally, there is a dependent relationship among the components of any activity in the same way that there is a dependent relationship among the behaviors of a child. A single element of media cannot be isolated without destroying the media — the value of the media is based on its components. For example, the emotional benefit gained from ball play is dependent on the neuromotor requirements, which, in turn, implicate perceptual-motor elements guiding the child's motor behavior.

The Other Services and Occupational Therapy

The therapist must obtain information about the child's treatment by other services so that he will be able to determine which objectives can be met best by occupational therapy and which by each of the other ancillary services. This process is relatively easy if the child's total treatment is being performed within one institution which has good communication. However, if the child attends public school, receives occupational therapy at an outpatient clinic weekly and physical therapy at home with monthly check-ups, the correlating of services most likely will be very difficult.

The content of the communication revolves around the specific treatment provided by each service. The therapist coordinates his treatment with other specialties to provide the needed developmental and dysfunctional treatment and to reduce the duplication of services. This is beneficial to the child because he receives unified and nonconflicting treatments — treatment which covers a broader range of behavior than otherwise would be possible. This fact does not mean that there is no duplication of services. It means that the services supplement one another without being repetitious in content. Recreational therapy may provide some of the gross motor tasks which are important to the child's development, but secondary to treatment. Occupational therapy may concentrate on perceptual-motor training and the emotional aspects of a one-to-one relationship. The social needs may be met in ward play directly supervised by volunteers, who are in turn guided by the nursing staff, occupational therapists, and recreational therapists. Some of the perceptual-cognitive needs may be treated in the special education classroom.

The *location of and time for treatment, personnel requirements,* and the *child's schedule* are the remaining factors about which data are collected. Frequently these factors are an integral part of the rehabilitation program over which the therapist has little control. Each will be discussed in the next section (Figure 3-5).

Objective 1: Develop dominance in left hand for unilateral function
    All materials are available for training except Alternative 5 (holding things for mother when helping in the kitchen). The child will remain in the hospital until training is complete, because of long distance between institution and the home. This alternative will be considered upon the child's return home.
Alternative 1: Coloring
    Comparison of the components of the media with the child's development and behavior:
        Neuromotor components: Weakness and incoordination of the left hand due to lack of its use as the dominant extremity. Susan will probably have some difficulty in grasping a crayon and manipulating it.
        Emotional elements: O.K.
        Sensory-perceptual elements: O.K.
        Social elements: independent function (another child is not required for treatment).
        Cognitive-language elements: not required.
    Handicapping factors: None on the left side. Susan may have a problem using her right arm and prosthetic hand to hold paper still. The positive factor is her young age and limited development of dominance on either side.
    Other services: P.T. 9-9:30 A.M. and 3-3:30 P.M. Susan is involved in the preschool group which is on a flexible morning and afternoon schedule of 10-12 Noon and 4-5 P.M.
    Location of treatment: Child's bedroom or occupational therapy department (occupational therapy room preferred).
    Occupational therapist's available time: 9:30-11 A.M. and 4:00-4:30 P.M.
    Time requirements: The preferred times for 30 minutes' treatment twice daily are 9:30-10 A.M. and 4-4:30 P.M. after physical therapy.
    Personnel requirements: One OTR is required who can be assisted by an OTS who eventually will do the treatment under supervision of the OTR.
    Child's schedule: Breakfast at 8 A.M.; physician's rounds 8:30 A.M. P. T. 9-9:30 A.M.; preschool group 10-12 Noon; lunch 12:00 Noon; nap 1-3 P.M.; P. T. 3-3:30 P.M.; preschool group 4-5 P.M.; supper 5:30 P.M.; bedtime 7:30 P.M.

FIG. 3-5. Collecting data on available resources. Alternative 1 illustrates the way in which data are collected on each alternative for Objective 1 in combination with all other data.

BUILDING TREATMENT MODELS

Building models is the process of organizing all the collected information in a variety of treatment programs in order to determine the approach which will hypothetically meet the treatment objectives most effectively. The variables found in the data may be combined in a variety of ways — with the constants always remaining the same. For example, in planning the treatment hour for Susan, certain facts are known: the physical therapy hour must be from 9-9:30 A.M. and 3-3:30 P.M. (*constants*). The occupational therapist has free time between 9:30 and 11:00 A.M. and 4-4:30 P.M. (the morning hours offer three variables, the afternoon offers one constant). Therefore, three treatment models can be built with three different morning treatment hours (Figure 3-6). Other data are analyzed in the same manner.

One of the first considerations in building models is the *scheduling of the treatment time*. The therapist must place his treatment hour within the schedule established by the particular institution (rest hours, meal times, and medical rounds, etc.). Within this framework, the therapist determines the frequency and length of the treatment sessions and the order or schedule for the presentation of treatment items within the specified hour.

The length of treatment time must be realistic for both the therapist and the child. The therapist determines the length of treatment time in relation to his other responsibilities. From the child's point of view, depending upon the kind of treatment and the type of relationship with the therapist, therapy can last from five minutes to five hours. The greater the length of treatment (up to the point of fatigue), the greater the probability of progressive change. This cannot be disputed, although it is seldom possible to give maximum time for treatment to one child. Sometimes the therapist who is working with social-emotional problems feels that *any* contact is therapeutic, even though it may last only five minutes. A few intense contacts with an emotionally disturbed child may be most effective; in the interim the child has time to think and work on various issues. Communication in terms of a deep exchange of ideas or feelings can only occur in the longer contact. Adequate time must be allocated for treatment to occur or for a change in behavior or attitude to take place. (This may be a temporary change necessary to the developmental process, but one which will disappear completely as the patient progresses; or it may become a permanent change in the form of an established new behavior.)

Treatment by facilitation techniques is done at least once daily for the children with neuromotor dysfunction for the repetition

Model I	Model II	Model III
Time: 30 minutes twice daily (9:30-10 A.M. and 4-4:30 P.M.)	Time: 30 minutes twice daily (10-10:30 A.M. and 4-4:30 P.M.)	Time: 30 minutes twice daily (10:30-11 A.M. and 4-4:30 P.M.)
Location: occupational therapy department—small room	Location: child's room	Location: occupational therapy department—small room
Personnel: 1 OTR, 1 OTS (observer)	Personnel: OTS	Personnel: 1 OTR
Individual treatment	Individual treatment	Individual treatment
Internal treatment schedule:	Internal treatment schedule	Internal treatment schedule:
Free play—(with dolls) 5 minutes	Free play—15 minutes	Coloring—15 minutes
Block building or other unilateral table play—10 minutes	Coloring—15 minutes	Unilateral table play with manipulative materials—10 minutes
Coloring—10 minutes		Free play—5 minutes
Ball throwing or gross motor activity 5 minutes		
	Lunch: 12:00 Noon—supervised by aide who may feed Susan herself to save time. No direction or supervision by OTR.	Lunch: 12:00 Noon—child's eating to be supervised by OTS with verbal instructions from OTR.
Lunch: 12:00 Noon—eating with spoon and drinking from cup. OTR supervises and teaches lunch room aide the procedure for encouraging the use of the left hand without weird adaptations of the right upper arm.		

FIG. 3-6. Building models for the treatment process to meet the first objective. The number of models built is dependent upon the number of variables.

which is necessary to learning. The desired goal is functional change which develops gradually.

A child with a perceptual deficit or an emotional problem also needs daily stimulation for corrective purposes. Depending upon his developmental age and ability to concentrate, he may be able to tolerate only short, frequent periods of stimulation (twenty to thirty minutes) at one time. On the other hand, the child may be very involved in treatment and have difficulty in ending the session.

In each of these cases, the therapist may see the child only weekly or monthly and may not perform the daily treatment. Instead, the therapist may supervise a school teacher, ward counselor or parent. As a result, the therapist probably would work for a longer period of time with the child and the supervising adult on the occasional contacts then he would on a daily treatment basis.

As he organizes the internal structure of the treatment session, the therapist plans treatment to match the child's natural order of behavior so that he will be able to gain maximum cooperation from the child. This includes the need for planning treatment at an optimum time within the child's total day. In activities of daily living training, for example, it is logical to teach a child dressing techniques (1) in the morning when he gets out of bed, (2) before, and (3) after his nap; and to train him in self-feeding at mealtimes.

Adults usually submit to practicing these skills at odd hours because they recognize the benefits for their rehabilitation. Young children do not understand peculiar schedules and may rebel; they understand only the "here and now" and not the value of treatment in relation to tomorrow. If the child is forced to perform at an undesirable time, the results of the treatment may be negligible.

The sequencing of tasks within the treatment session must be logical according to the needs of the child, his development, and his personality. Most likely, a toddler who is motor-minded will not sit still for half an hour of training in fine motor coordination with manipulative materials. He may sit still for a total of half an hour at three different times (ten minutes each) or slightly longer periods when he is a little sleepy or relaxed from previous physical activity. Thus, the treatment session for a toddler is interspersed with gross physical activities, such as running, wagon pulling, and push-and-pull play. On the other hand, a teenager may be able to concentrate easily on a difficult and even discouraging task for forty-five minutes with some encouragement from the therapist — alternating activities is not a problem.

It is desirable to choose the *physical facilities* for treatment which will meet the child's needs most effectively. For treatment sessions, it is preferable to have a bright, airy room rather than the small office-size room often used for evaluation. The type of room influences the attitude of the individuals, both child and therapist, within the room and consequently affects productivity. Bright spots of color mixed with nondistracting equipment and materials are important. A large, brightly painted mural on the walls might be very distracting to the hyperkinetic children, but blue and white checked curtains against a light blue wall with matching cabinets elicit a gay but restful feeling.

Again, the noncluttered effect is important: locked and unlocked cabinets with opaque doors; shelves for projects; hooks for aprons; a sink and counter for clean-up and so on. When treatment is done in the child's home, the ideal may not be possible. It is desirable, however, to have a space available for regular use that has limited distractions. This serves two purposes — it avoids disorganizing the whole household regularly and helps the child to develop and maintain a routine.

The physical facilities of the room are important but the emotional climate predetermined by the therapist is critical. There are some identifiable elements which enhance this climate. The consistency of the treatment hour gives the child certain expectations and helps him to prepare and feel secure during treatment. The preschool child, who lacks time concepts, knows he will see the therapist after his nap. The school-age child may anticipate the regular session, too, yet he can tolerate fluctuation in the treatment time if he is consulted about the change and given an opportunity to approve the new schedule.

Routine is important to children, particularly those who have been removed temporarily from their homes or for those who have unstable, erratic homes or families. The stability of a treatment hour, both the external schedule and the internal structure, reassures the child that someone cares about him. As a result of repeated consistency, the child can develop and maintain the trust in the therapist which is necessary to the successful therapeutic relationship.

In summary, by adding information on the scheduling and ordering of treatment to the previously gathered data, various possible models can be developed for the child's treatment schedule. In Susan's case, there are some variables which permit flexibility and some constants which are unchangeable and must be used in a consistent way in each of the models that is built. For example, one constant is the availability of only one OTR to treat the child (in another institution there might be two or more who are equipped to train the child.) Because of this constant, time, number and length of the training hours are automatically limited by the therapist's own schedule.

For purposes of simplification, the building of models will be based strictly on the sample of Objective 1: it has priority in treatment and can be explored independently of the other objectives. Once the child develops some coordinated function of her left hand, Objective 2 would be implemented, then 3 and so on until the total objectives are met. (See Figure 3-6 for the method of building three possible models.)

One point in relation to the building of models is exceedingly important in rehabilitation, "The models must meet a predetermined standard of performance selected for each objective. If the model appears to be inadequate, it is dismissed as a treatment approach." In the sample in Figure 3-6, the objective is for Susan to transfer the dominant functions from the right to the left hand. The standard of hand function which she must demonstrate in order to meet the objective adequately is hand function equivalent to the dominant hand function in a three-year-old child. The therapist must decide the degree to which Susan's function must match the average three-year-old's: how realistic is it to expect her to perform on a parallel basis? If the alternatives of block building, ball throwing, crayoning, or doll play do not meet the level of fulfillment for the objective, any or all of them may be dismissed.

It is difficult to set the same preselected standard of performance for each objective for each individual. As was noted in the discussion of the growth, learning, and other child development concepts, there is no predetermined guaranteed level of success for any individual. Therefore, the therapist or decision-maker can make only some educated judgments about the prognosis of treatment. In line with this, objectives were written for long-term rehabilitation. In addition, the therapist sets short-term objectives and watches for the cues in terms of their success, which will support or refute the possibility of attaining the long-term objective.

In some disabilities, it is probable that the objective will be attained, as in the case of Susan, because the objectives and prognosis are clear. Children with multiple handicaps, however, are at a disadvantage because the etiology, treatment and prognosis usually are hazy. There may be a question of the degree to which each is the causative factor which affects the setting of objectives according to priorities; and it in turn influences the prognosis. Depending upon the child and the cause, there may be a possibility of much further development or only negligible development.

Therefore, in setting the predetermined standard of performance, the therapist refers to competent resources which provide research on the treatment modality and its success with specific types of patients; the resources of the American Occupational Therapy Association (A.O.T.A.) or other professional groups which are using the modality; and the experience and success of the therapist himself (and his immediate associates) with the modality for the treatment of a particular kind of patient.

These comments are primarily applicable to the media which are built into the treatment model, since they are the core of treatment. The other units of the model are not as critical in determining a standard of performance, since they are the variables which influence the implementation.

THE WEIGHING OF COST AGAINST EFFECTIVENESS

This process, the weighing of cost of treatment against the effectiveness in terms of regaining health, is probably one of the

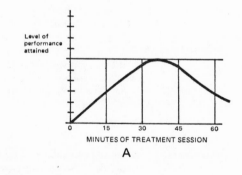

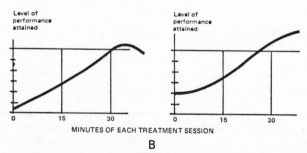

FIG. 3-7. Weighing the cost of treatment against the effectiveness. *A*, effects of increased fatigue on performance on a one-hour continuous treatment session; *B*, effects of increased fatigue on performance in two one-half hour treatment sessions.

most frequently overlooked factors in planning treatment in occupational therapy. The cost-benefit ratio may be applied broadly to the overall budgeting of a department, but seldom is each unit of the treatment model analyzed for its value in terms of cost.

Cost in occupational therapy may be in terms of money; it is much more likely, however, that cost will be in terms of the child's energy expenditure, the therapist's and child's time, or the child's overall development or health. (Emphasis may be placed only on the treatment of the dysfunction so that the child's overall development may lag or break down, while only the specific problem benefits from treatment.) An example of cost-benefit analysis is illustrated in Figure 3-7; the benefit of a one-hour

Model I	Results of Cost Analysis
Time: 30 minutes twice daily 9:30-10 A.M. and 4-4:30 P.M.	
Location: occupational therapy department—small room	This space is allocated for treatment; it is nondistracting and contains all needed treatment materials. Best choice.
Personnel: 1 OTR 1 OTS	OTR knows treatment procedure. He can supervise OTS's work with child after OTS has observed procedure for a period of time. Best choice.
Individual treatment Internal treatment schedule: Free play—5 minutes	Child can orient self to surroundings and therapist can observe the activities chosen to incorporate into treatment as appropriate.
Block building or other unilateral table play—10 minutes	Directly meets objective 1 without extending beyond child's ability to attend to the task. (Time can be increased or decreased as needed.)
Coloring—10 minutes Ball throwing or gross motor activity—5 minutes	Release of tension resulting from frustration with task or normal preschooler's need for activity.
Lunch: 12:00 Noon—eating with spoon and drinking from cup. OTR supervises and teaches lunch room aide the procedure for encouraging the use of the left hand without weird adaptations of the right upper arm.	OTR consults with aide periodically to make suggestions. This is not a time-consuming procedure, but gives aide support in encouraging new eating patterns and includes aide in treatment process. It gives the aide specific responsibilities. Best choice.

FIG. 3-8. Sample of cost analysis results for treatment Model I.

treatment block for Susan is compared with two one-half-hour blocks. Through this analysis it can be noted that a single block of one-hour treatment daily will probably not be as effective as two half hours because of the anticipated increased fatigue rate which correlates positively with the increased treatment time. Other variables which might be analyzed in determining the length of treatment sessions include: the type of treatment, the developmental needs of the child, and the degree of the dysfunction.

The monetary cost of one hour of continuous treatment is excessive compared with the benefits. The actual charge for treatment would necessarily increase because treatment time would have to be increased in order to meet the same standard of performance as found in the two one-half-hour sessions. This also would require increasing the length of the child's hospitalization, which would be psychologically and developmentally detrimental in addition to being exhorbitantly costly to the family. It is illogical for a child to remain in the hospital *only* for carelessly scheduled occupational therapy.

Model II	Results of Cost Analysis
Time: 30 minutes twice daily 10-10:30 A.M. and 4-4:30 P.M.	Morning treatment time is not directly after P.T.
Location: child's room	Competition for attention by other children wastes therapist's time for training Susan. Susan is distracted and doesn't meet standards for performance within the half hour.
Personnel: OTS	OTS is not experienced—would result in high cost of time for trial-and-error learning. Possible high costs in damage possible to prosthesis, which is unfamiliar to students.
Individual treatment Internal treatment schedule: Free play—15 minutes	Free play—high cost in money from time used on nonspecific treatment. Child might or might not use the free play time constructively to develop skills in left hand.
Coloring—15 minutes Lunch: 12:00 Noon—supervised by aide who may feed Susan herself to save time. No direction or supervision by OTR	No training is taking place during lunchtime so the cost of the service is high, with no benefit for the child who is in the hospital for treatment.

FIG. 3-9. Sample of cost analysis results for treatment Model II.

If the fatigue rate were the only factor under consideration, then Models I, II, and III each would be good choices for treatment (Figure 3-6). However, if number and quality of therapists were the primary factors, Model I would be superior as it contains one registered therapist and one student therapist. However, in the case of Susan (and most children who are treated in occupational therapy) there are many variables.

It can be noted in Figure 3-7B that the child begins the first treatment session at the same level of effectiveness as in Figure A; at the beginning of the second treatment hour, however, the effectiveness begins at a higher level because of the previous learning retained over the 4 1/2-hour interval between treatments. This indicates the gross discrepancy between the beginning of the second half hour of the continuous treatment in Figure A and the second half hour in Figure B.

When there are multiple variables, the cost-benefit comparison becomes difficult. A final decision must then be based on the relative importance of each variable. In comparing the use of personnel in Susan's case (the OTR versus the OTS) it is found that cost in terms of time (which is equivalent to money) is increased because of the ineffectiveness of the student who is still learning the mechanics of treatment. Although the OTR's time is more costly due to his skill, he requires less treatment time and usually has more effective results. Cost-effectiveness also can be in terms of risk to the child or the prosthesis, since the student does not know the materials with which he is working and may damage them. Cost analysis of Models I and II (see Figures 3-8 and 3-9), which resulted from the analysis of all these factors and others pertinent to Susan's treatment, indicates that Model I for Objective I probably will be the most effective overall treatment. It will be implemented in preference to the other models because it is most likely to result in successful treatment.

IMPLEMENTATION AND THE RESPONSIBILITIES OF THE THERAPIST, SUPERVISING ADULT, AND CHILD

An evaluation of the treatment model can be made only through implementation of treatment. Such an evaluation is essential in the iteration process within occupational therapy because of the variable which consists of the people involved: the occupational therapist, the supervising adult, and the child. These variables are in relation to the responsibilities taken by each member within the treatment process. Although implementation with consideration for individual responsibilities is not part of the method for organizing treatment, it is essential to the evaluation of the process. If ignored, the individual behaviors may negate all the effort expended on the systematic approach to planning treatment. These are the subtle behaviors which encourage the child's learning beyond the specific teaching unit.

Some minor variations in the treatment model are almost invariably necessary because of daily behavioral fluctuations in people. For example, Susan may be upset if her parents have not visited on the weekend and may be unable to tolerate any frustration at the 9:30 therapy session Monday morning. This may result in her being unable to cope with unilateral tasks and in her need for more free play and gross motor activity.

The purpose of the following three units is to identify some of the responsibilities which begin at the implementation of treatment and terminate at the end of treatment.

The Therapist's Responsibilities in Treatment

Initially, the responsibilities of the occupational therapist are to *motivate the child.* This is particularly necessary for the young child who does not understand the reason for his treatment and who cannot perform without some very close supervision from and interaction with the therapist. The older child may understand his problems and may be internally motivated to change his condition — in which case the therapist may serve a different function.

As a motivator, the therapist demonstrates some specific attitudes to gain and maintain the child's trust: honesty, directness and sensitivity. These attitudes are apparent throughout treatment. The therapist honestly and directly explains the facts of treatment to the child, who is capable of understanding what is to be done and how it will be done. The therapist is honest and sensitive in seeking cues about the child's immediate needs within each treatment session and must be ready to vary the program as necessary in order to encourage the child's development and learning. The therapist is direct in explaining the reasons for program changes to the child. Some children with severe cognitive limitations or within the early developmental years may not comprehend these comments in total; but will probably, through a nonverbal or single verbal expression gain a feeling or idea of the situation.

In addition, the therapist is *aware of the fluctuation in his own feelings* toward himself and the child — and the effect of these fluctuations on the child and his performance. This awareness includes being acutely sensitive to the situations which occur prior to the treatment period for both the child and the therapist. The child may have experienced trauma recently — as in the case of a spinal tap. Because of the child's emotional agitation, treatment in occupational therapy may be ineffective and the child may need his treatment hour rescheduled or the treatment objectives for that day changed. The therapist may have had an argument with another staff member and may be tempted to project his feelings onto the child but treatment is not rescheduled; instead, the therapist tempers his own behavior.

Discipline is used by the therapist as a positive means for changing the child's behavior — it is utilized for the benefit of the child, not as an emotional release of the therapist's anger. Discipline is "training which corrects, molds, strengthens or perfects. It is given with an attitude of guidance and direction along positive lines of building in the direction of acceptable behavior. It encourages positive responses."[5] The child has a right to know the therapist's feelings — but is *not* the scapegoat for the therapist. This is the process of feedback which gives both the adult and the child freedom to comment on and respond to one another's behavior honestly and openly. The therapist must not project his feelings toward personal problems onto the child and thus permit his anger to interfere with treatment.

Within the treatment setting, the therapist *avoids excess verbiage and listens* to the child. Initially, the therapist may need to converse with the child so that he will feel comfortable in the new surroundings. He modulates his voice to provide cues for the child and speaks casually, perhaps telling him about therapy or his project. The therapist asks only necessary questions in order to avoid increasing the anxiety level and keeps the verbal and nonverbal directions consistent to avoid giving mixed messages. As the child's security and comfort increases, he may begin to respond to questions, and, hopefully, begin to initiate conversation. At this point the therapist begins to withdraw from his role of initiator into his role of listener.

The therapist must know the treatment media thoroughly in order to *give consistent and accurate directions* while he continues to focus his attention on the child and his performance. This is true in both treatment and evaluation. The therapist cannot afford to get involved in the idiosyncrasies of the treatment media, which may result in his losing contact with the child. Occasionally, the treatment objectives specify that the child is to develop and show initiative — which may mean that the child is to be dominant in the teaching process; the child may learn with the therapist or teach him (see Chapter 2 for further discussion of giving directions).

Throughout the child-adult interaction, the therapist *switches between the roles of active and passive participant*. He works briefly with the child and then retreats in order to give the child the opportunity to perform. The therapist may demonstrate the stacking of blocks to the child. He may put one block on the pile and say, "You do it," the child places one, the therapist places one, and so on. This procedure may continue until the child has the concept of the task and the motivation to continue, at which point the therapist retreats (this means from giving assistance, not from the room!) until the next task is begun. In more complex tasks, the therapist may need to present a step-by-step demonstration with examples of each step to reduce the child's frustration. This is appropriate for the child who has a short-term memory and who cannot recall a total sequence — the therapist demonstrates one step, the child performs it, the therapist demonstrates the next step, and so on. Often this is used with complex structured tasks (tying a shoelace, or the buttoning process). At each new treatment session the therapist lets the child demonstrate his previous learning and assists him only if necessary.

The therapist is responsible for *teaching the child new behavior which is acceptable* within his home, the hospital, and so forth. If it is desirable to elicit an extreme and unusual behavior in the treatment session, the therapist must be sure that the child can discriminate between the places where it is acceptable and those where it is unacceptable. A physically handicapped child who has developed acceptable social, emotional, and language behavior at age nine or ten years discriminates between what is acceptable at home and what is acceptable in the institution in which he is being treated. The therapist must explain why one unit of behavior is acceptable in one situation but not in another. It may be all right for the child to splash fingerpaint on the floor or on the table in the occupational therapy unit because he can and will clean up the resulting mess after the treatment session; however, it is not acceptable for the child to splash fingerpaint at home on the kitchen table or on the kitchen carpet if they can be damaged by the paint.

The child must learn the appropriate behavior for different situations. If the child is incapable of distinguishing between appropriate and inappropriate behaviors, the therapist must plan treatment sessions which do not create conflict for the child. For example, all books and paper are removed from the sight and reach of a fifteen-month-old who likes to tear them up; in place of them, he is given nontoxic play dough to pull apart. The therapist does not permit the tearing of paper because the child probably would generalize this behavior to his home and it would not be acceptable for the child to tear up daddy's evening newspaper!

In *choosing the treatment modality* for the child, the therapist evaluates the long- and short-term requirements in relation to the child's abilities. With either media, the therapist is responsible for its completion within the designated period of time. This requires that the therapist know the child and the requirements of the activity: he must know the child's ability to attend to a task, the length of his hospitalization or the speed with which he works. The therapist then compares this information with her knowledge of the media in her planning.

After choosing the treatment modality for the child, the therapist gathers the tools which are appropriate to the child — those which are the right size and shape and which do not require skill beyond his developmental abilities. A three-year-old can manipulate clay but cannot use the potter's wheel; he may be given a stick or tongue depressor with which to work the clay, but would not be given a sharp tool with which he could hurt himself or another child.

The therapist must always be cognizant of the fact that activity is only the means to the accomplishment of the treatment objective. Treatment occurs in the process of the child's interacting with the nonhuman objects from which the end products result. A product may be very meaningful to the child; if he is not given the opportunity to complete it as he wants and expects, he may refuse to perform. This is particularly true of children of ten or eleven years of age who take pride in their craftsmanship, as compared with the preschool and early school-age children who build, construct and so forth for the sake of the activity itself and not for the end result. Preschool children enjoy clay because of its inherent qualities (manipulative stage of learning about the material), as opposed to the adolescents who want to make ceramic objects which can be fired in the kiln for permanency (creative-symbolic stage, which uses the materials for representation).

Once the child has behaved as desired and responded appropriately to the stimuli, the therapist is responsible for *rewarding or reinforcing* his efforts, which shows the child that his work is important, whether he is totally or partially successful. The therapist independently determines the appropriate rewards or chooses them with the child's assistance. Among them is permitting the child to choose a preferred task after the performance of a required task — a child often has a favorite activity and is motivated to work quickly in order to proceed with the special task. Another reward is the displaying of the object which the child has completed — through the comments and praise of others, the child gains confidence in his work. If the child's project is utilitarian, the therapist may encourage its being used and enjoyed.

Rewards are expected in our society. For a day of work a person receives money; for a well done volunteer task a person receives a thank you. It is realistic, therefore, that a child be rewarded for his work.

If the child already has his own internal reinforcement mechanism, the reinforcement of the therapist serves as an additional stimulus for further performance. External reinforcement is useful when it is sincere and given at deserved points of success. Only in a few pathological cases is it inappropriate to reward the child (see Chapter 5).

Responsibilities of Others: Adults and Peers

People outside the therapist-child relationship are always involved in treatment and many affect it in a positive or negative and direct or indirect way. One of the therapist's objectives is to involve them in a positive, direct manner whenever possible and to help them interact with the child therapeutically.

One of the objectives of development is for the child to become a social being who functions comfortably with people — including those within the family and those at work and play. The ideal is to involve the child's peers in the treatment program to the degree that is therapeutically appropriate. Toddlers are learning to function with peers in parallel play; preadolescents are interested in groups of their own sex.

Group treatment might be contraindicated for the individual who depends upon the group — the child or adolescent who forms superficial interpersonal relationships because he has no inner resources and must depend upon the group for stimulation. After one-to-one treatment and the development of inner strengths, the individual might be gradually reintroduced to group involvement. Large groups, however, are always contraindicated for the treatment of an individual since the individual's needs are lost in the attempt to meet everyone's needs.

Other individuals who are directly involved in treatment are the nonprofessionals, such as parents or aides. Parents carry out the treatment at home, following many of the same principles for therapy as are being used by the therapist. They are taught the techniques by the therapist and practice them under his supervision. In this situation they are encouraged to raise questions — in order to learn and understand the dysfunction, the treatment which they are performing and the prognosis. They should be told some of the whys of treatment — in order to diminish their anxiety or their "haloing" of the child's performance and to prepare them to evaluate change within the range of possible behaviors as the child progresses. The same or similar content is important to the occupational therapy assistant or aide to help them interact therapeutically with the child.

Parents also have some responsibility when their child is in an institution such as a school for the handicapped or a children's hospital. If the parents have not visited the child and watched his progress, they may be prepared neither for the changes in his behavior nor for their own work in continuing treatment. They should observe the child in treatment and talk with the therapist prior to the child's discharge so that they will learn about their role in follow-up treatment; it is seldom that a patient returns to his home environment with no follow-up care. If in no other way, personal-social changes have occurred in the normal developmental process because of the experience of illness and living away from home with peers. These changes may be beneficial or detrimental to the child.

The parents need to know the problems which have occurred, or those which might occur upon the child's return to the home. They need to know how these were handled by the staff and how they might continue to handle them. For example, the hospitalized infant may forget his parents and cry in fear of them as strangers for the first few days at home. The parents could interpret this as a rejection and be upset by the behavior, rather than realize that this is "normal" behavior which will cease after a period of adjustment for the infant.

In addition, the parents need to be informed of the child's developmental changes so that they will be able to keep pace with the child. This preparation will prevent their unintentionally encouraging him to regress to the level on which he performed upon his entrance to the institution. The *small* things make both parents and child better able to readapt to each other within the home and help home treatment to continue more smoothly than would be otherwise possible.

Responsibilities of the Child for his Treatment

The child, too, has responsibilities for his treatment and the place in which it occurs. The therapist encourages the child to continue his development at all times and helps him to develop appropriate behaviors secondary to the specific treatment goals. Secondary behaviors include his taking responsibility for his own behavior. In the preschool years, a child begins to receive work assignments within the home as a family member. The child within the institution is different only if his disability incapacitates him;

he is expected to accept responsibility at his developmental level. At home, he takes out and puts away his own toys and helps to keep his room tidy at about two and one-half to three years of age; in occupational therapy similar behavior is expected within the restrictions of the institution and the child's abilities. In unusual cases, responsibility in caring for the treatment room may be contraindicated. For example, in working with an emotionally disturbed child with a severe problem in the area of compulsive neatness, clean-up behavior might be de-emphasized for a period of time.

A basic rule in working with a child is: he is not to injure the therapist, himself, the equipment or the room. In the same way, he is to use tools appropriately, as in the case of a hammer which is for hammering nails and a saw which is for sawing wood. If the child does not comply with the basic rules, he is disciplined. He may be deprived of the use of the material which he used incorrectly or the part of his treatment hour in which he did not take responsibility. If it becomes apparent through the child's continuous lack of responsibility that he is attempting to avoid interaction with the therapist, the requirements of the therapist are reassessed as part of the testing for the sensitivity of the treatment model (Figure 3-10).

Children learn limitations and accept them with no more and no less grumbling than at home. A child sometimes recognizes his own need for responsibility and appoints himself a task, thereby maintaining some of the control and responsibility which he had when healthy and at home. Children seem to need some control or responsibility in situations (hospitals) in which they have lost almost total decision-making powers. Children can and should be expected to perform within the range of their functional and developmental abilities whenever possible.

TESTING FOR SENSITIVITY

By this time all theoretical preparations for treatment have been completed and reviewed and the actual treatment has been implemented. The testing for the sensitivity of the treatment is an ongoing evaluation of the treatment process over a specified period of time. It begins prior to the initiation of the treatment sessions, continues during treatment and ends with the making of decisions concerning the effectiveness of the model in meeting the treatment objectives. All aspects of the treatment process are evaluated. The schedule of the therapist is reviewed for its practicality. The internal organization of the treatment hour is checked for its

Theoretical Model I	Actual Situation	Sensitivity Testing
Time: 30 minutes twice daily (9:30-10 A.M. and 4-4:30 P.M.)	Same	Beginning to need other children for motivation. Less clinging to OTR. Plays with 3 other preschoolers (2½ to 4-year-old range). Susan willingly participates in therapy and uses her left hand. Increased success and accuracy is seen in feeding self and block stacking. Practice is needed for smooth performance. The internal 30-minute schedule must be flexible. Susan has multiple interests and is inclined to do different ones each time. She continues to use her left hand spontaneously.
Location: OT department—small room	Same	
Personnel: 1 OTR		
1 OTS observer	Same	
Individual treatment	Presently the same, Susan regularly asks for Tommy.	
Internal treatment schedule:	Organization of internal structure varies to meet Susan's immediate needs.	
Free play—5 minutes		
Unilateral type of table play—10 minutes		
Coloring—10 minutes		
Gross motor play—5 minutes		
		Nursing staff is cooperating in supervision and OTR no longer participates.
Lunch: 12:00 Noon—eat with spoon and drink from cup.		

FIG. 3-10. Testing for sensitivity.

accuracy in meshing the theoretical needs with the actual needs of the child. The sensitivity measure might be visualized as illustrated in Figure 3-10. It compares the original treatment model with the actual situation and identifies those factors which are satisfactory and those which need to be changed.

QUESTIONING ASSUMPTIONS

Each of the units in the treatment model are re-evaluated in terms of the child's success or failure. If the child is making gains, treatment is continued following the same model with, perhaps, some additional treatment alternatives. If a unit is not eliciting satisfactory results, it is further evaluated for the cause of its failure. If the assumptions on which the unit was based appear inadequate or incorrect, the objectives must be changed. For example, in the planning of treatment, it was assumed that Susan had only a single dysfunction and no other physical problems. If another problem had been discovered in the process of treatment (during the sensitivity testing), the original treatment objective(s) might need to be revised to incorporate this previously unrecognized problem.

All assumptions made in the preparation for treatment are questioned daily, weekly, monthly and so forth. The question is "Is the treatment model meeting the criteria for treatment?" (Figure 3-11).

How much individual one-to-one supervision does Susan actually need in learning to use the left hand now that the basic pattern is established?

1. In 4 hours of treatment time, the child began to use the left hand automatically—awkwardly, but functionally.
2. Now 8 hours later (in total) she uses it without prompting.
3. She usually accepts suggestions for easiest way to perform a task, such as the position in which to hold the crayon.

Can Susan tolerate other children?

1. She asks for Tommy (roommate on the ward) during treatment.
2. She plays with 3 other preschoolers on the ward.

Is there need for supervision by the OTR at lunch?

1. With occasional prodding and assistance from the aide Susan eats with her left hand and drinks milk. Minimum accidents.

FIG. 3-11. Questioning assumptions relevant to the sensitivity testing for Model I.

RE-EXAMINING OBJECTIVES

The objectives are re-examined in light of new information which states that the child has regressed or progressed at a rate different from the one originally anticipated or has plateaued in his development. The alternatives chosen for each objective are then analyzed in order to determine whether the problem is in the objective itself or in the analysis prior to the building of the models. If treatment appears to be effective in meeting the chosen objectives it is continued. The objectives which were temporarily ignored are re-examined in light of their applicability to the situation at the present. Is the child ready for the new and sequentially advanced behaviors? The new information from the re-examined objectives may appear as illustrated in Figure 3-12.

Objectives	Re-Examination
Primary objectives:	
1. Develop dominance in left hand for unilateral function.	This objective is no longer number 1. Practice with some support should be continued. Encourage drawing as prewriting skill.
2. Develop right hand (prosthesis) in reach, grasp, and release for assistive functions.	Implement training for Nos. 2 through 6. With left hand ready as dominant, child is ready to learn mechanics of special training (stump also is ready for prosthesis).
3. Develop transfer between left and right hand.	
4. Develop bilateral hand function.	
5. Develop functional independence in ADL skills appropriate to Susan's developmental level.	
Secondary objectives:	
6. Develop self-confidence during mother's absence.	Nos. 6 and 7 are partly accomplished, secondarily to treatment in occupational therapy.
7. Develop peer relationships	
Additional objective:	
8. Assist child in coping with reactions to prosthesis	No. 8 resulted from No. 7. Child needs some help in play with other children and the handling of their reactions to the stump and prosthesis.

FIG. 3-12. Re-examining objectives.

OPENING NEW ALTERNATIVES

Opening of new alternatives to meet the objectives has already been explained and continues the cycle of iteration. At this time, one of the possible treatment alternatives for Susan is nursery school. It would provide additional developmental experiences and the opportunity to practice skills with the left hand and the right prosthetic hand (reinforcement of her in-hospital training in a normal setting). This alternative would also be effective in meeting objectives 6, 7, and 8. It is recommended only because the child has developed the basic skills necessary to participation in nursery school since the beginning of treatment.

Alternatives are added or deleted at the beginning of the new cycle, which will continue until the law of diminishing returns takes over. This means that the effort put into the treatment of the child is no longer worth the benefits gained by the child; in spite of treatment, the child can no longer develop or learn — as in the case of the severely retarded child who develops to a degree, plateaus, and then continues no further over a period of years. The indication is that the child has reached his maximum potential and must be maintained at that level. The occupational therapist is of no value to the child in helping him develop further — although the therapist *may* give *other* staff members suggestions for maintaining some function, such as positioning or visual stimulation. The therapist may have done all he could to help the child develop — as in teaching Susan the technicalities of the prosthetic hand. The therapist must then decide whether he will continue to assist in the child's general development or whether there are others who can perform the task better, perhaps the child's mother or nursery school teacher. At this point, the value of occupational therapy for the child is minimal and the value of nursery school appears to be maximal (Figure 3-13).

---

i. Nursery school to assist in reinforcing objectives 1-8.
Selection of new alternatives to meet additional objective 8:
1. Speak for child as comments are made about her prosthesis to help the child develop adequate responses (3 years old may be too young to handle this verbally).
2. Teach tasks which are the same for other preschoolers to reduce discrepancy between normal and abnormal.
3. Reinforce "talents" or behaviors of child which are not associated with the dysfunction—singing, dance, verbal games, and so forth.

FIG. 3-13. Selection of new alternatives to meet each of same objectives.

118

SUMMARY

The scientific decision-making process in occupational therapy is a detailed approach to the planning, implementation, and analysis of therapy as diagrammed in Figure 3-14. It is a process through which the therapist can develop a logical framework for the treatment of each patient by raising the kind of questions and collecting the information relevant to cost-benefit comparisons of alternative ways of treatment. Once the therapist learns and makes the process automatic through practice, he does not write it down as illustrated in the example of Susan's treatment. The costs in terms of the therapist's time would far exceed the benefits from the resulting treatment; only in making major decisions would the formalized analysis be worthwhile.

It must be re-emphasized that the illustrative case has been oversimplified for the purpose of demonstrating the scientific decision-making process. Children treated by the occupational therapist generally have multiple problems, which offer no easy resolution. The multiple variables and uncertainties resulting from institutions, the rapidly changing methods of evaluation and treatment, and the varied capabilities of therapists require highly specific planning for each child. It is the responsibility of each therapist to be scientific in his approach to each child's problem — for without quality input in terms of complete and accurate information gathering, there can be no quality output in terms of treatment.

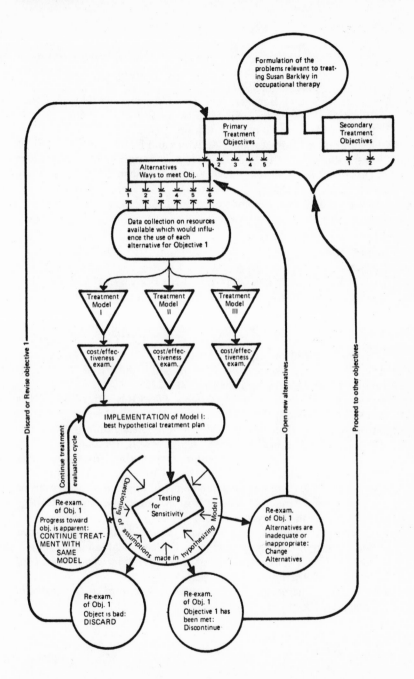

FIG. 3-14. Summary diagram of the iteration process used in occupational therapy with Susan Barkley. The same procedure would be applied to primary objectives 2 through 5 and secondary objectives 1 and 2.

References

1. *Report of Workshop on Application of Educational Objectives in Curriculum Construction* (New York: American Occupational Therapy Association, 1967).
2. Quade, E.S. and Boucher, W.I. (eds.) *Systems Analysis & Policy Planning* (New York: American Elsevier Pub. Co., 1968).
3. Cooper, M. Personal communication, 1970.
4. Maurer, P.A. "Prevocational Activities and Evaluation for the Child and Adolescent." In Hislop, H.J. and Sanger, J.O. (eds.) *Chest Disorders in Children* (New York: American Physical Therapy Association, 1968).
5. Schad, C.J. Personal communication, 1961.

Bibliography

Anthony, E.J. "The Child's Discovery of His Body." In Hislop, H.J. and Sanger, J.O. (eds.) *Chest Disorders in Children* (New York: American Physical Therapy Association, 1968).

Fehr, M.J. (ed.) *Normal Growth and Development with Deviations in the Perceptual Motor and Emotional Areas* (St. Louis: Washington University School of Medicine, 1966).

Frank, J.D. "The Therapeutic Use of Self." *American Journal of Occupational Therapy* 12(1958), pp. 215-225.

Hartley, R.E. *Understanding Children's Play*, Revised edition (New York: T.Y. Crowell, 1963).

Hartley, R.E. and Goldenson, R.M. *The Complete Book of Children's Play*, Revised edition (New York: T.Y. Crowell, 1963).

Kiernat, J.M. (ed.) *Perceptual-Motor Dysfunction, Evaluation and Training* (Madison, Wisconsin: University of Wisconsin, 1966).

Report of Workshop on Organization and Administration for Registered Occupational Therapists (Boston: Boston University, Sargent College of Allied Health Professions, 1969).

West, W.L. (ed.) *Occupational Therapy for the Multiply Handicapped Child* (Chicago: University of Illinois College of Medicine, 1965).

Weston, D.L. "The Dimension of Crafts." *American Journal of Occupational Therapy* 15(1961), pp.1-5.

Weston, D.L. "Therapeutic Crafts." *American Journal of Occupational Therapy* 14(1960), pp. 121-122, 133.

NOTES

NOTES

Chapter Four
Neuromotor Development

Doris A. Sukiennicki, O.T.R., R.P.T.

(July 1971)

NEUROMOTOR DEVELOPMENT

Watching the baby explore himself and his surroundings is fascinating. During the first few years the baby learns to use his body. Neuromotor development is concerned with this maturation of the nervous system and the parallel acquisition of control over the muscular system. Every species of higher organism has a maturation process which is genetically determined. Gesell states:

Behavior has shape. Environmental factors support, inflect, and modify, but they do not generate progressions of development. Growth is an impulsion, and a cycle of morphogenetic events is uniquely a character of the living organism.[1]

Predictable patterns of motor behavior begin to emerge at birth. These inborn patterns exist as a potential and are subject to reduction or slight modification in form by environmental forces.

There are four principles concerning the *anatomical directions of development* which the occupational therapist must consider when evaluating or treating a child. First, maturation starts in the head regions and proceeds toward the feet (the cephalocaudal direction). For example, the baby can lift and turn his head before he can volitionally move his feet. The baby learns to control the joints which are closest to the central axis of the body — the proximal joints before the outward or distal joints. For example, he controls his shoulder joints before his wrists. Maturation proceeds from the front surfaces of the body, expanding to the back surfaces, or ventral to dorsal. Finally, control spreads from near the midline in the anatomical position outward or in the ulnar to radial direction. This may be seen in the early grasp patterns in which there is a shift from the little finger side of the hand to the thumb and index fingers.

Two maturation patterns occur in man. The first is *phylogenetic progression*, which refers to the repeating of primitive patterns derived from the evolutionary development of man as a vertebrate. The newborn baby or neonate placed in water makes well-coordinated swimming movements that diminish after a few months, showing a primitive behavioral pattern. The second is *ontogenetic progression*, which refers to more recently evolved traits, such as the ability to stand erect, in the biological development of the individual.

The baby's earliest movements are generalized and massive in nature, later becoming more localized and specific. The newborn's movements are likely to be uncoordinated and abrupt as he responds in an undifferentiated and total fashion. He gradually learns to control his body. As he interacts with his surroundings he masters the dynamically opposed components of motor skills such as left and right, ipsilateral and contralateral, bilateral and unilateral, and bending and straightening. This control does not develop smoothly. First one, then another, dominates in fluctuating modes with periods of greater and lesser maturity and coordination until fully balanced development is achieved. Smooth motor performance is dependent on the balance and interaction of these antagonistic components. This process is called *reciprocal neuromotor interweaving.* [2,3] For example, the baby of 44 weeks is less successful grasping a small object than he was eight weeks previously. He is in a transitional stage in achieving a more advanced type of grasp and suffers a functional regression. [4] Neuromotor development is continuous; all areas do not develop simultaneously or at the same rate. Each area has spurts and dormant periods. Each child establishes an individual rate and pattern of development.

Physical Growth and Development

An understanding of the patterns of growth and development and the variations in expression of these dynamic processes is fundamental to any comprehensive understanding of children. This knowledge is useful both in observing the child with neuromotor deficits, and in the interpretation of his individual mode of development to his parents. Emphasis should be placed on the individuality of the child rather than on the parents' unfulfilled expectations. Even severely handicapped children progress, although perhaps very slowly. The therapist and the parents must attune themselves to the individual rate of progress.

Growth is defined as an increase in dimension or as tissue accruement. Development refers to a temporal process usually involving a progression from a relatively simple to a more complex structure or organization. Development refers to the process of growth rather than the end product. Maturation conveys both growth and differentiation and includes the aging processes.[5] Physical growth is affected by nature in terms of heredity and nurtured by the physical and emotional environment.

The child's height, weight and age are the most conspicuous indicators of physical growth. Circumferential measurements of the head, chest, abdomen and limbs, as well as limb lengths, are other common indicators. The extent of the skeletal ossification, called the bone age, as well as the extent of dental development determined by the number of teeth that have erupted, are used to appraise physical development. Comparisons of the measurements, by cross-sectional methods, of large numbers of children related to the chronological age has yielded average growth figures useful for reference. The keeping of sequential records of measurements and observations of a child provides an individual mode of progression or longitudinal expression of growth. Visiting the local grammar school, noting the tallest and the smallest child of the same age in a classroom, gives a perspective on the scope of individual variation. The rate and final outcome of growth is least predictable during the late adolescent period, even using the longitudinal method.

Most of the body growth has been accomplished by late adolescence. The period from birth to adolescence is usually divided into three stages: one, from birth to the beginning of the third year, called infancy; second, from the third to the tenth year, termed childhood; and third, from the tenth year until adult stature is reached from sixteen to nineteen, called adolescence. Certain aspects of growth may predominate a particular stage of development. The various systems of the body each have their unique patterns and rhythms of growth. Growth in height, weight, bones and muscles follows a general pattern of rapidly accelerated growth during infancy, a slowing during childhood, and a resumption of growth during adolescence. The bones, providing the structural basis for the body, have their own maturational curve. The skull achieves most of its growth during the first seven years, accounting for the loss of the baby look at that age. The vertebrae have achieved half to two-thirds of their entire growth by the end of the third year. The bone age (maturity of bony structure) is determined from roentgenograms observing the state of ossification of the growth centers. Osseous maturation is considered to be one of the better indices of general growth.

Calcification of the skeleton begins before birth and continues until maturity. The wrist and hand bones are useful as indicators during the entire period of childhood.[6]

The body proportions change considerably from birth to maturity. At birth, the baby's head constitutes one-fourth of his total height whereas at maturity it will only constitute one-eighth of his height.[7] There is also a marked change in the limb-to-trunk lengths. The young baby sucks his toes with ease. The adult usually cannot duplicate this feat. These proportional changes also result in shifts in the center of gravity of the body. It may be more difficult or at least different for an older child to repeat the early increments of development in remedial treatment. Other variations in bodily proportions may be attributed to the body build. Three types of body build have been described by Sheldon: the endomorph, the mesomorph and the ectomorph.[8] The endomorph usually has a stocky build with a large viscera and a soft roundness of the body and accumulations of fat. The mesomorph is characterized as the ideal athlete with a predominance of muscle, bone and connective tissue. His physique is usually rectangular in shape. The ectomorph has a linear fragility with thin muscles and less subcutaneous tissue. He has a low body weight compared to body length, and a light bone structure. The body type may predispose the child to a particular growth style or typical body posture. Most people are a combination of types. Although these types may be readily identifiable in childhood, they frequently may not be manifest until growth has stopped.

The growth and development of the central nervous system varies from the cycle of height, weight, bone and muscle previously mentioned in that it is more accelerated with growth nearly complete by the sixth year. The central nervous system includes the brain, spinal cord and the cervical and spinal nerves. It is not fully developed at birth. The posterior portion of brain, the phylogenetically older part, is proportionately larger and shows greater detail of development than the forebrain or cerebral hemispheres. In the adult the forebrain is the largest and heaviest portion of the brain. It is thought to have integrative functions in the conscious and voluntary processes. The nerve fibers of the cerebral hemispheres or white matter have not developed their outer membranes or myelin. The development of the central nervous system that started in the uterus continues in the infant for the first few years. At birth, the brain is one-third its adult mass. By the end of the second year it has achieved four-fifths of the adult size. At six years it is nine-tenths of the adult size. The brain grows rapidly during the first six years and then imperceptibly until late adolescence. The development of the motor skills closely parallels and is dependent on the physical maturation of the nervous system. Neuromotor development is nearly complete by two years and refined at six. The structures of the brain mature in the order that they were formed phylogenetically and ontogenetically. The lower, older portions of the brain which are concerned with regulation of vital functions mature first. The outer layer of the forebrain called the cerebral cortex is thought not to be functioning appreciably at birth.[9] The baby's early stereotyped behavior is regulated by the lower nervous centers and lacks the integrating and restraining influences of the higher centers.

Maturation of the Reflexes

In comparison with the young of most other animals, the human newborn is extremely helpless and unable to cope with environmental stresses. He lies helpless and unable to oppose gravity. His behavior is involuntary and based on inborn stimulus-response mechanisms called reflexes. The earliest reflexive responses are generated by the internal and external stimuli of pain, cold and hunger and are protective in nature. The baby can do what is important in order to survive: breathe, eat, eliminate, and call his mother by crying. Reflexively he sucks, vomits, swallows, urinates, defecates, cries, sneezes, coughs, yawns, hiccoughs, and carries on peristaltic activity. Already he possesses some reflexes of position and movement. These early primitive reflexive responses reflect the relatively undeveloped state of the nervous structures and the domination of the lower centers concerned with the regulation of vital functions. The relationship of the reflexes with anatomical levels of the nervous system has been established. The ascending structural maturation is accompanied by the emergence of more postural and movement reflexes. From the total and relatively undifferentiated responses of the newborn, partial patterns arise. These become increasingly specific and localized. As the reflexes interact, more complex motor patterns evolve. Gradually, the child gains a sense of equilibrium, permitting him to move from the static postures and permitting greater interaction with his surroundings. As the highest nervous centers mature, some of the early primitive reflexes, referred to as transient reflexes, are assimilated and gradually inhibited. The reflexes form the substrata to voluntary movement. Hellebrandt[10] cites indirect evidence of the influences of the tonic neck reflexes, one of the so-called transient reflexes, in the golf swing and other instances of physical stress in the adult. The specific reflexes to be discussed are selected either because of their importance in the evolution of motor skills or because of their significance clinically to the occupational therapist in evaluation and remedial treatment. Most of the experimental studies of reflexes have used animals as subjects. The following discussion relates to human responses.

There are two categories of general static reactions: the *attitudinal reflexes* and the *righting reflexes*.[11,12] The attitudinal reflexes are postural reactions which function automatically to maintain the upright position through changes in muscle tone in response to the position of the body or parts of the body. There are three principal groups of attitudinal reflexes: *local static reactions, segmental static reactions* and *general static reactions*. The attitudinal reflexes are proprioceptive — they arise from the stimulation of receptors of position and movement located in the muscles, tendons and inner ear. Local static reactions involve one part of the body such as a limb. Two types of static reactions are the *stretch reflex* and the *supporting reactions*. The passive stretch of a muscle induces a reflex contraction of that muscle resisting the extending force called a stretch reflex. The stretch reflex is considered the basic postural reaction. Passive stretch refers to the stretching of a muscle by an outside force such as an opposing muscle or gravity. The *positive supporting reaction* occurs when the sole of the baby's foot is pressed against a supporting surface or the toes of the foot are bent backward, causing the leg to develop supporting tone, turning it into a pillar-like structure capable of supporting the body weight for a short period. A similar response can be elicited in the arms. The *negative supporting reaction* is the loosening of the limb following the positive supporting reaction. This relaxation begins at the most proximal joint of the limb which is the hip or shoulder.

The segmental static reactions involve whole segments of the body. Included is the *crossed extension reflex* which involves the legs. When a painful stimulus is applied to a leg it causes a protective withdrawal or flexion reaction in that leg and a straightening or extension of the other leg.

The general static reactions start in one segment and affect other segments of the baby's body. Two general static reactions are the *tonic neck reflexes* and the *tonic labyrinthine reflexes*. The tonic neck reflex manifests itself in an asymmetrical and a symmetrical form. When the baby rotates his head, the arm and leg on the jaw side extend, and the arm and leg on the skull side flex. This response is more pronounced in the arms and is termed the *asymmetrical tonic neck reflex* (Figure 4-1). When the head is flexed forward, there is an increased flexion tone in the arms and an increased extensor tone in the legs. When the head is dorsiflexed (bent back), there is a reversal of the above response with an increased extensor tone in the arms and an increased flexor tone in the legs. Both patterns are manifestations of the *symmetrical tonic neck reflex.* When the infant is lying on his back (supine), there is an increased extensor tone in his arms and legs. When he lies on his abdomen (prone), there is an increased flexor tone in his limbs. Both are variations of the tonic labyrinthine reflex.

    The second category of general static reactions is the *righting reactions.* The righting reflexes function to keep the top part of the body uppermost and to maintain the head and body in their proper relationship. The righting reactions include: the *labyrinthine righting reflexes acting on the head, body righting reflexes acting on the head, neck righting reflexes acting on the body, body righting reflexes acting on the body,* and the *optical righting reflexes.* The labyrinthine righting reflexes acting on the head function to maintain the head's orientation in space and arise from stimulation to the inner ear. The head tends to seek the horizontal position in space regardless of the position of other parts of the body and independent of vision. The body righting reflexes acting on the head act to keep the head oriented with respect to the body. When the infant lying on his side has his legs grasped and turned to the opposite side, rotating the pelvis, the trunk and head follow. The neck righting reflex acting on the body functions to keep the body oriented to the head and is complementary to the righting reflex mentioned above. If the infant's head is turned while he is lying on his back, the rest of his

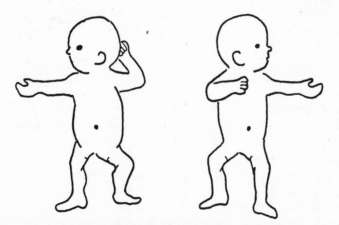

FIG. 4-1. Asymmetrical tonic neck reflexes.

body will follow. The body righting reflexes acting on the body tend to keep the body oriented. They involve a segmental rotation of the trunk between the shoulders and the pelvis. The optical righting reflex acts to maintain the individual's head in its proper orientation in space through vision.

A group of *kinetic* or *movement reactions* include the *Moro reflex*, the *Sprungbereitschaft* and the *Landau reflexes*. The Moro reflex (Figure 4-2) is commonly elicited by striking the pillow under the baby's head. The baby responds by straightening and spreading his arms and spreading his fingers. The response is less distinct in the legs. The Sprungbereitschaft or protective extension of the arms is the extension of the arms and extension and spreading of the fingers by the child to protect his head when he is held in the air and thrust downward head first. Milani-Comparetti and Gidoni include the Sprungbereitschaft as part of a group of protective limb extension reactions, *parachute reactions*,[13] in response to sudden displacement of the erect trunk. The Landau reflexes are a combination of the tonic and righting reflexes. When the baby is lifted, supported under the chest, his head assumes a vertical position and his back and legs extend with the back sometimes arching upward. When the head is pressed into forward flexion, the tone in the legs and back is lost and they collapse.

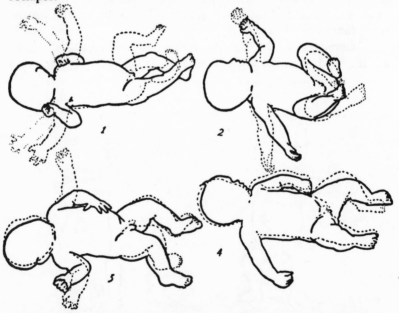

FIG. 4-2. The somatic movements in the several phases of the Moro reflex. (From McGraw, M. B. *The Neuromuscular Maturation of the Human Infant* (New York: Hafner Publishing Company, 1969), p. 25.

Two important *spinal segmental* reflexes are the *flexor withdrawal* and the *extensor thrust*. Spinal segmental reflexes involve whole body segments such as the legs and are mediated at the spinal level. The flexor withdrawal, also called the *avoidance reflex*, is elicited by a painful stimulation to the leg causing flexion of the ankle, knee and hip and withdrawal of the limb. The extensor thrust is the strong transitory extension of the infant's leg elicited by stimulation of the ball of the foot when the infant's leg is flexed.

The following reflexes are seen in the very young baby and are clinically significant to the occupational therapist. The newborn has a *suckling reflex* that is elicited by contact to the lips, gums or the front of the baby's tongue. Reflex swallowing usually follows suckling, coughing, sneezing and hiccoughing. Swallowing is also evoked by stimulation in the mouth or at the back of the tongue. The *rooting reflex* is elicited by touching or stroking around the baby's lips or on the cheeks. The baby responds by moving his head from side to side, attempting to follow the stimulus. The rooting movement helps the baby find the mother's nipple. The *stepping reflex* is a rhythmic alternate stepping response elicited by contact of the baby's foot against a surface. The *grasp reflex*, also called the *tonic palmar reflex* (Figure 4-3), is the flexing and gripping of the baby's fingers when the palm of his hand is contacted. Galant's reflex, also called the *trunk incurvation reflex*, is evoked by stroking the side of the baby's low back (the lumbar area). This elicits an arching or curving of his trunk sideways with the hollow or concavity towards the side being stroked. The final reaction to be discussed, the *hopping reaction*, depends on the cerebral cortex for full attainment. When the infant is moved in the horizontal plane (forward, backward, sideways, etc.), he makes hopping movements to restore the center of gravity and to maintain his balance.

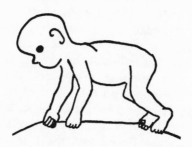

FIG. 4-3. Palmar and plantar grasp reflex.

The *equilibrium reactions* are the automatic balancing responses. The evolvement of equilibrium reactions and their mature forms as evoked by tipping a rocking table with the subject in the lying, sitting, quadruped and standing positions were described by Zador.[14] More recently, Martin[15] described them, preferring to call them *tilting reactions*. (See reflex timetable, Table 4-1.)

The Reflexive Substrata to Motor Development

The general pattern of reflexive development has been discussed. How the reflexive maturation provides the postural framework from which the motor developmental tasks emerge will be considered in lying, sitting, kneeling, standing, walking and grasping. Bobath has clearly described the postural reactions and their importance in motor development.

Prone   In the abdominal lying posture, the newborn tends to keep his arms and legs drawn up under his body. He can turn his head from side to side which prevents him from suffocating. He usually lies with his head turned to the side. Gradually the early pattern of total body flexion in all positions subsides. At about two months the labyrinthine righting reflexes acting on the head emerge, functioning to maintain the head in its normal position in relation to gravity, and the baby lifts his head from the surface. Head lifting is a very important acquisition which later functions to lead the body to the erect posture. In the older infant the optical righting reflex will reinforce the head lifting. The raised position of the head evokes the neck righting reflex, so that the upper part of the trunk raises up bringing the body into its normal alignment with the head. The extensor tone extends down the baby's back and into his legs, so that when the head is raised, the legs extend at the hips, knees and ankles. This interaction of the reflexes is called the *symmetrical chain reflex in the abdominal position*. In the infant of seven or eight months, the raised head, arched back, and extended legs persist even when the child is suspended in the abdominal position, supported under the thorax. This is called the Landau reflex. If the head is pushed down, the legs loosen, and this response disappears, demonstrating the dependence of this response on the labyrinthine righting reflex acting on the head. It can no longer be observed in the second year. The arms begin to support the upper body off the surface; initially, the elbows are flexed and the forearms rest on the supporting surface. Later the upper body is supported on the extended arms. The positive supporting reaction acts to stiffen

TABLE 4-1

Reflex Timetable

Responses	Weeks					Months							Years			Source
	1-4	2	3	4	5	6	7	8	9	10	11	12	2-3	3-5	After 5	
Moro	+	+	+	±	±	±	±	±	±	−						Peiper
Asymmetrical TNR	+	±	±	±	±	±	−									Peiper
Symmetrical TNR	+	+	+	+	+	+	−									Fiorentino
Tonic labyrinthine	+	+	+	+	−											Fiorentino
Grasp	+	+	+	±	±	±										Peiper
Neck righting	+	+	+	±	±	±	±	±	±	±	±	−				Bobath
Labyrinthine righting		+	+	+	+	+						±	±			Bobath
Optical righting					+	+	+	+	+	+	+	+	+	+	+	Fiorentino
Body righting on the body													±	±	+	Bobath
Protective extension of the arms						+	+	+	+	+	+	+	+	+	+	Fiorention
Equilibrium reactions in																
Prone						+	+	+	+	+	+	+	+	+	+	Bobath
Supine							+	+	+	+	+	+	+	+	+	Bobath
Sitting								+	+	+	+	+	+	+	+	Bobath
Quadrupedal											+	+	+	+	+	Bobath
Standing												+	+	+	+	Bobath

first the upper arm, and then the entire arm. At eight months, the emergence of the protective extension of the arms augments the support of the upper body by the arms. The commonly observed posture of the baby lying on his abdomen, with his head and chest raised off the surface, supported by his arms, shows the interaction of the labyrinthine righting reflex, the optical righting reflex, the Landau reflex, the positive supporting reaction and the protective extension of the arms. This is a clear example of reflexive evolvement from a simple to a more complex response. Later the body righting reflex acting on the body aids the baby to come to the sitting position from the abdominal lying posture. It has a segmental rotary action so that when the hips or shoulders are turned, the other segments come into alignment.

Supine   The newborn infant (Figure 4-4) in the *back-lying position* usually lies with his shoulder and hips rotated outward and his arms and legs spread, with the knees and elbows flexed. The back-lying posture is again predominantly one of flexion, and reflects the prenatal curled-up position of the baby in the uterus. The head is usually turned to the side and the influences of the assymmetrical tonic neck reflex, which extend the jaw limbs and flex the skull limbs, are frequently observed. At four to five months, the tendency toward asymmetrical posturing diminishes, and the head is frequently held in the midline position under the influences of symmetrical tonic neck reflex. At six months, the tendency to react in massive patterns of flexion and extension diminishes so that the baby, lying on his back, can play with his feet, bending his hips, while keeping his legs straight (Figure 4-5).

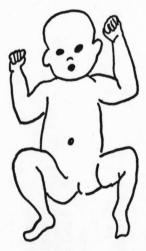

FIG. 4-4. Newborn.

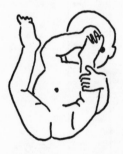

FIG. 4-5. A baby of six months playing with his feet (breakup of total patterns).

The *labyrinthine reflex* is absent when the infant lies flat on his back. If it were not extinguished in this position, it would not be possible to sleep on one's back.

Rolling   The newborn infant sometimes rolls (Figure 4-6) involuntarily from his back to his side, because of the curve in his back. The earliest reflexive rolling is in response to the head being turned, and the body following; this is the neck righting reflex acting on the body. At seven to twelve months, the pattern of the whole body rolling in response to the head turning has been modified. Segmental rolling appears. When the hips or shoulders are turned, the other segments follow, manifesting the body righting reflex acting on the body. At the same time, the first voluntary rol'ing begins. Initially, it is from the abdominal-lying position to the back-lying position. Later the baby will roll from back-lying to abdominal lying.

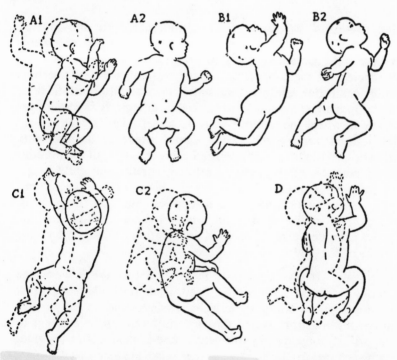

FIG. 4-6. Four positions involved in rolling from a supine to a prone position. Phase A, newborn; Phase B, spinal extension; Phase C, automatic rolling; Phase D, deliberation. (From McGraw, M. B. *The Neuromuscular Maturation of the Human Infant* (New York: Hafner Publishing Company, 1969, p. 45.) (Reprinted by permission of Columbia University Press.)

Sitting   When the newborn infant is pulled to the sitting position (Figure 4-7), his head sags backward, and only falls forward on the chest after the vertical position is reached. Subsequently, the labyrinthine reflex attempts to orient the head to its normal position, causing the head to strain forward when the child is pulled from the back-lying position to sitting. At about seven months he sits with his arms braced in front of him. The receptive zone of the positive supporting reaction has spread to the buttocks, giving the back extensor tone. It also provides extensor tone to the arms and is reinforced by the protective extension of the arms. The breakup of the total responses of flexor or extensor patterns coincides with the emergence of sitting. Sitting involves extension of the back with flexion of the hips. Later he will be able to flex his hips and extend his knees in the long sitting position. As the equilibrium reactions develop, the child can respond to shifts of his body. The arms are liberated from the necessity of propping the body, enabling him to reach out.

Crawling and creeping   Crawling refers to moving by dragging the body along the surface by arm and leg movements (Figure 4-8). Creeping refers to progression with the abdomen lifted clear of the supporting surface. Although the symmetrical tonic neck reflex reinforces the static postural pattern of the head lifted up and extended arms and flexed legs, it is no longer apparent when the child begins to creep. Persistence of the symmetrical tonic neck reflex would prevent the necessary extension of the legs when the head is erect. At about ten months, the interaction of the righting reflexes enables the child to get onto his knees from the back-lying or abdominal-lying positions. The positive supporting reaction supplies extension to the arms. The protective extension of the arms provokes forward reaching of the extended arm, as well as augmenting the support of the weight of the body.

Standing   It was previously mentioned that the labyrinthine righting reflex, as it acts on the head, leads the body to the erect posture (Figure 4-9). Early in the baby's development, the positive supporting reaction, acting through the feet, enables his legs to support his body. The evolvement of the Landau reflex provides extensor tone to the back and legs, also augmenting standing. When the infant is standing, the righting reflexes act to maintain the normal alignment of the head and body. The development of equilibrium reactions allows automatic responses to postural shifts. The protective extension of the arms acts to protect the body during falls.

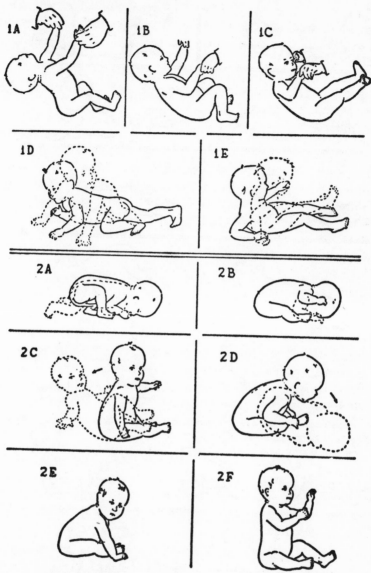

FIG. 4-7. Five phases of the rising aspect and six phases of the resistive aspect of neuromuscular development in achieving a sitting position. Phase A, the newborn or passive; Phase B, the orthotonic; Phase C, voluntary flexion; Phase D, the ventral push; Phase E, the dorsal push. Phase A, newborn; Phase B, incipient resistance; Phase C, exaggerated resistance; Phase D, trunkal resistance; Phase E, sustained resistance; Phase F, independent sitting. (From McGraw, M. B. *The Neuromuscular Maturation of the Human Infant* (New York: Hafner Publishing Company, 1969), p. 64.) (Reprinted by permission of Columbia University Press.)

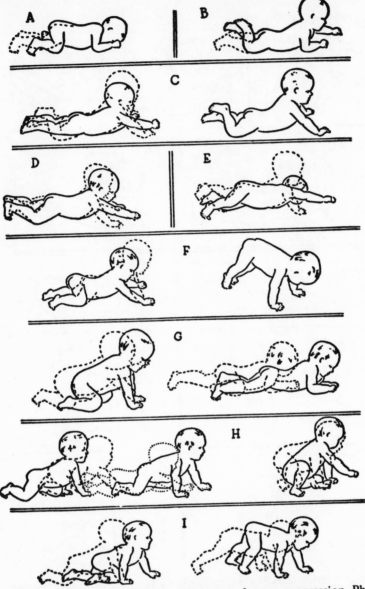

FIG. 4-8. Nine phases in the development of prone progression. Phase A, newborn; Phase B, beginning spinal extension; Phase C, advanced spinal extension; Phase D, incipient propulsion in superior region; Phase E, incipient propulsion in inferior region; Phase F, assumption of creeping posture; Phase G, deliberate but unorganized progression; Phase H, organized progressions; Phase I, integrated progression. (From McGraw, M. B. *The Neuromuscular Maturation of the Human Infant* (New York: Hafner Publishing Company, 1969), p. 51.) (Reprinted by permission of Columbia University Press.)

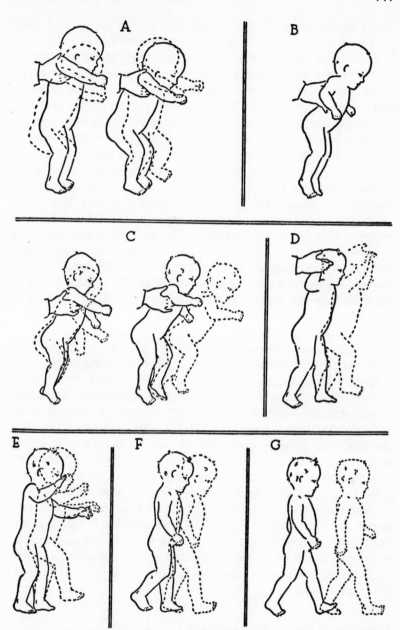

FIG. 4-9. Seven phases of erect locomotion. Phase A, the newborn or reflex stepping; Phase B, inhibition, or the static phase; Phase C, transition; Phase D, deliberate stepping; Phase E, independent stepping; Phase F, heel-toe progression. (From McGraw, M. B. *The Neuromuscular Maturation of the Human Infant* (New York: Hafner Publishing Company, 1969), p. 77.) (Reprinted by permission of Columbia University Press.)

Grasp and Release   The evolvement of the patterns of grasp have been described by Twitchell,[16] Halverson [17, 18] and Castner.[19] The arms of the newborn are flexed with the hands fisted, reflecting the early pattern of total body flexion (Figure 4-10). When the newborn baby's arms are pulled so that the shoulder adductors are stretched, a strong synergistic flexion occurs in all the joints, resisting the stretch, in a *traction response*. While the newborn baby's arms are usually held flexed, they extend when he is startled, as part of the Moro reflex. At the age of about one month, the traction response can be evoked by contact stimulation to the hand. The grasp reflex begins as a tactile response but is immediately reinforced by proprioceptive impulses. The grasp reflex is present until about the sixth month. The *instinctual grasp response* appears at five to ten months. At four to five months a contact stimulus to the medial side of the hand causes hand supination orienting the hand to the stimulus. At the same time eye-hand coordination begins to develop. The baby becomes fascinated by the movements of his hands, and also begins to engage his hands in the midline. Soon, as the instinctual grasp response develops, the hand will not only orient to an object, but will follow and grasp it. Gradually the infant's grasp becomes increasingly differentiated with the digits responding singly. True voluntary grasp begins to emerge from about nine months to a year. Voluntary release of objects begins at ten months. The infant of one year continues to have difficulty releasing small objects. In early grasp patterns, the whole hand is used. At about six months the first real grasp occurs with the fingers pressing the object against the palm. The first opposition grasp occurs about seven months and is fully developed by eight months. By one year the grasp is delicate with the fingers exerting the appropriate amount of force to hold the object. The developmental sequences of grasps are illustrated in Figures 4-10 through 4-12. Although the grasp pattern is well developed during the first year, functional accomplishments in the seated position will be hampered until the equilibrium reactions in the seated position are well developed. (See Table 4-2.)

Schedule of Motor Development

During the first two years the baby will learn to roll, sit, crawl, stand and walk. The baby attains these skills in a sequential and predictable manner. Normal motor development has been investigated and described in detail by Gesell,[20] Illingworth,[21] McGraw[22] and others. Although discrepancies in the timing of the appearance of some motor skills occur among the schedules, the schedules agree on the general rate. The most celebrated studies of infant development are those by Gesell and his associates at the Yale Clinic of Child Development. Scales have been devised for the motor, adaptive, language and personal-social behavior areas. Some of the variations relate to the lack of criteria for evaluating a particular item, such as: the child sits briefly, or the child sits with slight support. It is advantageous for the occupational therapist to use a motor developmental schedule that has many items at the various age levels. Table 4-3 is derived largely from the schedules of Gesell,[23,24] Illingworth[25] and others.

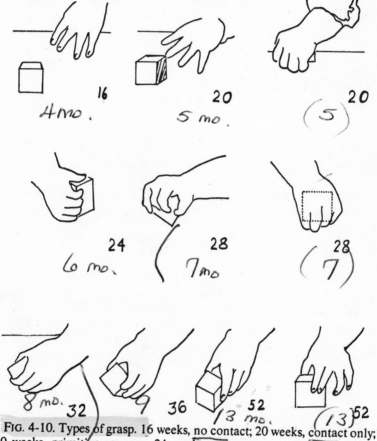

FIG. 4-10. Types of grasp. 16 weeks, no contact; 20 weeks, contact only; 20 weeks, primitive squeeze; 24 weeks, squeeze grasp; 28 weeks, hand grasp; 28 weeks, palm grasp; 32 weeks, superior palm grasp; 36 weeks, inferior forefinger grasp; 52 weeks, superior forefinger grasp. (From Halverson, H. M. "An Experimental Study of Prehension in Infants by means of Systematic Cinema Records." *Genetic Psychology Monographs* 10 (1931), pp. 212-215.) (Provincetown, Massachusetts: Courtesy of the Journal Press.)

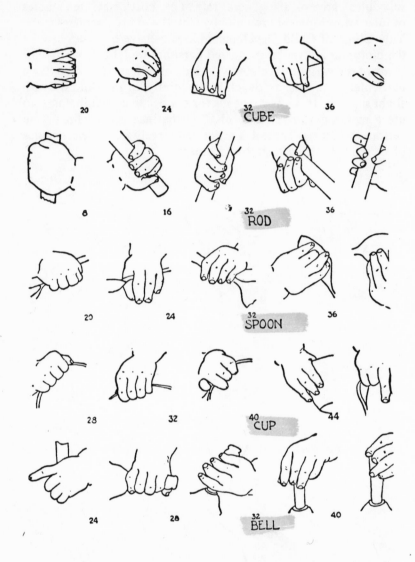

FIG. 4-11. Showing a series of grasps in developmental sequence for each of five objects: cube, rod, spoon, cup, and bell. The numbers below each drawing indicate the age at which that grasp occurs. (From Halverson, H. M. "A Further Study of Grasping." *The Journal of General Psychology* 7 (1932), p. 41.)

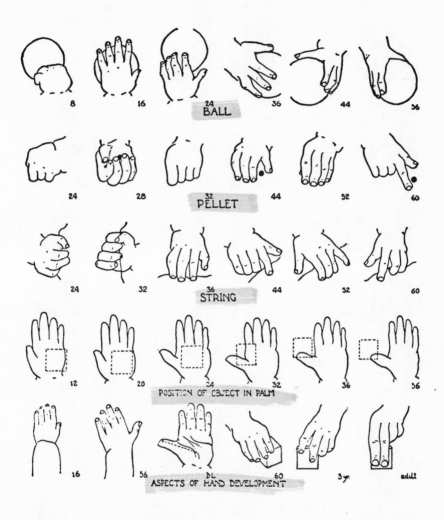

FIG. 4-12. Illustrating a series of grasps in developmental sequence for each of three objects: ball, pellet, and string. This figure also shows the six successive positions on the palm against which the fingers press objects, such as cubes. Under the caption "Aspects of Hand Development" appear in order: the forearm of a 16-week infant, the forearm of a 56-week infant, the developmental line (note broken line) of opposition in grasping and digital grasping by a 60-week infant, by a 3-year-old child, and by an adult, respectively. (From Halverson, H. M. "A Further Study of Grasping." *The Journal of General Psychology* 7 (1932), p. 44.)

TABLE 4-2

Sensorimotor Developmental Chart

Age	General Responses	Oral Reflexes	Gross Motor Skills	Upper Limb	Sensory
1-4 weeks	Moro: strong Asymmetrical TNR Symmetrical TNR Neck righting Withdrawal reflex Tonic Labyrinthine Positive and negative supporting reactions Infantile stepping* Extensor thrust	Suckling Rooting Swallowing Vomiting Tongue protrusion	Prone infantile crawling movements Asymmetrical postures predominate	Grasp reflex Traction response Both hands fisted	Pain: present Tactile: touch and pressure Temperature: hot, cold Smell: present Taste: sweet, sour, salty, bitter Hearing: poorly developed Vision: functioning
2 months	Moro: present TNR: diminishing Neck righting Labyrinthine righting Withdrawal reflex* Extensor thrust* Crossed extension reflex* Positive and negative supporting	Suckling Rooting	Holds head up to 45° prone lying	Grasp reflex	Eye follows less than 90° Attends to bell by diminished activity
3 months	Moro: diminishing TNR: diminishing Neck righting Labyrinthine righting Positive and negative supporting reactions	Suckling Rooting	Holds head up 45-90° prone lying Bears weight on forearms	Grasp reflex Hands open Plays regarding hands	Tickle reaction Eye follows to 180°

4-6 months	Suckling* Rooting*	Moro and TNR: diminishing* Neck righting Labyrinthine righting Positive and negative supporting reactions* Protective extension of arms (6 months) Landau Equilibrium prone Optical righting	Supine head control Symmetrical postures predominate Rolls prone to supine	Grasp reflex: diminishing 1st voluntary grasp Hands come together in play Plays with hands and feet in supine Control elbow extension	Turns head towards sound
7-12 months		Neck righting* Labyrinthine righting Optical righting Protective extension of the arms Landau Equilibrium supine, quadrupedal Body righting acting on the body	Pulls to standing Rolls supine to prone Pivots (7 months) Sits (8 months) Crawls (9 months) Creeps (10 months)	Grasp reflex: diminished First opposed pinch First voluntary release (9 months) Control supination-pronation of forearm	
12-14 months		Labyrinthine righting Optical righting Landau Protective extension of arms Body righting acting on body Equilibrium kneeling, sitting, standing,	Cruises sideways holding furniture (11 months) Stands alone (1 year) Walks (13-18 months)		

TABLE 4-3

Motor Developmental Schedule

One Month
  Head usually turned to side.
  Hands fisted.
  Stares vacantly.
  Infantile crawling movements.
  Supine: Legs flexed, externally rotated, heels on supporting surface. When pulled to sitting head sags backward and then falls forward onto chest.
  Mass motor activity reaction to stimuli.

Two Months
  Direct regard.
  Head bobs when sat erect.
  Eye follows object past 90°
  Prone: Holds head up to 45° with chest up.
  Supine: When pulled to sitting, head sags less.

Three Months
  Holds head steady in upright posture.
  Hands begin to open.
  Plays by regarding hands.
  Eye follows to 180°.
  Prolonged fixation on light or person.
  Prone: Bears weight on forearms.
         Face held $45\text{-}90^\circ$ with hips straight and knees bent.

Four to Six Months
  Supine: Head predominantly held in midline and symmetrical posture.
          Hands engage.
          Visually pursues lost toy (5 mo.).
          Grasps feet (6 mo.).
  Prone: Props on extended arms (5 mo.).
         Pulled to sitting with no head lag (5 mo.).
         Rolls prone to supine (6 mo.).
         Lifts head and assists when pulled to sitting (6 mo.).
  Rotates head to inspect surroundings (4 mo.).
  Perceives 8 mm. pellet on table (4 mo.).
  Reaches with palm facing downward (forearm pronation).
  Uses Excessive grip strength (6 mo.).
  Rescues toy dropped within reach (6 mo.).
  First voluntary grasp of palmar type (fingers against palm) (6 mo.).
  No voluntary release.

Seven to Twelve Months
  Supine: Brings feet to mouth (7 mo.).
  Prone: Pivots (8 mo.).
         Crawls (9 mo.).
         Creeps (10 mo.).
  Sitting: Bounces actively when sitting (7 mo.).
           Sits alone for one minute (8 mo.).
           When leans forward can re-erect self (9 mo.).
           Sits for 10 minutes (9 mo.).

TABLE 4-3 (continued)

Motor Developmental Schedule

Seven to Twelve Months (continued)
    Standing: Pulls to knee stand (9 mo.).
               Cruises sideways holding onto furniture (11 mo.).
               Pulls to standing using furniture or rail (10 mo.).
    Hand use:First opposed pinch (7-10 mo.).
               First voluntary release (9-12 mo.).
               Grasps pellet using thumb in scissors grasp (9-11 mo.).
               Reaches extending arms for toys out of reach (8 mo.).
               Holds one object, regards, and grasps another (8 mo.).
               Brings one toy against another (9 mo.).
               Grasps with neat pincer grasp (12 mo.).

Twelve to Eighteen Months
    Creeps quickly with good coordination.
    May creep with elbows and knees extended (12-14 mo.).
    Creeps upstairs (14-16 mo.).
    Pivots sitting (12 mo.).
    Stands alone momentarily (12 mo.).
    Rises independently without supports (15 mo.).
    Goes from standing to sitting by falling (14-16 mo.).
    Assumes and maintains kneeling posture (12-14 mo.).
    Walks (13-17 mo.).
    Grasps using fingertips in opposition to thumb (12 mo.).
    Falls by collapse (15 mo.).

One Year and a Half
    Walks: Sideways, backward.
    Ascends stairs holding onto hand or rail.
    Runs stiffly.
    Walks into a ball, doesn't kick.
    Looks out of window at people, plane, moon.
    Piles three blocks.
    Seats self in small chair.
    Hugs doll.

Two Years
    Walks: Using heel-toe gait.
               On tiptoe. (2½)
               Kicks ball on direction.
               Runs better.
    Stairs: Up and down using two feet per step.
    Picks up object from floor.
    Rhythmical responses bending knees, bouncing, nodding, swaying, swinging arms.
    Gets down from adult chair.
    Squats in play.
    Jumps from 12″ height (One foot leads).

TABLE 4-3 (continued)

Motor Developmental Schedule

Two Years (continued)
    Reach and Grasp: Turns door knobs (forearm rotation).
                  Tower of six to seven.
                  Overgrasps and over releases. (2½)
                  Imitates vertical and circular stroke.
    Vision: Enjoys watching moving objects.

Three Years
    Hand use: Tower of nine to ten.
              Copies circle, imitates cross.
              May shift handedness or use non-dom. hand (3½).
              Mild tremor in fine motor coordination (3½).
              Feeds self well and unbuttons front buttons.
    Jumps: From one foot height with both feet together.
              From one and a half foot height with one foot leading.
    Stairs: Up with alternate foot placement without support.
              Down using two feet on one step without support.
    Throws ball without losing balance (3).
    Walking: Swings arm with opposite leg.
              Walks chalkline heel-toe pattern.
              Hops on one foot three times (3½).
    Stands on one foot momentarily.
    Catches large ball with arms extended.

Four Years
    Very active.
    Enjoys balance activities.
    Throws ball overhead.
    Uses scissors and tries to cut straight line.
    Stands on one foot four to eight seconds.
    Can vary speed running smoothly turning corners, stopping and starting quickly.
    Standing broad jump (8-10″).
    Running broad jump (23-33″).
    Somersaults.
    Bounces ball awkwardly.
    Names heavier of two weights.
    Stands on one foot with eyes closed.
    Copies square, draws triangle.
    Gains strength, ease in leg use.

Five Years
    Stands on one foot more than eight seconds.
    Coordination reaches new maturity—greater control of body with economy of
        movement.
    May walk with feet pronated.
    Large muscle control advanced over small muscle control.
    Jumps from table height.
    Places fingers on piano keys, may experiment with chords.
    Skips alternately.
    Down stairs using feet alternately without support.

TABLE 4-3 (continued)

Motor Developmental Schedule

Five Years (continued)
Tries roller skates, jump rope, stilt use.
Interested in bicycle rather than tricycle (5½).
Hops on one foot ten or more times.
Running broad jump (28-35").
Frequent change of posture from sitting, standing, squatting.
Likes to climb fences.
Beginning to use hands more than arms catching small ball but often misses.
Can walk a straight line.

Six Years
Almost in constant motion.
More deliberate.
Sometimes clumsy.
Spends time wrestling, tumbling, crawling, climbing, swinging.
Tries roller skates and stunts on bars.
Cuts, pastes, hammers, uses tools.
Jumps from 12" landing on toes only.
Stands on alternate feet with eyes closed.
Likes balance activities.

Seven Years
Repetitious in activities such as soft ball, roller skates, etc.
Boys manipulate tools.
Learning to bat and pitch ball.
More cautious in gross motor activities.
Likes to run.
Pencil tightly gripped often close to tip.
Pencil pressure may be heavy.
Both hands used playing piano but with unequal pressure.

Eight Years
Interested in team sports.
Body movements more rhythmic and graceful.
Eye-hand coordination improved in speed and smoothness.
Girls can run into moving jumprope but cannot alter step.
Less tense hold on pencils, brushes, tools.

Nine Years
Some timidity of speed as in skiing, cars.
Interested in strength and lifting things.
Works and plays hard tending to pursue one activity until tired.
Great team sport interest.

Adolescence
May be awkward due to acceleration and asymmetries of anatomical growth, such
as arm length to trunk length.

NEUROMUSCULAR DYSFUNCTION

Neuromuscular dysfunction pertains to abnormal, incomplete, or impaired functioning of the nerves and muscles. The disorders to be discussed include dysfunctions of the motor system. The motor system includes that portion of the nervous system that relays impulses from the nerve centers out to the body tissues. Motor dysfunction may result from involvement of the central nervous system, the peripheral nerves relaying impulses from the brain stem or spinal cord to the muscles, the nerve and muscle junction called the myoneural junction, or the muscles. Disorders that impair the motor system are classified in various ways. Lesions of the motor system are commonly divided into *upper motor neurons* and *lower motor neurons.* Lower motor neuron lesions occur somewhere in the final common pathway in the motor cell bodies of the brain stem or spinal cord, or in the axon passing to the skeletal muscle motor end plates. The lower motor neuron lesion produces a characteristic clinical picture. Since the impulses from the brain and spinal cord cannot reach the skeletal muscle fibers, the muscles shrink or atrophy. The muscle tone is lost and the muscles become limp or flaccid; the lower motor neuron paralysis is commonly referred to as *flaccid paralysis.* The reflexes are diminished or absent. The disturbance of motor power produced by upper motor neuron lesions depends on the site of the lesion. Upper motor neuron lesions cause little or no muscle atrophy, hyperactive deep reflexes and absent superficial reflexes, and pathologic reflexes. These lesions may be manifested in decreased muscle tone which is called *hypotonicity,* increased muscle tone which is called *hypertonicity* or *spasticity,* or *fluctuating muscle tone.* The physician must make a differential diagnosis between delayed motor development without pathology, a lower motor neuron lesion, and central nervous system lesion.

Recently attention has been focused on early detection of medical problems in infants and children. Early detection is especially essential in children with central nervous system lesions. During early infancy most of the maturation of the nervous system occurs, the relatively fixed movement patterns evolve, the organization of motor coordination takes place, and most of motor development and motor learning is accomplished. Symptoms may be detected during the routine examination of the infant by a physician. The mother may seek advice because the baby is difficult to feed, unusually irritable, does not achieve the expected motor skills, assumes unusual postures, is unresponsive, or does not use parts of his body. The parents will want to know what is wrong with the child, what can be done about it, why the problem happened, and whether future children will be normal (Figure 4-13).

Motor development is delayed or retarded in some children without a pathologic cause. The quality of the motor tasks is within normal limits, but the timing is delayed. Possible causes of delayed or retarded motor development are: delayed maturation of central nervous system structures; prematurity or shortened gestation; emotional deprivation; prolonged illness resulting in debilitation; marked obesity; lack of opportunities to practice motor skills because of illness or physical deprivation; a familial characteristic; or an individual developmental response.

Etiologic Factors

The upsurge of interest in the field of preventive medicine offers new hope for many unborn children. Current research efforts are shedding new light on factors operant in the parents prior to conception, and factors affecting the mother and baby after conception. Efforts are being made to offer prenatal medical care to all segments of the population. Sources of neuromotor dysfunctions will be considered in three stages: the prenatal period from inception until the beginning of labor; the perinatal period from the beginning of labor until birth occurs; and the infancy period from birth to about five years of age.

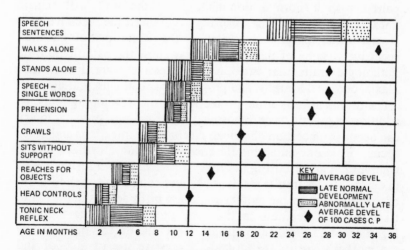

FIG. 4-13. Normal development compared with average development of 100 cerebral palsied. (From Denhoff, E. and Holden, R. H. "The Developmental Ladder in Cerebral Palsy." In *The Crippled Child* (Chicago: Courtesy of Crippled Children and Adults of Rhode Island, Inc., October, 1951).)

Prenatal Factors

Most of the prenatal factors can be grouped under three headings which include environmental factors which affect intrauterine life, chromosomal aberrations, and genetic abnormalities. Human cells normally contain 23 pairs of chromosomes, with the exception of certain reproductive cells. At conception each parent contributes one 23-chromosome reproductive cell. One pair determines sex, and 22 pairs control the structure and function of the body. The chromosomes have a number of genes located on them. Genes are the basic units of heredity that determine all the inborn characteristics. Some pathologic traits are hereditary. These traits may be expressed or unexpressed in the parents. Some pathologic traits are sex-linked, carried on the female sex chromosome. Although these sex-linked traits are unexpressed in the mother, they are transmitted to the male offspring. Sometimes chromosomal defects occur accidentally during the formation of the reproductive cells. A dominant pathologic trait is expressed in the parent carrying it, although occasionally a generation is skipped. Generally, only one parent is affected as dominant traits are relatively rare. Half the offspring would be expected to express the dominant trait. Pathologic traits that may be transmitted dominantly are myotonia dystrophica, Huntington's chorea, and muscular dystrophy of the facioscapulohumeral type. Some traits may be carried dominantly, or recessively. When a recessive gene for a pathologic trait is paired with a normal dominant gene, the trait will remain unexpressed. Some of the offspring may inherit the recessive trait. If the other parent also carries the same pathologic trait recessively, some of the offspring may show the pathologic trait. Pathologic traits that are carried recessively are Friedreich's ataxia, peroneal atrophy, and progressive spinal muscular atrophy.

The uterus affords some protection to the developing fetus. In addition to genetic or chromosomal abnormalities, prenatal injury can occur from certain chemical, mechanical, infectious and other agents. Environmental interference is the most critical in the embryonic period during the first trimester. Severe insults result in death. Milder insults result in changes compatible with life. Use of certain drugs by the mother can cause birth defects in the child. Examples are deafness in the baby produced by the mother's ingestion of quinine, and multiple congenital defects produced by the mother's use of thalidomide. Excessive use of alcohol and tobacco affect the baby. Irradiation of the mother is especially critical during the early stages of pregnancy and may cause genetic damage to the baby. Some maternal infections may be passed to the developing baby, such as German measles, chicken pox, measles, mumps, tuberculosis, and syphilis. If the mother contracts German measles during the first three months of her pregnancy the baby often suffers visual, auditory, and mental defects. Malnutrition of the mother affects the baby, as seen in anemia. An injury to the mother in the form of a blow, or fall on the abdomen, or a pelvic fracture, may injure the developing baby. Incompatibility of the blood between the mother and the child, the Rh factor or ABO factor, causes oxygenation problems in the baby and may result in brain damage. A protective injection is now available to prevent buildup of Rh antibodies in the mother's blood. If the mother suffers metabolic disturbances such as diabetes or myasthenia gravis the baby is affected. Recently there has been more concern about the relationship of environmental pollutants and birth defects such as high mercury levels in the soil where food is grown. In this area many questions remain unanswered.

Perinatal Factors

A high correlation exists between prematurity with a low birth weight and defective babies. During labor and delivery lack of sufficient oxygen to the baby is a potential cause of brain damage. This oxygen deficiency may result from maternal anesthesia, infant mechanical respiratory obstructions, delayed delivery of the baby's head as in a breech delivery, or premature separation of the placenta. Birth injuries may also result from a difficult labor caused by the position or size of the baby, or problems of the mother's pelvic size and shape, or uterine problems. Artificial means of delivery such as use of forceps to effect the birth may also be a factor. All the etiological factors mentioned often cause impaired functioning in the emotional and mental spheres as well as the physical spheres.

Infancy Factors

Damage may occur from infections contracted during the child's early years such as encephalitis, brain abscesses and meningitis. Viral and bacterial invasions may result secondary to the childhood diseases or otitis media, sinusitis, osteomyelitis, or tonsillitis. Another source of brain damage is the premature closing of the growth areas between the skull bones, called craniostenosis. Children may suffer brain damage from many environmental causes, from falls, or in automobile accidents. Young children ingesting lead or mercury or breathing excessive carbon monoxide often suffer residual damage.

Neuromuscular Weakness in Infancy

Diseases of the lower motor neuron and diseases of the skeletal muscles seen in infancy and childhood are included in Table 4-4. Almost *any metabolic disorder, endocrine disorder, or infectious disease can result in neurological abnormalities* and affect the neuromuscular apparatus. Some examples include hypothyroidism, renal insufficiency and adrenal dysfunction. Some central nervous system diseases are manifested by a lack of motor activity or muscle weakness. Seizures are a common complication in these diseases. Examples include leukodystrophies, lipid storage diseases and Wilson's disease. The anterior horn cells are the cell bodies of the motor nerve fibers located in the anterior portion of the spinal cord. Diseases of the anterior horn cells produce a motor rather than a sensory deficit. Examples are infantile spinal muscular atrophy and poliomyelitis. The children affected may have severe muscle weaknesses, but their eyes are generally not affected. The peripheral nerves are the nerves originating in the base of the brain and the spinal cord that supply the muscles and glands. Two peripheral nerve disorders are

TABLE 4-4

Causes of Congenital and Infantile Neuromuscular Weakness*.

A. Metabolic and infectious disorders which may secondarily affect the neuromuscular apparatus.
B. Disorders of the central nervous system including myelopathies.
C. Disorders of anterior horn cells.
 1. Infantile spinal muscular atrophy (Werdnig-Hoffman).
 2. Poliomyelitis and related viral disorders.
D. Disorders of peripheral nerves.
 1. Guillain-Barré syndrome.
 2. Familial forms of peripheral neuropathy.
E. Disorders of the neuromuscular junction—myasthenia gravis.
F. The primary myopathies.
 1. Muscular dystrophies.
 2. Inflammatory myopathies.
 3. Congenital nonprogressive myopathy syndrome.
 4. The myotonic syndrome.
 5. The periodic paralyses.
G. Skeletal, tendinous, and ligamentous disorders.

*Table 4-4 reprinted by permission from Munsat, T. L., and Pearson, C. M. "The Differential Diagnosis of Neuromuscular Weakness in Infancy and Childhood." Developmental Medicine and Child Neurology (1967), p. 222.

Guillain-Barré syndrome, infectious polyneuritis, and Charcot-Marie-Tooth, also called peroneal muscular atrophy. The *primary myopathies* are due to functional and structural derangement of the skeletal muscle fibers. The pathology is in the muscle fibers. Two examples of *inflammatory myopathies* are polymyositis and childhood dermatomyositis. The *congenital nonprogressive myopathies* are manifested by proximal symmetrical weaknesses with depressed reflexes. They are nonprogressive or progress slowly.

Various systems of classification of the *muscular dystrophies* exist. A primary distinction between the types is the generally rapid progression of the *Duchenne type* in contrast to the slower progression, and greater localization of the fascioscapulohumeral and limb-girdle varieties. The Duchenne type, also called the *generalized familial* muscular dystrophy or *pseudo-hypertrophic* muscular dystrophy is the most common form seen in childhood. It is inherited in a sex-linked pattern. Onset is prior to the sixth year. There is an apparent enlargement of the muscles of the scapula, upper arms, calves and the shoulders because of fatty infiltration of the muscles. Later muscle wasting occurs. The disease is characterized by changes in muscle size, an early waddling walk, and a characteristic way of coming to the standing position by using the arms to walk up the thighs pushing the body into the erect position. When the patient becomes bedridden, contractures of the elbows, knees, and increased lateral curvature of the back frequently occur. Occupational therapy is aimed toward maintenance of as much function as possible, prevention of deformities, and diversional activities.

In the *limb-girdle* type of muscular dystrophy onset is commonly between eight and twelve years of age. It progresses more slowly and is milder than the Duchenne type. The pelvic girdle is affected early, and the child has difficulty ascending and decending stairs. In the following months or years, weakness and wasting of the proximal muscles of the arm occurs. The child's life span is somewhat shortened. In the *fascioscapulohumeral* type, also called the *Landouzy* and *Dejerine* type, the onset is between the ages of six and twenty. Transmission is hereditary with both sexes equally affected. The mode of transmission is dominant. Weakness and wasting occur initially in the face and shoulder girdles. A characteristic symptom is the inability to raise the arms above the head. The face assumes a mask-like expression and the muscle wasting spreads to the shoulders and upper arms. The juvenile form (Erb type) does not affect the facial musculature and progresses more slowly, sometimes remaining dormant for years. Two other forms are the *ocular* muscular dystrophy, also called *progressive dystrophic ophthalmoplegia* and *distal* muscular dystrophy, also called *myotonic dystrophy* or *myotonic atrophica.* Drooping of the eyelids and facial, shoulder, and shoulder girdle weakness are characteristic of the ocular type. In the distal type there is weakness of the face, eyelids, neck, jaw and distal limbs. The occupational therapy program depends on the symptoms, the rate of progression and prognosis. In the slower progressing forms of muscular dystrophy more emphasis is placed on maintaining or increasing function, sometimes through the use of adapted equipment. Since inactivity is commonly accompanied by increasing disability, deformity, and obesity, it is important to keep these children active, utilizing their remaining abilities.

Joint laxity and muscular weakness because of skeletal, tendinous and ligamentous disorders may cause a motor developmental delay.

Central Nervous System Disorders

Moore,[26] in 1968, stated that approximately half of the case loads in any given hospital or clinic involve patients with neurological deficits. Those central nervous system disorders which involve the motor sphere and are commonly seen in occupational therapy will be discussed. Abnormalities of the skull and vertebrae, with defects in the closure of the bones, may permit portions of the spinal cord or brain to herniate through the defect. Classification of these disorders depends on what structures have herniated and the extent of the herniation. Some examples include the spina bifida occulta, spinal meningocele, meningomyelocele and myelomeningocystocele. In some children the skull bones close prematurely. Premature bone closure during the first seven years may result in compression and damage to the brain. *Hydrocephalus* is an excessive enlargement of the head because of obstruction of the cerebrospinal fluid circulation. The increased pressure damages the brain structures. *Cerebral neoplasms* are not infrequent in children. The prognosis is usually poor, but depends on the site and type of tumor. Occupational therapy is determined by the prognosis and the presenting symptoms. It is frequently diversional and maintenance-oriented, rather than rehabilitational.

Examples of progressive lesions of the central nervous system are Friedreich's ataxia and dystonia musculorum deformans. These disorders are rare and infrequently seen in occupational therapy.

Very few neurological disorders produce isolated disturbances of motor power. Most of the central nervous system lesions produce associated visual, auditory, sensory, perceptual, intellectual, emotional and psychological disturbances. Normal motor activity is dependent on an intact sensorimotor system. The sensory system provides continuous information vital to coordinated voluntary movements. Although this chapter emphasizes the motor sphere, the occupational therapist must think in terms of sensorimotor function. Isolated consideration of the motor system is artificial. Assessment of the sensorimotor system is useful in analyzing the deficit and in organizing a total occupational therapy program.

Cerebral Palsy

Cerebral palsy is defined as abnormal brain function or syndromes of cerebral dysfunction present from birth or occurring during the early formative years because of a nonprogressive central nervous system lesion with a predominant component of motor dysfunction. It is an inclusive term used to describe groups of children with nonprogressive motor handicaps. The motor dysfunction manifests itself in abnormalities of movement and posture. The impaired neurological functioning is expressed in various body systems such as defective vision, hearing, intellectual functioning, perception, and sensation. The child is frequently subject to seizures and may have accompanying emotional or psychological disturbances.

The two most common lesions encountered are congenital malformations and destructive brain lesions. Dekaban[27] cites congenital malformations as the second leading cause of infant mortality during the first year. Cerebral palsy is one of the major crippling diseases of childhood. Although the neurological lesions of cerebral palsy are nonprogressive, the manifestations are dynamic, especially during infancy. The expression of the lesions relates to the maturational stage of the nervous system. During early infancy when behavior is dominated by the lower central nervous structures, largely the brain stem and subcortical mechanisms, symptoms may be absent or masked. Later, as the higher centers are activated, the disorganization of the nervous system becomes more apparent. The very young baby is often delayed in motor development and may lack muscle tone or be floppy. Many months later the baby develops increased muscle tone in the form of spasticity, rigidity or involuntary movements. The transient reflexes that are normal in the young baby persist in the older child. The lack of integration of reflexive behavior, resulting in abnormal postural responses, abnormal sensory input, faulty feedback from the body and purposeless motor output, form a vicious repetitive cycle interfering with normal motor development and acquisition of the motor milestones.

Classification of cerebral palsy is based on clinical findings rather than etiology or pathology. Several systems of classification exist. A commonly used system in the United States was devised by the American Academy for Cerebral Palsy in 1956.

CLASSIFICATION OF CEREBRAL PALSY (Minear)

Physiologic (motor)

A. Spasticity
B. Athetosis
  1. Tension
  2. Nontension
  3. Dystonia
  4. Tremor

C. Rigidity
D. Ataxia
E. Tremor
F. Atonia (rare)
G. Mixed
H. Unclassified

Cerebral palsy is commonly described by the distribution or parts of the body that are involved. In *monoplegia,* which is unusual, a single limb is involved. *Paraplegia* refers to involvement of the legs. In *hemiplegia* involvement is limited to one side of the body. *Triplegia* refers to involvement of one arm and both legs; this is unusual. *Quadriplegia* refers to involvement of all four limbs. In *diplegia,* all four limbs are involved, but the legs are more severely affected. In *double hemiplegia* both sides of the body are involved, but one side is more involved. The majority of cerebral palsy cases can be classified under spastic quadriplegia, spastic diplegia, spastic hemiplegia or athetosis.

Spastic Quadriplegia

Spasticity refers to increased muscle tone. Quadriplegia reflects the involvement of the whole body. The impairment is usually asymmetrical on one side of the body; the two sides of the body seldom are equally involved. The newborn baby frequently seems normal. A careful examination might reveal diminished muscle tone (hypotonia) with a paucity of movements. In the next few months, the neck, and then the back and limbs, stiffen when the baby is startled or handled. In the late stages of symptomatic evolvement the initial extensor spasticity is supplanted by flexor spasticity. Total patterns of flexion or extension predominate. A marked increase of extensor muscle tone occurs in the back-lying position. Because of the retraction of the head and shoulders the child cannot raise his head or reach out with his arms. If the effects of the tonic labyrinthine reflex are strong, an increase in flexor tone will occur when the child is turned to his abdomen. In the *abdominal-lying* position the child is often totally flexed at the hips, knees and arms, and the hands are fisted. In some cases the upper limbs are flexed and the hips and legs are extended. In some children the extensor tone predominates, persisting even in the abdominal lying position. If this is the case, the extensor tone is relatively less in the abdominal position than the back-lying position. Because of the positive supporting reaction acting through the buttocks, the spastic quadriplegic child has difficulty bending his hips in order to sit. He sits with his hips forward and his body leaning backward. To compensate for the position of the lower trunk, the upper back and neck strain forward. The spastic adductor muscles bring his legs together producing a narrow sitting base. Balance is further jeopardized by the poor head control. If the head control is severely impaired, the child will be unable to sit independently. When the child stands, the pressure on the soles of his feet elicits extension of his legs, back and neck. He tends to be thrown off balance backward. It is not possible for the child to walk until he gains some control of this neck extension. He stands and walks with his trunk and head leaning forward and his chin jutting forward. He walks on his toes with his knees bent, his thighs coming together or his legs crossing one in front of the other, called scissoring. His hips roll inward. As his foot strikes the ground, the extensor tone tends to throw him backward. The crossed extensor reflex sometimes causes a reflexive relaxing of the opposite leg. The child's ability to sit, stand, and walk depends on the severity of his condition, and whether he can support himself with his arms. Reach and grasp patterns remain primitive with a palmar grasp, the fingers pressing the object against the palm. Typical deformities occur in spastic quadriplegics, and the therapist needs to constantly monitor and try to counteract them. These include lateral curvature of the spine (scoliosis) and antero-posterior deviations of the upper spine (kyphosis); flexion deformities of the hips, knees, fingers, and forearm pronation; shortening of the heel cords with the foot turning inward or outward (equinovarus, equinovalgus); and subluxation of the hip.

Spastic Diplegia or Paraplegia

In the *spastic diplegic*, spasticity predominates, with the legs more involved than the upper body. The *spastic paraplegic* has minimal upper body involvement. Children in these categories have better head control, use of the upper limbs, and speech. The symptomatic freedom of the upper body and limbs and the ability to support with the arms enhances the child's function appreciably. The child tends to have hip and knee flexion. To compensate for the hip flexion which would throw the upper body forward, he has an increased compensatory low back curve (lordosis). His primary disability is in locomotion. The following deformities frequently occur: increased antero-posterior deviations of the back (kyphosis and lordosis), hip subluxations or dislocations, flexion contractures of the hips and knees, tight hip inward rotators and adductors, and heel cord shortening with foot rotation (equinovarus or equinovalgus).

Spastic Hemiplegia

The *spastic hemiplegic* has a spastic paralysis of one side of his body. The arm is more involved than the leg. The involved side is smaller because of a stunting of growth. The arm is held in a characteristic posture with the shoulder rolled inward and the arm held close to the body. The elbow, wrist, and fingers are flexed, and the forearm pronated with the thumb adducted across the palm. Spastic hemiplegia is often recognized earlier than other forms of cerebral palsy because of the asymmetrical picture. The baby may not kick that leg, reach with the arm, or may hold his head to one side. Motor development is usually delayed and patterns are abnormal because of the impairment. The baby crawls, dragging his involved side behind. He usually avoids that side, developing the intact portions of his body. He sits with his weight on the good side. He uses the uninvolved upper limb for manipulation. When using his good hand, an overflow occurs into the affected side, exaggerating the flexed position of the limb. The overflow from the sound side to the involved limb, or other parts of the body, is called *associated reactions*. The involved upper limb usually suffers sensory losses and circulatory disturbances. The child only uses the involved arm when bilateral holding or stabilization is essential. The grasp pattern in the involved hand remains primitive. When the child with spastic hemiplegia stands, he maintains his weight on his uninvolved leg. His whole physical orientation tends to become one-sided. Initially, the spastic hemiplegic child lacks tone in the leg and it will not support him. As he begins to bear weight on the involved leg, the extensor tone increases until finally he walks on the toes of his involved leg. When standing on the involved leg, it tends to roll inward, flex somewhat at the hips and knee, and stiffens so that he is standing on his toes on that side. To overcome the extensor spasticity in order to step, as he puts his weight on the involved leg, the knee hyperextends, allowing the body to move forward in relation to the leg. Other gait disturbances are attributable to the inequality in leg lengths. The spastic hemiplegic often develops secondary muscle weakness, probably from disuse. He drags his involved side behind, with his arm held in marked flexion. Typical deformities that should be monitored and counteracted when possible are: contractures of the distal parts of the involved arm, wrist and finger flexion, forearm pronation, thumb adduction, heel cord shortening with foot rotation (equinovarus or equinovalgus) and lateral deviations of the spine (scoliosis) with the hollow of the curve towards the involved side, because of the growth differences and muscle shortening on the involved side.

Athetosis

Athetosis is characterized by fluctuating muscular tone, purposeless involuntary movements, and diffuse postural instability. The distribution is usually symmetrical and involves the whole body with the upper body commonly more involved. During the first year the baby may be hypotonic, having deficient muscular tone. The initial symptom is exaggerated extension of the head, back and limbs when the child is handled or startled. At this stage, the symptoms are similar to those in the young spastic quadriplegic child. Gradually the generalized extensor reactions diminish as involuntary localized movements occur. The involuntary movements are intensified by volitional exertion and movement. These involuntary movements disappear in sleep. Residuals of the generalized extensor reaction remain, particularly in the legs.

The athetoid suffers from an excess of movement and from deficit postural fixation and control of voluntary movement. The cooperative action of the muscles around the joint, called co-contraction (which is essential for postural fixation), is impaired. Deficient feedback through the nervous system and impairment of reciprocal function of opposing muscles result in a lack of guidance and control of movements. The persistence of the tonic reflexes results in stereotyped reactions, dependent on the position of the head and body. Head control is usually poor. The more advanced righting and equilibrium reactions may be severely retarded in development or may not develop. The child's ability to balance is compromised. As the child stands, the pressure through the feet causes extension of the legs and trunk. When this response is exaggerated it is called an extensor thrust, and thrusts the child backward. The athetotic child usually cannot use his arms to support himself. It may take years for the child to learn to stand or walk. As the child steps, reducing the extensor tone, he **may** collapse. To avoid collapsing the athetoid leans his trunk back to reinforce the extensor tone needed to maintain him erect. He tends to use his less involved legs to initiate rolling and to come into the quadrupedal position. Ability of the athetotic child to stand and walk depends on the severity of leg involvement and the amount of head control present. The involuntary movements and laxity of the joints result in very few deformities. Occasionally the hips, fingers or lower jaw subluxes. Sometimes a lateral deviation of the spine (scoliosis) occurs.

ASSESSMENT OF MOTOR DYSFUNCTION

Testing Procedures

Rarely will the occupational therapist have the sole responsibility for assessing the status of motor performance in the child. He will share this responsibility with the physician, the physical therapist and, perhaps, the speech therapist. The precise areas of responsibility of each evaluator, and the portion of the assessment he conducts, depend on the structure of the particular work situation and his individual abilities, as well as the time he has available. Each member of the allied health professions has developed special skills. Some overlapping of skills occurs, especially in the area of physical disabilities. Some flexibility in roles is desirable, and areas of responsibility should be defined in each work situation to avoid duplication of efforts using identical means. Many of the assessments of the child become shared efforts.

Each occupational therapy department should have the proper neuromotor evaluative tools including books, manuals, journals and forms. A minimum of diagnostic equipment is needed. This equipment should include a means of measuring joint motion (goniometers) and miscellaneous items to measure sensation. The principles for evaluation, described in Chapter Two, apply equally to the testing of motor behavior. Formal tests should be dated and the examiner identified. All testing should be administered accurately, using standardized methods of examination when possible. When using new types of tests or test formats, the source should be identified. In devising new tests, the source of the standards should be noted. The test results, from correctly administered tests, should be reproducible. The information gained from the tests and evaluations should be carefully recorded and filed so that they are readily available to add to the composite record shared by the medical team, in treatment planning, to determine progress and to check the efficacy of treatment. Scoring should be in a form that is subject to statistical analysis whenever possible. Graphic representation of the results is highly desirable.

The evaluation and testing of motor dysfunction in the presence of neuromotor dysfunction presents special challenge. It is an attempt to evaluate nervous system disorganization, which cannot be directly observed, from the indirect clinical manifestations. The external manifestations do not provide a simple map of the pathology; they are connected in complex and indirect ways. The purpose of the motor screening is to identify the problem areas. Several areas of motor functioning should be appraised. The level of motor performance and its relation to the child's age should be determined. The quality of movement should also be considered. The presence of abnormal postural reflexes and abnormal muscle tone should be recorded. Any habitual postural patterns that may lead to deformities and developing contractures of the bones and muscles should be noted. Unfortunately, a comprehensive test covering all of these aspects is not available.

Tests and Evaluations

Motor Tests

Motor performance may be appraised by use of portions of a general developmental examination designed for normal children, or by tests specifically designed for examining children with neurological deficits. The general developmental examinations, of which Gesell's schedules are the most celebrated, have the advantage of being standardized. The tests designed for impaired children, although they largely use normative data from Gesell, are for the most part not standardized. The advantage of the specially designed tests is that they tend to organize the material under clinically useful categories, and have rating systems that yield more information about the performance, the quality of movement, and whether bracing or assistive devices are used. More detailed definitions occur in tests designed for impaired children. For example, the following item is in a developmental examination for normal children: at twenty-eight weeks the infant sits briefly, and leans forward on his hands. A corresponding item occurs in a test designed for impaired children: at seven months, the infant sits on the floor for one minute without support in the tailor or long sitting position. Both types of tests include self-help activities. After the initial evaluation, problem areas that have been identified, such as the child's inability to feed himself with a spoon, may need careful analysis in terms of developmentally required skills. Appraisal of the developmental status is usually a shared endeavor involving the occupational and physical therapist. The physical therapist usually assesses the gross motor skills leading to erect posture and locomotion. The occupational therapist commonly administers the remaining portions of the general tests. In motor developmental tests, the occupational therapist appraises the upper limbs and their purposeful activities.

The Developmental Schedules of Gesell describe the characteristic behavior of infants during the first three years at eight key ages under four categories: motor, adaptive, language, and personal-social. These schedules are standardized. The book entitled *Developmental Diagnosis*[28] includes a procedural manual.

The Developmental Screening Instrument[29] by Knoblock divides the items into five behavior categories: adaptive, gross motor, fine motor, language, and personal-social. The occupational therapist will find the division of motor activities, according to whether they are gross or fine, a useful distinction.

A Graphic Method for the Evaluation of Motor Development[30] by Zdanska-Brincken and Wolanski comprises thirty-four test items describing the sequential stages of motor development in normal children which lead to locomotion. Four grids pictorially record the stages of head and trunk movement, development of sitting position, development of standing, and locomotion in relation to age. A nomogram summarizes the more important stages of motor development. The examination covers the development from one month until the child walks. This test is included in this series because it provides a rapid graphic means of recording the stages of motor development which have been attained.

A developmental test compiled by Jones[31] for the appraisal of cerebral palsied children includes four scales: locomotive development, self-help development, speech development, and personal-social development. A summary chart of growth and achievement combines the four developmental ages derived from the above scales with the mental age, the social maturity rating, and measurements of physical growth including the dental age, the height age, weight age, and head and chest circumferential ages. Data from retesting can be recorded on the same chart. The chart of growth and achievement presents a comprehensive view of the developmental levels in many areas and indicates the rate of development as well as the child's chronological age.

A Cerebral Palsy Activity Record[32] by Ingram et al., was devised to assess the progress and developmental level of cerebral palsied children. The test items are grouped under two categories: social and motor. The test covers the period from one month to five years. Scoring only indicates those items that have been successfully accomplished. The scores yield a motor quotient (M Q) and a social quotient SQ). These quotients may be plotted on a graph showing the successive developmental levels and indicating the rate of development. The authors state that there are insufficient items at some levels. In this test the occupational therapist usually tests the items under the social behavior category.

The Motor Development Test[33] is the fourth revision of a test compiled at the New York State Rehabilitation Hospital. The test is divided into two parts: *Motor Development Test for Upper Extremities* and *Motor Development Test for Posture and Locomotion.* The developmental levels extend from infancy through the sixth year. The upper extremity section, administered by the occupational therapist, has sixty-six items. The areas of development considered in the upper extremities test are hand use, feeding, dressing, grooming, and prewriting. Scoring reflects the level of functioning, e.g., whether the child needs assistance, whether he can perform independently but is awkward or slow, and whether performance is normal.

A test battery described by Zausmer and Tower[34] divides the motor tasks into thirteen units, e.g., sitting, standing, head control, rolling, crawling, prehension, fine manipulation, etc., according to the age levels. The rating scale describes eight levels of performance, from no attempt being made to a normal pattern with notable skill and speed. A numerical score is obtained by assigning points to each of the items, based on the age intervals between the test items. A percentage of the individual test item score is determined, based on a formula derived from the performance rating. A motor quotient is obtained by dividing the total score by the chronological age in months. The authors suggest that the motor quotient can be used as an index of motor development in the same way as the intelligence quotient (IQ).

The Preschool Functional Activity Test[35] by Footh and Kogan is not a developmental test but indicates the level of function. It is divided into four parts: General Motor Development, Ability to Manage a Wheelchair, Activities of Daily Living, and General Activities. The test is designed for the young child. The test has high instrument reliability. A procedural manual is available. The test was devised to assess the effectiveness of physical therapy in

TABLE 4-5 *Test Items with Administration and Scoring Procedures*

Upper Extremities

1. *Alternate finger-to-nose, finger-to-finger.* The child was instructed to touch the *end* of his nose and the *tip* of the examiner's finger alternately. The examiner's finger was held at the child's eye level and at the child's arm's length. The score was the number of times the child could fully complete the cycle in ten seconds. One cycle required the child first to touch the end of his nose and then the examiner's finger. If he missed either one, the cycle was not counted.

2. *Opposition.* The child was instructed to touch the tip of his index finger to the tip of his thumb on the same hand. The score was the number of times the child could successfully complete the task in ten seconds.

3. *Pronation-supination.* The child, seated on a straight-back or folding chair with his hands on his thighs, was asked to turn his palms alternately up and down on his thighs. The score was the number of times the child could successfully complete the task in ten seconds.

4. *Patting.* The child, seated at a table with his forearm and hand resting on the surface, was asked to pat his hand on the table without lifting his forearm from the surface. The score was the number of pats in ten seconds.

5. *Finger wiggle.* The child, seated as in Task 4, touched his fingers in sequence on the table surface as if idly drumming, beginning with the little finger and moving in rapid succession to the ring, middle, and index fingers, without moving the thumb. The score was the number of complete cycles in ten seconds.

6. *Finger tapping.* The child, seated as in Task 4 with his hand flat on the surface, palm down, tapped only his index finger; the other fingers and thumb remained flat on the table. The score was the number of taps in ten seconds.

Lower Extremities

7. *Alternate heel-to-knee, heel-to-toe.* The child was placed on his back. The tip of the examiner's index finger was placed on the child's knee. The child bent his toes back on that foot toward that knee, keeping the knee straight. The child then touched the examiner's finger and his big toe alternately with the heel of his other foot. The score was the number of cycles successfully completed in ten seconds. Successful completion consisted of the child's being able to touch the examiner's finger and then his big toe. If he missed either, the cycle was not counted.

8. *Foot patting.* The child, seated on a chair with his feet flat on the floor, patted the ball of his foot without raising his heel off the floor. The score was the number of pats in ten seconds.

9. *Heel-toe tapping.* The child, seated as in Task 8, tapped the floor first with the heel and then with the toes of the same foot. The score was number of cycles in ten seconds.

Balance

10. *Modified station.* The child stood with one foot directly in front of the other so that the heel of the front foot touched the big toe of the back foot, and raised both arms fully extended over his head. The score was the length of time the child could remain in this position up to thirty seconds. (The clock was stopped only if the child moved either foot from the starting position.)

11. *One leg stand.* The child placed his hands on his hips and stood on one leg with the opposite leg bent to 90 degrees at the knee joint. The score was the length of time the child could remain in this position up to thirty seconds. (The clock was stopped only when the child moved the foot on which he was standing or if he touched the floor with the nonweight-bearing leg.)

12. *Heel-toe walking.* The child walked a line with one foot directly in front of the other, heel-to-toe. The score was the number of steps he took in ten seconds.

*From DeHaven, G., and Mordock, J. "Coordination Exercises for Children with Minimal Cerebral Dysfunction." Reprinted with permission from *Physical Therapy*, Volume 50:0, 339, March 1970.

cerebral palsy. The scores on each item reflect five levels of performance, 0-4. The scores of each of the four sections are totaled separately. The scores provide a means of comparing data from periodic testing. The *Children's Hand Skill Survey*[36] by Tyler and Kogan was devised to measure the functional performance of the upper limbs. The scales appraise manipulative and self-help skills in children from birth to seven years.

The *Devereux Test of Extremity Coordination* (DTEC)[37] was designed by DeHaven, Mordock and Loykovich to evaluate coordination deficits for children with minimal cerebral dysfunction. It is recommended for use in treatment planning for children over six or seven (Table 4-5).

The *Test of Motor Impairment*[38] by Stott, Moyes and Headridge is derived from the Gollnitz revision of the *Oseretzky Test of Motor Ability*. It is a general test of motor abilities and is designed to screen children for minimal neural dysfunction. The test is divided into five categories: balance items, upper limb coordination, whole body coordination, manual dexterity, and simultaneous movement. Test items are grouped under yearly age levels from under five to over thirteen. The test is scored on a pass or fail basis: two points are given for failure of an item and one point is given when arms or legs are tested separately at the child's age level or below.

The *Bobath Test Chart of Motor Ability*[39] measures the child's ability to control or move away from his abnormal postures in eight key positions based on the developmental sequence. The quality of the performance is rated on a 0 to 6 scale.

A *Cerebral Palsy Assessment Chart*[40] by Semans, Phillips, Romanoli, Miller and Skillen, (Figure 4-14) was devised to assess the basic postural controls. A series of test postures in the supine, prone, sitting, kneeling, squatting, standing and walking positions are utilized. Performance is graded using values from 0 to 5. The test yields information about muscle tone, the severity of the condition, limitations of range of motion and their source, how abnormal patterns of movement interfere with motor development and the quality of movement. This test is included, although it is administered by physical therapists, because it combines the important aspects of range of motion testing, reflexive testing and quality of movement, as well as how the abnormal postures interfere with the assuming and holding of key postures in sequential steps leading to erect posture and locomotion. Semans refers to the desirability of developing a similar test to appraise the mechanisms underlying the sequential development of prehension.

CEREBRAL PALSY ASSESSMENT CHART
BASIC MOTOR CONTROL

Name:_____ Birthdate:_____ Diagnosis:_____

Test Postures and Movements	Examiner:	Name:		Name:		Name	
		Date	Remarks	Date	Remarks	Date	Remarks
Supine 1. Hips and knees fully flexed, arms crossed, palms on shoulders.							
2. Hips and knees fully flexed. (a) Extend right leg. (b) Extend left leg.		R. L.		R. L.		R. L.	
3. Head raised.							
Prone 4. Arms extended beside head. Raise head in midposition.							
5. Arms extended beside body, palms down.							
6. (a) Flex right knee, hips extended. (b) Flex left knee, hips extended.		R. L.		R. L.		R. L.	
7. Trunk supported on forearms, upper trunk extended, face vertical.							
8. Trunk supported on hands with elbows and hips extended.							
Sitting erect 9. Soles of feet together, hips flexed and externally rotated to at least 45°.							
10. Knees extended and legs abducted; hips 90°–100°.							

FIG. 4-14. Cerebral palsy assessment chart. From Semans, S., Phillips, R., Romanoli, M., Miller, R., and Skillen, M. "A Cerebral Palsy Assessment Chart." Reprinted with permission from *Physical Therapy*, Volume 45: 463-468, May 1965.)

CEREBRAL PALSY ASSESSMENT CHART
BASIC MOTOR CONTROL

Name:_____ Diagnosis:_____ Birthdate:_____

Test Postures and Movements	Exami er:	Name:		Name:		Name:	
		Date	Remarks	Date	Remarks	Date	Remarks
11. Legs hanging over edge of table. (a) Extend right knee. (b) Extend left knee.		R. L.		R. L.		R. L.	
Kneeling 12. Back and neck straight (not hyperextended). (a) Weight on knees. (b) Weight on hands.		a b		a b		a b	
13. Side sitting, upper trunk erect, arms relaxed: (a) On right hip. (b) On left hip.		R. L.		R. L.		R. L.	
14. Kneeling upright, hips extended, head in midposition, arms at sides.							
15. (a) Half kneeling: weight on right knee. (b) Half kneeling: weight on left knee.		R. L.		R. L.		R. L.	
Squatting 16. Heels down, toes not clawed, knees pointing in same direction as toes, hips fully flexed, head in line with trunk.							
Standing and components of walking 17. Standing, correct alignment.							
18. Pelvis and trunk aligned over forward leg. Both knees extended. (a) Right leg forward. (b) Left leg forward.		R. L.		R. L.		R. L.	
19. Bear weight on one leg in midstance. (a) Shift weight over right leg. (b) Shift weight over left leg.		R. L.		R. L.		R. L.	
20. Heel strike. Rear leg extended and externally rotated, heel down. Both knees straight: (a) Right heel strike. (b) Left heel strike.		R. L.		R. L.		R. L.	

Fig. 4-14 *(continued)*

A revised chart for *Routine Developmental Examination in Normal and Retarded Children,*[41] by Milani-Comparetti and Gidoni (Figure 4-15), is divided into two sections. The top section contains a behavioristic scale modified from Koupernik. The lower section includes the primitive reflexes and the righting, parachute and tilting reactions. In the behavioristic section the chronological age in months is recorded in the block corresponding to the functional finding. In the bottom section a notation is made of presence or absence of the reflexes. The reflex patterns necessary for each motor task appear below the motor task in the vertical column. The test directly correlates the reflexive maturation with the sequential developmental motor performance culminating in locomotion. It is presented because of its unique approach which correlates reflexive and motor development although it would not ordinarily be administered by an occupational therapist. It provides a rapid means of screening children.

Muscle Testing

The standard muscle test, described in *Muscle Testing: Techniques of Manual Examination,*[42] is an unreliable tool in measuring muscle strength in patients with neurological deficits. It is recommended as a manual (rather than mechanical) means of determining the amount of muscle weakness resulting from disease, injury, or disuse. It is an effective tool when used to measure muscle weakness in lower motor neuron pathology. In the presence of neurological deficits, the ability to use the muscles depends on the position of the body, the relationships of the body segments, and the relative limb positions. Brunnstrom[43] cites the example of the adult hemiplegic who could not straighten his elbow in the abdominal lying position, but could fully straighten his elbow while back-lying. The standard muscle test administered to children with neurological deficits gives equally distorted results. To overcome this problem, Brunnstrom[44, 45] developed motor testing procedures based on the typical recovery stages of hemiplegics which indirectly indicate the state of recovery of the central nervous system. Although this test is not directly applicable to children with neurological deficits, it merits the attention of the occupational therapist because of its unique approach to motor testing in dealing with a specific neurological problem.

Range of Motion Tests

Present methods of measuring range of motion include visual estimation, radiography, photography, schematography, outline tracing and goniometry.[46] The visual method, although probably

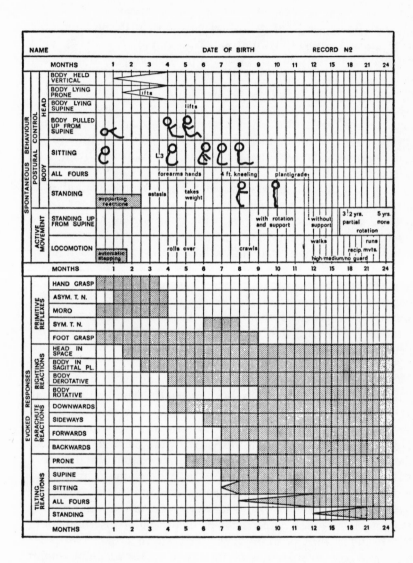

FIG. 4-15. Developmental chart. (From Milani-Comparetti, A. and Gidoni, E. A. "Routine Developmental Examination in Normal and Retarded Children." *Developmental Medicine and Child Neurology* (1967), p. 637.)

the least accurate, is the starting point for further measurements. The radiographic method using x-ray films is the most accurate. The physician utilizes the radiographic method to monitor problem areas. A method being explored measures motion by photographing the joint in several positions or through multiple exposures. Photography and cinematography are being used extensively in the clinical setting to provide graphic records not only of joint range of motion, but to record the child's patterns of movement. Goniometry is the most commonly used form of manual examination by physicians, physical therapists and occupational therapists. A protractor is used as a measuring instrument. The axis is placed at the center of the joint, and the arms lie parallel to the long axis of the joint segment. Usually one arm of the protractor is stationary, and the other moveable. There are a variety of goniometers available. The goniometric method of measuring joints is relatively reliable in patients with lower motor neuron problems. In patients with neurological deficits, the fluctuating muscle tone distorts the measurement of active and passive joint motion. Patients with a neurological deficit often lose the full range of joint excursion and then develop joint contractures. In spite of the measurement problems, the occupational therapist must take the responsibility for keeping some type of record of joint mobility in the upper limbs for use in treatment planning and in order to stay alert to impending problems.

Sensory Testing

A test for sensory loss must accompany the neuromotor testing as the two systems are inseparably linked. The message to the nervous system through the sensory system must be accurate in order to get the appropriate response. If the message is garbled, the response may be disorganized. Accurate testing of the sensory system is very difficult. Sensation is critical to normal hand function, and the occupational therapist is intimately concerned with the development of hand function. The various tests usually evaluate light touch, superficial pain, two-point discrimination, temperature, joint position sense, and asterognosia. Two-point discrimination refers to the minimum distance at which two-point contact stimuli can be distinguished from one. Position sense refers to nonvisual recognition of the position of a joint. Asterognosis is the ability to recognize common objects by feel. Some definitions of asterognosia also include shape and form as well as object recognition. The problem of measuring sensation in the hand and upper limbs has been investigated by Werner and Omer,[47] Kent,[48] Van Prince and Butler[49] and others.

Reflex Testing

An assessment of reflex activity is essential to understanding the way in which a neurological lesion expresses itself. Fiorentino[50] provided a useful clinical tool in her illustrated procedural manual for examining and recording reflexive development (Table 4-6).

Selection of Tests

Acquiring a clear understanding of the underlying disorder of movement in children with neurological deficits involves skill and effort. The areas of motor function of most concern to the occupational therapist are: those of the face, eye, and mouth musculature; neck control; the upper limbs; and those automatic balancing actions such as propping and tilting reactions which accompany prehension, particularly in the sitting and standing positions. A battery of tests is necessary to yield information about sensation, joint mobility, muscle tone, reflexive behavior, the quality of movements, achievements of the motor developmental self-care tasks, as well as to pinpoint the inequalities and asymmetries in body growth and motor function.

A variety of tests are mentioned, as none is singly capable of measuring all the aspects of neuromotor dysfunction. The specialized tests which measure motor development cover a wide range of motor behavior from birth to six years of age when the normal child has attained the motor skills necessary for normal functioning. They do not cover children from birth to twelve or thirteen or the mild and severely affected child equally well. If the neuromotor dysfunction is very severe, the evaluative instrument must be calibrated to accommodate the dysfunction. If the problem is minimal, the measuring graduations must be very fine to discern it. The following procedures are intended only as a starting point: they include tests that have been described earlier in the chapter and have been published in the last few years.

Recommended for the child with minimal cerebral dysfunction are the *Test of Motor Impairment* by Scott, Moyes and Headridge and the *Devereux Test of Extremity Coordination* by DeHaven, Mordock and Loykovich. Complementary information critical to motor functioning in minimal dysfunction children may be obtained from perceptual-motor testing such as the standardized *Ayres Space Test,*[51] which includes a perceptual-motor test battery. In addition, it would be worthwhile to administer a general developmental test with a motor component such as the *Gesell's Schedules,* or Knoblock's *Developmental Screening Instrument,* which separates fine and gross motor activities.

TABLE 4-6
Newington Hospital for Crippled Children Occupational Therapy Department
Reflex Testing Chart*

Name:

B.D:

Date:

Reflexes	+	−	Comments:
1. Level One–Spinal:			
a. Flexor Withdrawal			
b. Extensor Thrust			
c. Crossed Extension			
2. Level Two–Brain Stem:			
a. Asymmetrical Tonic Neck			
b. Symmetrical Tonic Neck			
c. Tonic Labyrinthine-supine			
prone			
d. Associated Reactions			
e. Positive Supporting Reaction			
f. Negative Supporting Reaction			
3. Level Three–Midbrain:			
Righting Reactions:			
a. Neck Righting			
b. Body Righting acting on the Body			
c. Labyrinthine Righting acting on the Head			
d. Optical Righting			
e. Amphibian			
4. Automatic Movement Reactions:			
a. Moro Reflex			
b. Landau Reflex			
c. Protective Extensor Thrust			
5. Level Four–Cortical:			
Equilibrium Reactions:			
a. Prone-lying			
b. Supine-lying			
c. Four-foot kneeling			
d. Sitting			
e. Kneel-standing			
f. Standing-hopping			
dorsiflexion			
see-saw			
g. Simian posture			

*From Fiorentino, M.R. *Reflex Testing Methods for Evaluating CNS Development* (Springfield, Illinois: Charles C Thomas, Publisher), 1970.

For the mild to moderately severely involved child the following areas of testing are recommended. Fiorentino's *Reflex Testing Methods* yields precise information about the stage of reflexive maturation, and includes some of the equilibrium reactions. The *Revised Chart* for Routine Developmental Examination in Normal and Retarded Children, by Millani-Comparetti and Gidoni, correlates the reflexive maturation with the stages of motor development. For the moderately or severely involved child, *A Cerebral Palsy Assessment Chart* by Semans et al. yields information about the child's ability to assume basic postures, how abnormal postures interfere with the assuming or holding of postures, and the source of limitations of joint movements. The last two tests would ordinarily be administered by the physical therapist. For the mild to moderately involved child under five, either of the following motor development tests is suggested: *The Preschool Functional Activity Test* by Footh and Kogan, which includes a section on wheelchair management and whose ratings are descriptive of the degree of accomplishment observed; *The Cerebral Palsy Activity Record* by Ingram, Wither and Speltz, which yields pass-fail information. The authors of this test state that it is weak in the motor zones above three years. One of the tests of sensation should be administered to the hands.

For the severely involved child the following tests are suggested: reflexive testing in the manner suggested for the moderately involved child, or Semans' chart. In the severely involved child it is essential to try to prevent deformities. A means of identifying and monitoring joint mobility in the severely involved child is essential. Often in these children there are irregularities of swallowing and breathing, sucking, drooling, and mouth closure problems that need to be carefully analyzed by the occupational therapist.

Other motor tests of interest to the occupational therapist are the *Motor Age Test* [52] of Johnson, Zuck and Wingate; the *Dallas Motor Development Test* [53]; and *A Code Method for Evaluating Function in Cerebral Palsy* [54] developed at the Detroit Orthopedic Clinic. There is a lack of uniformity of testing throughout the United States in treatment centers serving children with neuromotor dysfunction. Many evaluation forms and tests are being used in occupational therapy and physical therapy departments. New tests are being developed in an attempt to condense and simplify the testing procedures while still presenting a comprehensive view of motor function. Improved tests are needed to evaluate how the child moves his upper limbs in reach and grasp, the compensatory trunk reactions accompanying prehension, and the interrelations of the evolution of eye-hand coordination, sensation, and prehension. Administering batteries of tests is time-consuming. Some of the tests, such as the Milani-Comparetti and Gidoni developmental chart and the Zdanska-Bricken and Wolanski graphic method of evaluation, can be administered in a very short time with practice. In some of the motor developmental tests, not every item is administered. The examiner often starts with the items one level below the estimated functional level. A careful evaluation saves time in the long run, permits the occupational therapist to make a cogent approach to treatment, contributes to understanding the whole child, provides a basis for treatment planning and a means of monitoring progress, and checks the efficacy of treatment techniques. The book *The Result of Treatment in Cerebral Palsy,*[55] by Wolf, is concerned with these problems. After the completion of the evaluation and an intradisciplinary sharing of information, the therapist is ready to begin treatment.

TREATMENT OF NEUROMOTOR DYSFUNCTION

Classical Treatment Techniques

Conditions causing neuromotor dysfunction have been recognized and illustrated since ancient times. Most of the classical treatment procedures used to educate the motor apparatus of the child who has central nervous system impairment are derived from procedures successfully used for other pathological conditions. In a broad sense, they constitute a peripheral approach to treatment which attempts to treat the external manifestations of the impairment.

Following are some of the classical treatment procedures used. Treatment often begins with *passive movement* — the therapist moving the body part. When possible, the child assists with the movement; this is *active assistive motion.* The treatment progresses from *active movement* by the child, to *movement resisted* by the therapist. A program of relaxation is carried out by teaching *conscious relaxation,* usually starting at the head and descending. Muscle training is initiated starting with a single unit such as an isolated muscle or single joint, and expanded to larger patterns of movement, thus organizing the individual muscle contractions into more complex patterns. In order to prevent contractures and deformities, to provide function and stability, and to control the motions that expend the child's energies, bracing methods, such as body braces, leg braces, corsets, and special chairs, etc., are used. Surgical intervention is another means commonly used to enhance function and correct deformities. For example, weighted cuffs on the shoes, wrists, and crutches are used to promote sensorimotor feedback and to stabilize and assist in body control. Massage, manipulations, and baths are used to improve muscle circulation, to increase the tone in weak muscles, or to decrease the muscle tone in hypertonicity. Although many of the above techniques are still used, concepts of treatment have changed and newer techniques have been developed. Before discussing the more recent treatment approaches, some basic information about the nervous system will be reviewed.

Brief Review of the Nervous System

The *central nervous system* consists of the *brain* and the *spinal cord*. The *peripheral nerves* carry impulses in both directions between the central nervous system and other body tissues such as skeletal muscles, smooth muscles and glands. The nervous system can be considered as a system of multiple-linked neural loops. The *neuron* is the basic structural and functional unit of the nervous system. It consists of a cell body with processes such as the dendrite and axon projecting from it. The *sensory* or *afferent neuron* relays impulses toward the central nervous system. The *motor* or *efferent neuron* relays impulses from the central nervous system to the periphery, glands and muscles. The motoneurons pass to specialized terminations in the muscles and glands called myoneural junctions. A single neuron supplies a number of muscle fibers called a motor unit in skeletal muscles, with each branch ending as a motor end plate. Harris[56] speaks of the levels of the brain such as the spinal level, midbrain level and cortical level. He says they are "subunits tied together to form functional packages, often through multiple, reciprocal, interconnecting pathways." *Nerves* are composed of sensory and motor nerve fibers. A *nerve fiber* is the elongated process of the nerve cell, or neuron. The autonomic nervous system is by definition a motor system, a division of the peripheral nervous system which supplies the smooth muscles, glands and conducting tissue of the heart. The *somatic motor system* is a division of the peripheral nervous system which supplies the skeletal muscles. In the somatic motor system the cell bodies of the motoneurons are located exclusively in the central nervous system, in the anterior portions of the spinal cord or in the brain stem. In autonomic outflow the cell bodies are situated in ganglia outside the central nervous system with one exception, the adrenal medulla. The *reflexes* have been previously mentioned as *inborn stimulus-response mechanisms* which produce a relatively fixed pattern of response for any given stimulus. The neural pathway consists of sensory or *afferent neurons* which relay the impulses arising in the sensory receptors to the spinal cord; connections are made within the cord by the *intercalated* or *internuncial neurons*. Motor or *efferent neurons* transmit the impulses to the periphery. The reflex arch can function at the spinal level independent of higher nervous centers. *Reflexes* may be classified as superficial or deep, somatic or *autonomic* or *pathologic*. Peripheral nerves are also classified by their size in either a number or letter system. The letter system classifies the peripheral nerves in a descending order of size (circumference) as *A, B,* or *C fibers*. The A fibers have the largest diameter and conduct impulses at the greatest speeds. It follows that the C fibers are smaller and conduct impulses more slowly. There are four subgroups of A fibers: *alpha, beta, gamma* and *delta.* The alpha motoneurons are the larger neurons which go to the regular muscles. The gamma motoneurons pass exclusively to some specialized muscle fibers called *intrafusal* fibers, which are located in the muscle spindle. The *muscle spindle* is a *stretch receptor located within the muscle.* Impulses passing over the gamma motoneurons contract or relax the intrafusal fibers and influence the stretch receptors which are mounted on these fibers by increasing or decreasing the muscle spindle's susceptibility to discharge. The gamma activation may be strong enough to cause the muscle spindle to discharge, but when the activation is too weak to discharge the spindle, the contraction of the intrafusal fibers causes a lowering of the threshold necessary to discharge the spindle. The gamma loop system is activated through stretch, pressure, temperature, touch, etc.

The sensory and motor systems are inseparably linked. All information comes through the sense organs. Simple motor acts are initiated through the sensory organs and complex acts are controlled by means of the sensory organs. *Sensory receptors* are specialized endings of sensory neurons. Sensory receptors may be classified in several ways. They may be classified for clinical use in terms of the sensation and its disturbances: *special senses, superficial* or *cutaneous sensations, deep sensations,* and *visceral sensations.* Sensory receptors are sometimes classified by the agent or energy which stimulates them such as *chemoreceptors, mechanoreceptors,* etc. A commonly used system is *Sherrington's classification* based on the source of the stimulus and the location of the receptor, i.e. *interoceptors, teleceptors, proprioceptors,* and *exteroceptors.* The teleceptors receive information from a distance from the special sense organs such as the eyes, nose and ears. The proprioceptors are located in the tendons, muscles, and joints, and are stimulated by the body itself. They provide information about the length and tension of muscles, joint position, and the acceleration or deceleration of a joint. The perception of movement, weight, and position are known as kinesthesia and are dependent on cutaneous and visceral sensations as well as proprioceptive sensations. The labyrinthine receptors are located in the inner ear and provide information about the position and movement of the head. The labyrinths of the vestibular system activate the postural reflexes which act on the neck, trunk and limbs to maintain posture or equilibrium. They also set up reflexes involving the eye muscles to keep images on the retina. The proprioceptors, the cutaneous receptors, and the visceral receptors and the eyes also provide information about the position and movement of the head. The eyes play a very important role in man, enabling him to compensate for vestibular dysfunction more fully than other animals. The exteroceptors are located in the skin and mucous membranes and signal information regarding pain, temperature, touch and pressure.

Motor activity can be influenced by sensory stimulation in various ways. Motor output can be affected by *spatiotemporal summation*; by increasing the sensory input from central and peripheral sources so that the input converges on common motoneurons more or less simultaneously, the sum effect may be sufficient to exceed the motoneuron threshold and cause a discharge when a single input was insufficient. Sherrington observed and described another process called irradiation. Irradiation is the spreading of excitation to greater numbers of motoneurons in specific patterns when a stimulus is gradually increased in strength. *Recruitment* is the increased activation of larger numbers of motoneurons when a prolonged stimulus of unaltered intensity is applied. *Reciprocal innervation* is the simultaneous relaxation of the antagonist or opposing muscles when the agonist muscle contracts. *Adaptation* is the gradual diminution of receptivity of the receptor to the stimulus. The discharges decrease and may cease in response to the stimulus. Some techniques to facilitate motor expression through sensory input that may be utilized in occupational therapy include: muscle stretch; resistance; synergistically linked movement patterns; bilateral activities; traction and compression, visual, auditory, gustatory, and olfactory stimulation; touch; pressure to the skin; thermal applications; movement; the position of the head and body in space; and the postural reflexes.

Systems of Treatment

A number of treatment systems are used by occupational therapists, physical therapists, and speech therapists in treating children with neuromuscular disorders. Experimental data from neurophysiologic research complemented by clinical investigations have generated new treatment approaches in the last few decades. These systems provide a neurophysiologic basis for treatment utilizing the sensory mechanism to activate, facilitate, or inhibit motor responses. The most celebrated treatment systems which are used for children with dysfunction of the neuromuscular mechanism will be briefly described and include those of: Temple-Fay, Doman-Delacato, Rood, Bobath and proprioceptive neuromuscular facilitation (PNF).

Temple-Fay System[57, 59]

Fay, a neurosurgeon, developed a system of treating cerebral palsied children using *reciprocal patterning* in primitive patterns of movement. He noted the similarity of locomotor patterns between the newborn human infant and the fish, amphibian and reptile. The child, in treatment, repeats the phylogenetically older patterns of movement starting at his lowest level of mobility: the undulating movements of the fish, one of the earliest patterns seen in the baby; the *homolateral pattern* with the limbs on the same side moving together; the *homologous pattern* with the lower or upper limbs moving together, seen in the amphibian and baby; and the *diagonal-cross pattern* seen in the reptile with the right arm and left leg moving simultaneously and the left arm and right leg moving together. Reflexes, which are normally present in the young baby but pathologically persist in the older child, are used to initiate the semiautomatic movements. For example, the tonic neck reflex can be used by turning the head from side to side to produce a homolateral pattern of movement in the child with the limbs on the same side working together. Selective stimulation of the defense mechanisms is used to facilitate muscular responses. For example, eliciting the withdrawal reflex of the legs produces movements that are similar to stepping. Sequences of reflexive activity are used to elicit walking movements. Many methods of breaking up unwanted reflexes called *unlocking reflexes* are described by Fay. The importance of development of cerebral dominance is stressed. This system uses a recapitulation ontogenetically of phylogenetic developmental sequences in treatment to bring movement under voluntary control. A thorough knowledge of the phylogenetic and ontogenetic developmental sequences and specific techniques is prerequisite to using this system of treatment.

Doman-Delacato System[60, 62]

Doman, a psychiatrist, Doman, a physical therapist, and Delacato, an educator-psychologist, have adapted and expanded many of the theories and methods of Fay into a system of treatment for brain-injured children. Treatment at the Institutes for the Achievement of Human Potential (IAHP) in Philadelphia, Pennsylvania, is based on neurological organization. Neurological organization is defined as "the dynamic balance between excitatory, inhibitory, and feedback systems in the brain,...which enables the individual to adapt successfully to his environment."[63] Treatment is aimed at the brain, the source of neurological dysfunctioning, rather than at the peripheral manifestations. Treatment sometimes includes brain surgery. The *Neurological Developmental Profile* is administered to the child to determine the areas of neurological disorganization. This profile is a developmental scale of three important sensory functions—visual, auditory and tactile competence—and three important motor functions—mobility, language and manual competence. The essential tasks described in these areas delineate seven brain stages that are correlated with the chronological age at which these tasks have normally been accomplished. The test yields an average developmental stage expressed as a neurological age (NA).

The concept that integration of the higher levels of neurological functioning is dependent on the integrity of the phylogenetically older neuromotor system on a hierarchal basis is emphasized in treatment. Nonsurgical treatment provides opportunities for normal development in the unimpaired areas of function and attempts to reorganize neurological functioning in the areas of dysfunction.

There are twenty-two nonsurgical treatment procedures listed under five basic principles. The five treatment procedures under the first basic principle are devised to supply the basic sensory stimulation to the brain and include visual, auditory, tactile, gustatory, and olfactory information. The second basic principle includes four procedures to program the brain including tactile programming, which passively superimposes the primitive movement patterns at the child's functional level, and the next successive higher level. It also includes auditory programming at the child's level of language competence and the next higher level. Visual programming for manual competence culminates in handwriting. Procedures for developing eye, foot, ear and hand dominance are included. The third basic principle includes five procedures that demand an immediate response. The fourth basic principle includes six sensorimotor procedures which provide opportunities for the brain to functionally use the programming included under the second principle. The last principle includes two procedures to increase the circulation, oxygen and nutrients to the brain and to prevent an overaccumulation of cerebrospinal fluid and cerebrovascular compression.

A home program is devised for each child. This system insists on parental participation and the conscientious following of the home treatment program. The importance of early prone crawling and creeping sensorimotor experiences is emphasized, and these activities make up a large part of the home program. Passive reciprocal patterning is advocated in the severe child to provide sensorimotor information to the brain rather than to exercise the arms and legs. It takes several people to passively pattern the severe child. A typical program might include patterning four times daily for five minutes. The Doman-Delacato system of treatment emphasizes sensory stimulation, development of body image, development of cortical hemispheric dominance, breathing techniques, the use of reflexes as initiators of reciprocal movement patterns and combinations of reflex chains to produce walking.

Rood System[64,65]

Rood, a physical therapist and occupational therapist, developed treatment procedures based on neurophysiologic theories to activate, inhibit or facilitate motor expression through the sensory receptors. The exteroceptors are stimulated, using squeezing, pressure, pain, vibration, touch, brushing, stroking, or thermally through the use of ice or neutral warmth. The proprioceptors are influenced through the position of the head, through stretch, muscle contraction, muscle contraction plus stretch or outside resistance, and joint compression. The exteroceptors of the special senses are stimulated by light, various tastes, sounds, odors, etc.

A dermatome is the sensory mapping on the skin of a single segment of the spinal cord. The dermatomes of adjacent segments of the cord overlap. The therapist stimulates the dermatome of the skin that corresponds to the same segment supplying the muscle he wishes to influence. Frequently the dermatome lies over the muscle but there are important exceptions.

Rood considers both the rate of conduction in the various peripheral nerve sensory fibers as well as whether they go to the regular muscles or to the muscle spindle, smooth muscles, etc., the stimuli that activates them, and the total response evoked. Rood has stimulated interest in the gamma motor system.

Stimuli are applied in order to evoke muscle patterns of action in the developmental sequence.

Rood describes a developmental sequence of four phases of muscular responses. In the earliest phase the muscle shortens or lengthens with its antagonist, or opposing muscle, relaxing. An example is the contraction of the posterior neck muscles when the prone lying baby bobbingly lifts his head off the surface. The second phase involves muscles working together to stabilize the body, agonist and antagonist. The third phase involves movement superimposed on the co-contraction patterns. Examples are the shoulder and hips when the baby in the creep position rocks backward and forward. In these heavy work patterns movement takes place at the proximal or origin end of the muscles. Finally, muscles work in light work patterns with movement at the distal end of the muscle, producing refined skilled movements. Muscles can be divided into two groups, depending on whether they routinely function in heavy work patterns or light work patterns. The long narrow skeletal muscles, flexors and muscles that pass two joints primarily act in light work patterns. The deep, more powerful muscles that only pass one joint such as the abductors and one-joint extensors usually function in heavy work patterns. Some muscles work in both heavy work patterns and light work patterns.

Patterns of muscular responses seen in the infant are evoked automatically, i.e., nonvolitionally, in the patient in their developmental sequence (Figure 4-16).

The sequence of application of stimuli is important in this method. The exteroceptors are stimulated first because they are slower to respond. Brushing precedes icing. The muscle patterns of phasic activity and co-contraction patterns precede light work patterns and skilled movement. Bilateral activities precede unilateral activities. Flexors are stimulated before extensors, and adductors before abductors.

The Rood treatment system includes procedures to affect the autonomic, somatic and branchial motor systems. The treatment regime includes programs for impairment of the vital functions including respiration, sucking, swallowing fluids, phonation, chewing, swallowing solids and speech articulation.

The occupational therapist using the Rood techniques should have a strong neurophysiologic background, understand the developmental sequence and the muscles and their actions, the dermatome distributions, and understand precisely how and when to use the treatment procedures. Indiscriminate use of sensory stimulation such as icing or brushing to the head and trunk may be harmful. The novice is safer using the proprioceptive techniques that the Rood system advocates.

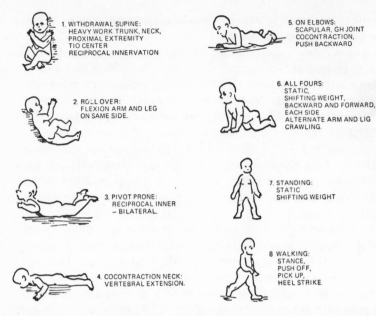

1. WITHDRAWAL SUPINE:
   HEAVY WORK TRUNK, NECK,
   PROXIMAL EXTREMITY
   TIO CENTER
   RECIPROCAL INNERVATION

2. ROLL OVER:
   FLEXION ARM AND LEG
   ON SAME SIDE.

3. PIVOT PRONE:
   RECIPROCAL INNER
   – BILATERAL.

4. COCONTRACTION NECK:
   VERTEBRAL EXTENSION.

5. ON ELBOWS:
   SCAPULAR, GH JOINT
   COCONTRACTION,
   PUSH BACKWARD

6. ALL FOURS:
   STATIC,
   SHIFTING WEIGHT,
   BACKWARD AND FORWARD,
   EACH SIDE
   ALTERNATE ARM AND LIG
   CRAWLING.

7. STANDING:
   STATIC
   SHIFTING WEIGHT

8. WALKING:
   STANCE,
   PUSH OFF,
   PICK UP,
   HEEL STRIKE.

FIG. 4-16. Ontogenetic motor patterns according to Rood. (From Rood, M. "Approaches to the Treatment of Patients with Neuromuscular Dysfunction," Study Course VI, Third International Congress, World Federation of Occupational Therapists, 1962, published by Kendall/Hunt Publishing Company, p. 34.)

Bobath System [66,69]

Bobath, a neurologist, and Bobath, a physical therapist, developed a system known as *neurodevelopmental treatment* for cerebral palsied children. The Bobaths founded the Western Cerebral Palsy Center in London, England. The neurodevelopmental approach acknowledges the developmental and pathological deviations from normal motor behavior evident in the cerebral palsied child. Bobath observed the release of postural and movement patterns in cerebral palsy from the higher inhibitory control of the nervous system. The cerebral palsied child has abnormal postural activity with abnormal postural tone. The persistence of the infantile reflexive patterns limits the range of selective movement patterns. The development of the normal postural reactions that are adaptive and protective in nature, such as protective extension of the arms and the equilibrium reactions, are prevented or underdeveloped.

Neurodevelopmental treatment emphasizes inhibiting the abnormal postural patterns and promoting the development of normal postural reactions. The hypertonic muscular activity is suppressed or more nearly normalized through the use of *reflex inhibiting patterns* (RIPS). When the tone is more nearly normal, spontaneous movement occurs, or movement is facilitated. A series of postures has been developed that suppresses the reflexive activity that is preventing normal movement which is fundamental to head control, sitting, kneeling and erect posture. The sensorimotor aspects of motor learning are stressed. It is very important for the child to feel normal movement, affording the child's nervous system an opportunity to reintegrate normal sensory inflow with motor output.

Another phase of treatment involves developing the normal postural reactions. Some minor deviations from the normal developmental sequence are made to avoid overdevelopment of patterns that are characteristic in cerebral palsied children. For example, Bobath advocates the development of protective extension of the arms sideways or backwards initially rather than forward, which is the earliest pattern in the normal infant, to avoid exaggerating the undesirable arm patterns such as extension with inward rotation and adduction of the arms. The normal postural reflexes are developed through stimulating the automatic responses by shifting the body weight and disturbing the body balance in many positions.

When the child's muscles have low postural tone against gravity, or are weak because of muscle imbalance, facilitory techniques using proprioceptive and tactile stimulation are used. These stimulative techniques are often used in conjunction with the inhibition patterns to avoid stimulating spasticity and abnormal postural responses. These techniques are used more frequently with ataxic and athetotic children, but may be used with spastics in the presence of low postural tone and in the absence of the tonic reflex activity. These techniques include weight bearing, with or without pressure, and resistance. Weight transfers are evoked in a variety of positions and cover a rather large range of motion for the spastic child and a smaller range of motion accomplished more slowly for the athetoids and ataxics.

The technique of placing and holding develops the child's ability to stop movement at any stage. Placing and holding are defined as the automatic adaptation of the muscles to changes of posture. The ability to place and hold is prerequisite to controlled smooth voluntary movement.

Tapping is used to "place" the limbs and body. It is used to increase postural tone of muscles—usually to stabilize and fixate the body in sitting, kneeling, standing, etc., postures so that voluntary selective movements can take place.

The neurodevelopmental approach stresses the importance of very early treatment of the infant before abnormal patterns are set, prior to the development of secondary contractures and deformities, and while the nervous system is the most plastic. Neurodevelopmental treatment attempts to counteract the development of abnormal postural reactions and tone, and to mobilize the child, helping him to develop control over the abnormal sensorimotor patterns, and to facilitate normal development building the functional patterns that the child needs for normal activities. This system systematically assesses each child and starts treatment at his level. The treatment program is planned and taught to those who care for the child. The mother with the cerebral palsied child must learn to handle her baby with skill to help him experience more nearly normal sensorimotor experiences, rather than abnormal patterns of movement which he will later try to use for functional activities. The Bobath system focuses on integration of automatic patterns of movement and postural adjustment. The Bobaths do not advocate the use of restraining apparatus such as braces, with the exception of temporary use of short leg braces or casts.

The Bobaths suggest that their treatment not be combined with other regimes that advocate wearing braces for long periods of time. They also feel that the results will be limited if irreversible structural changes have occurred. The occupational therapist using these techniques must know the Bobath system, understand normal sensorimotor developmental sequences and the substrata of reflexive maturation, and understand the normal sequential development of the baby as well as the abnormal motor behavior in the cerebral palsied.

PNF[70-72]

A well organized system of treatment known as proprioceptive neuromuscular facilitation provides a complete therapeutic exercise regime. PNF techniques are defined as "methods of promoting or hastening the response of the neuromuscular mechanism through stimulation of the proprioceptors."[73] The original concepts expressed by Kabat, a physician, have been implemented and the scope of application broadened by Voss and Knott, physical therapists. The treatment goal of PNF is "to promote motor learning."[74] The rationale for treatment is a neurophysiologic approach based on the works of Sherrington and others.

The techniques are based on normal responses of the neuromuscular mechanism reinforced by sensory stimulation and reflexive patterns. Mass movement patterns of a diagonal-spiral character are utilized in treatment. The stretch reflex is used to initiate and facilitate the movement pattern. The automatic reflexes such as the tonic neck, labyrinthine and righting reflexes that reinforce movement in healthy subjects are used in treatment. The less involved parts of the body are utilized to facilitate the impaired parts and to promote a balanced response. Optimal response resulted from the muscles contracting from their elongated positions to the maximally shortened state. Resistance is applied throughout the movement range to demand a maximal muscular response. Stimulation is applied by the hand placement through pressure to the skin over the muscles, tendons and joints. The joint proprioceptors are stimulated by application of traction or approximation (compression) during the movement. Traction enhances movement, while compression promotes the stabilizing muscular responses. Approximation or compression is also used to stimulate the postural reflexes. Voluntary effort is called forth to reinforce the patterns. The subject is asked to visually follow the movements. The three components of the movement patterns are flexion-extension, movement across and away from the midline and rotation. In PNF treatment techniques, two types of muscle contractions are utilized: isotonic contractions that involve movement and isometric contractions that are responsible for stabilizing a part.

Some specific techniques used in the movement patterns are *repeated contractions*, based on the need for repetition in motor learning. *Rhythmic initiation* of a movement pattern facilitates the ability to initiate movement. This technique is used in patients who cannot initiate movement because of rigidity or spasticity. Rhythmic initiation involves relaxation, followed by passive movement of the part by the therapist. The body part is returned to the beginning point. When the pattern is repeated the patient is asked to assist. *The reversal of antagonists* technique is derived from normal activities and can be seen in the many movement patterns of chopping wood, hammering, and in grasp and release. This technique develops the normal reversal of muscle actions and helps to develop coordination, strength, endurance and balance movements. *Slow reversals* followed by *holding techniques* are used to gain range of motion, or to develop strength or endurance. The slow reversal employs *isotonic contractions* and *slow reversal-holds*, using both isotonic and isometric contractions. *Rythmic stabilization* employs isometric contractions or co-contraction of the muscles to stabilize the body. Relaxation is promoted through *reciprocal innervation*, the relaxation of the opposing or antagonistic muscles during the contraction of the muscle (agonist). Relaxation techniques are used to gain range of motion instead of passive stretching.

An example of a facilitation pattern for an upper limb is the *flexion-abduction-external rotation pattern*. This pattern is composed of finger and thumb extension, wrist supination and extension towards the thumb side, the elbow remaining extended, the shoulder flexed, abducted, and externally rotated, with the scapula rotating, adducting, and elevating, and the clavicle rotating and elevating away from the sternum. A preparatory direction is given describing the movements. The command for action is given as stretch is gently applied to the muscles. The movement normally starts distally and moves toward the proximal joints. In the described facilitation pattern, the therapist's right hand is placed over the back and toward the thumb side of the fingers and wrist of the patient. The left hand placement varies, depending on the part of the pattern to be emphasized. The return to the beginning position involves the antagonist pattern of extension-adduction-internal rotation (with elbow extension). These patterns are combined into the motor skills of rolling, sitting, standing, etc., and the self-care activities.

Treatment involves assessment of the neuromuscular deficit. The specific way the treatment techniques are employed depends on the precise nature of the neuromuscular deficit of the patient. These techniques form a complete therapeutic exercise regime that can be adapted to different disabilities and age groups. The facilitation patterns are combined to develop the motor skills of rolling, sitting, standing, etc., and the functional self-care activities.

In children with central nervous system deficits the particular problems are analyzed. Some characteristic manifestations mentioned by Knott are deviations from normal patterns of movement, for example, in reach and grasp. The child may start in one pattern and end in another. Characteristic wrist movements in extension and flexion in the cerebral palsied are opposite of those used in the PNF faciliation patterns. The reflexes are hyperactive. The neck and trunk motions are impaired by muscle weakness or incoordination. The face, tongue and breathing apparatus are disturbed. The primitive patterns are sought first. Knott notes that in the upper limbs this pattern is the extension-adduction-internal rotation with wrist flexion toward the ulnar side seen in the prenatal positions. In treatment, this pattern is mastered before proceeding to other patterns. Resistance may be used to smooth and coordinate muscle patterns when there is no muscle weakness. The hyperactive stretch reflex is used to initiate movement. The head and trunk movements are concentrated on first, using primitive patterns initially. The best coordinated groups are used to reinforce the weaker, more impaired groups. Mass flexion or extension may be used, depending on which should be stressed. Simple activities are developed before the more complex ones. Approximation maneuvers at the shoulder or pelvis stimulate the postural responses. The righting reflexes are evoked when resistance is given to achieve balance. Balancing techniques precede movement. Guided manual resistance in the facilitation patterns is used to reduce incoordination. Cold is frequently employed in the form of ice to reduce hypertonicity.

It is recommended that the occupational therapist planning to use this system read *Proprioceptive Neuromuscular Facilitation, Patterns and Techniques,*[75] by Knott and Voss. This book recommends that the novice gain experience in the treatment patterns with normal subjects. When beginning with patients the novice should start with the total patterns such as the mat activities.

Contributions of the Treatment Systems

Ayres[76] speculates that in the next twenty years a neurophysiological approach to treatment of patients with motor dysfunction will be well developed. She suggests a single, well-developed theory of motor behavior and treatment will emerge. Solutions will occur from a composite of fragments of knowledge derived from the clinical field and from basic research. Evidence in the form of controlled studies is already demonstrating the ability of the environmental factors to modify, accelerate or depress motor patterns. The exact nature of the plasticity of the central nervous system and how amenable the patterns are to modification remains unanswered. Unfortunately, the physical and occupational therapist cannot wait for the ultimate solution, but must treat patients now using the best empirical methods, utilizing the neurophysiological information available, and hypothesizing where the clinical information deviates or where there are gaps in information. The systems of treatment are not static. They are evolving as clinical experience is gained and therapists are applying the new information from basic scientific investigations. The various theoretical schools are not mutually exclusive; there are parallel development and exchange of ideas. An example of growth is the rather recent incorporation of proprioceptive and tactile stimulation procedures into the neurodevelopmental treatment of the Bobaths. Some major contributions of the systems using a central approach or neurophysiological approach rather than a peripheral approach follow.

The majority of occupational therapists use an eclectic approach, selecting from the various treatment systems and scientific data. (Refer to Table 4-7 for a comparison of the major and contributing facilitation mechanisms used in the major treatment systems.) The Fay and Doman-Delacato systems of treatment have used reflexes as initiators of movement. Both systems use the recapitulation of the phylogenetically older patterns of movement in treatment in order to achieve the ontogenetic patterns and the higher integrated levels of motor functioning. Fay contributed significantly by his recognition and description of the phylogentically early levels of sequential motor development in the neonate or newborn. Kabat advocated the use of the concept of mass synergistic patterns of diagonal movement facilitated by proprioceptive stimulation. Diagonal movement

TABLE 4-7

Facilitation Used in Systems of Therapy

	Phelps	Deaver	Brunnstrom	Fay-Doman	PNF	Bobath	Rood
Stimulus	*		*		*	*	†
Labyrinthine Reflexes	*		*			*	*
Tonic Neck Reflexes	*		*			*	
Righting Reflexes	*		*		*	*	*
Postural Reflexes	*		*	*	*	†	*
Synergic Patterns	*		†				
Orientation	*		*		*	*	*
Strength	*	*			†		
Range of Motion	*	*			*		
Ontogenetic Patterns	*				*	*	*
Phylogenetic Patterns				†			
Bracing	*	†	*				

* Contributory facilitation mechanism
†Major facilitation mechanism

*From Gillette, H.E. *Systems of Therapy in Cerebral Palsy* (Springfield, Illinois: Charles C Thomas, Publisher), 1970, p. 47.

patterns are reinforced by facilatory procedures of voluntary effort, visual following of the movement and parts, the postural reflexes, the stretch reflex and other tactile and proprioceptive mechanisms. Brunnstrom also used synergistic muscle patterns in treatment. Brunnstrom[77] has developed a system of treatment for adult hemiplegics to produce purposeful movement using synergistic patterns of movement in therapy. The treatment goals involve gaining control over the predictable flexor and extensor synergies so that multiple combinations of these movement patterns can be used in purposeful activities of self-care, locomotion and manipulation.

Rood has focused attention on the gamma motor system and stimulation of the nervous system, particularly through the exteroceptors. All systems now recognize the importance of how a child is handled and focus on the importance of hand placement by the therapists. Rood also defined muscle action in terms of heavy work patterns and light work patterns. She described the evolution of muscle activity from phasic action with reciprocal relaxation of the opposing musculature, development of co-contraction patterns, and finally the evolvement of the refined skilled patterns involving voluntary use of the distal parts, particularly the arms and legs.

Bobath focused attention on the need for inhibition of the undesirable motor activity as well as activation and facilitation of balanced skilled patterns. Bobath's exquisite understanding and feeling for movement and her techniques for handling the child have added to the repertoire of therapist skills. The Bobaths also contributed techniques for developing the postural and equilibrium reactions by automatically stimulating the desired responses by gently shifting the child off balance.

The above examples are just a few of the major contributions of the theoretical schools of treatment toward development of a unified neurophysiological approach to treatment, and illustrate how the systems are complementary.

Areas of disagreement exist. Major disagreement among the systems exists in the area of using the more primitive reflexes as innovators of movement. The systems focus on and emphasize different aspects of normal development in treatment. The systems developed with different patient populations. Brunnstrom's system of treatment was devised for the adult hemiplegic. The Bobaths developed their technique after years with cerebral palsied children who frequently suffer from hypertonicity of muscles. Kabat originally developed his techniques for muscle weakness from paralysis. Knott has extended the application and adapted treatment to other patients with neuromuscular deficits.

Rood's system of treatment has also been adapted and extended from the cerebral palsied to other neuromuscular deficits. The Doman-Delacato system treats children with neurological deficits and offers a multidisciplinary approach to the manifestations of neurological disorganization including reading, behavioral and perceptual, not just the sphere of motor impairment. Prominent in the treatment procedures of Knott and Rood is the use of ice. They use it in different ways to stimulate or inhibit tone. Knott primarily uses ice to decrease hypertonicity. Rood uses ice, applying it in a different fashion, to stimulate muscle responses. Knott, Rood and Bobath use compression through the limbs to obtain postural responses. Knott uses cortical and automatic responses while Bobath and Rood concentrate less on cortically directed activity, emphasizing the subcortical automatic responses. *The occupational therapist will often find it necessary to use her hands to place demands on the child's motor system in addition to her traditional use of purposeful activities.*

Occupational Therapy for Neuromotor Dysfunction

The child, the boy, the man, should know no other endeavor but to be at every stage of development wholly what that stage calls for. Then will each successive stage spring like a new shoot from a healthy bud, for only the adequate development of man at each preceding stage can effect and bring about adequate development at each succeeding stage.[78] (Friedrich Froebel).

The occupational therapist strives to help the child maximize his developmental potential. Cognizant of the specific deficits, he organizes a treatment approach supporting the natural maturation process and uses neurofacilitation techniques to try to inhibit abnormal motor behavior and to bring out more advanced motor behavior. He tries to provide an emotional climate which supports growth and affords opportunities for success even for severely afflicted children. The occupational therapist presents stimuli and challenges provoking the child to interact with his surroundings, and supports these efforts. He plans with the family and others caring for the child so that there is ample opportunity for the child to practice accomplishments.

Purposeful Activities

The occupational therapist has traditionally used purposeful activities as treatment. Curran [79] defines purposeful activity as focusing the conscious effort toward the object of movement rather than to the movement itself. Since the brain does not know muscles, only movement and purpose, the occupational therapist is in an ideal position to influence motor behavior through the manipulation of activities of self-care and play. This technique is neurophysiologically sound. The earliest years of infancy and childhood are devoted to relating to the environment through the sensorimotor system. The earliest development tasks, after the achievement of physiological balance, are to learn to move and fixate the eyes, ingesting liquids and progressing to solids, and the acquisition of locomotor skills.[80] The occupational therapist supports the achievement of these normal developmental tasks. They are natural to the child at each stage of development. The child takes great pleasure moving and balancing as he perfects his righting and equilibrium reactions. The trampoline, stilts, dodgeball and swings are all pleasurable means of exercising these abilities in therapy.

The child should not focus on what he is therapeutically achieving, since the desired response is subcortical, or beneath awareness. Most of our movements are automatically controlled by the lower nervous centers. For example, when walking one thinks about where he is going, with the senses monitoring the ground and automatically modifying the walking pattern. No attention is focused on making muscles work, or directing segments of the body such as moving the leg forward volitionally. Walking is so automated that therapists who need to teach patients to walk must be taught the mechanics of walking. Directing the many motor activities we engage in during each day would exhaust our energy and attention.

The occupational therapy approach to motor learning is through *doing*. He presents the stimulus in the form of sights, shapes, textures, and through handling and positioning the child. Having presented the challenges the therapist encourages and praises the efforts of the child. Increments should be small enough to allow success. The child learns through new experiences which are reinforced by success. The early motor developmental tasks which should be monitored by the occupational therapist are head control, eye fixating and following, sucking and swallowing, ingestion of solids, gross arm movements, eye-hand coordination, trunk control, emerging grasp patterns, propping and equilibrium reactions in the sitting position, refinement of the grasp pattern, sensory discrimination, and later the higher equilibrium reactions and perceptual motor development. In children with motor impairment due to neurological disorders, the therapist tries to facilitate normal patterns of movement using selective sensory input that supports neural integration into the functional patterns that constitute voluntary movement. Treatment begins at the developmental level of deficit.

Communicating

The occupational therapist functions as a facilitator of those aspects of normal development of the child about which he possesses special knowledge and skills. This facilitation of development takes place through interaction with the child-patient, his family, the multidisciplinary team, and frequently others who closely associate with the patient. All members of the team must develop effective communicative skills in writing and speaking. Shared information is greater than the sum of its parts. Each specialist views the child from his own vantage point. Each member of the multidisciplinary team must avoid a myopic view of the child. The recent tendency is toward a global approach to the child. Through communications with the various specialists working with the child, shifting priorities of emphasis must be determined so that a coordinated and unified treatment approach can be implemented.

Ongoing communications must be established with the parents. The parents should understand the goals of treatment. They need to know the present level of functioning of the child, and the next developmental steps sought. The parents with their intimate knowledge of how their child responds often can find means of initiating therapeutic activities, and can provide opportunities for practice of recently learned skills. The parents are in an optimal position to judge when the child is ready to move forward, and to support the child's natural impetus. The occupational therapist can often help the parents solve some of the physical problems they may encounter in handling the child. It is important that the child be handled in a manner that facilitates the desired neuromuscular responses, and avoids the development of deformities. Communicating with the parents affords a chance to support their efforts, and to exchange those positive bits of information about the child that please the parents.

Most important, the therapist must develop rapport and open communications with the child. The child functions as a positive or negative force in his own habilitation. Children can help themselves. The child of seven or eight should learn to assume some of the responsibility for caring for himself. As he becomes older, he should have the opportunity to learn about his disability. He should understand his own treatment program and take a part in the setting of treatment goals. The untreated intelligent child often learns ways of controlling his abnormal motor behavior to enhance function. For example, he may purposely avoid the influences of an exaggerated asymmetrical tonic neck reflex by directly facing activities and keeping them near the midline of his body. The child's efforts to discover and practice ways of enhancing purposeful movement should be supported, although the young child must be discouraged from using pathological reflexive activity to achieve function.

The emergence of the occupational therapist as an educator has evolved through necessity. The child receives occupational therapy for thirty to sixty minutes daily at most. Often he only receives treatment one to three times during the week. The treatment session, out of necessity, becomes a laboratory for evaluating and setting treatment goals, for finding the best ways of accomplishing goals, and monitoring and measuring progress. The first step in attempting to integrate the specific treatment techniques from the formal occupational therapy session into the child's everyday functioning involves communicating with and teaching the child, his parents, and those who surround him during the day.

A Developmental Approach to Treatment

Treatment of motor dysfunction in the child with a neurological deficit should follow the inherent orderly sequences of normal motor development. Treatment generally should proceed cephalocaudad, starting at areas of dysfunction in the upper regions of the body and descending. For example, facilitation of eye following or neck control should precede facilitation of trunk musculature for sitting. Treatment should proceed proximal to distal. Procedures to control shoulder musculature should precede fine finger activities. The occupational therapist is in a strong position ontogenetically as she works with the head regions in swallowing, sucking, biting, neck control, and the shoulders and arms. The visual development is one of the primary motor tasks for the young baby. In the early months the baby spends most of his waking hours exercising his ocular functions. Later visual information is correlated with other sensory information, especially touch and kinesthesia. Treatment should progress from gross activities to fine motor skills. Mastery of gross motor patterns is prerequisite to refined control. In treatment, consideration should be given to the phylogenetic and ontogenetic evolvement of patterns of movement. Postural stability provides the foundation for voluntary movement. Emphasis in treatment should be placed on developing the heavy work patterns that secure posture through co-contraction, moving in those heavy work patterns, and then seeking the refined light work patterns.

An example of a co-contraction movement pattern for the hands and wrists would be sawing or using a screwdriver. Isolated muscle contractions do not occur in functional and automatic movements, although it is possible to have an isolated muscle contraction, especially in the fingers. Muscles work together in synergistic groups in movement. Movement and muscle action of the distal parts of the body such as the hands should be considered within the whole pattern of muscular response that occurs, including muscular activation at the wrist, elbow, shoulder and trunk. It is important to understand the contribution of specific muscle groups to the various patterns of movement. Whenever feasible the sequential phases of development of motor tasks should be followed. For example, reaching in the side-lying and back-lying positions should precede reaching from the sitting position. Free sitting with knees and hips flexed or in the long sitting position should precede chair sitting postures. The control gained in the earlier patterns merge into and provide the basis for further refinement. Application of the above principles of treatment is easier, and the results of therapy more effective in treating the young infant during his first few years when his nervous system is the most plastic. As the child reaches five or older, the cultural pressure to achieve motor tasks becomes greater. It is important in treatment to afford the older child the opportunities to practice at lower levels of motor development even though he may, for example, be fastened into a chair for portions of the day. Finally, one of the most important factors in motor learning is the need for repetition. It has been recognized for a long time that action repeated will deepen into a kind of groove down which future behavior will tend to run. Current ncepts of the nervous system speak of neuronal integration or ᴍotor learning by establishing new patterns of sensorimotor organization that are dependent on repetition for reinforcement. Learning motor skills is a long and repetitious process. Therapeutic attempts to alter motor behavior may be just as long and repetitious as those experienced by the baby learning those skills for the first time. It takes a year for the baby to learn to voluntarily grasp and release. When the above principles are incorporated into an occupational therapy program, they provide a developmental approach to treatment especially suited to the child with a disorder the neuromotor mechanism.

Treatment Planning

Upon completion of the evaluation, the planning of the individual occupational therapy program begins. The most important aspects of planning involve the setting of treatment goals, devising ways of implementing these goals, and means of measuring their accomplishment. The long range goals should be determined. Next, the long range goals must be divided into well defined consecutive steps, or short term goals. These consecutive steps or short term goals define how the child can reach the long range goals and provide standards necessary to measure progress. An equally critical function of the short term goals is to afford the child opportunities for success. It has been said that nothing breeds success like succeeding. It is vital that the child have the reinforcement of success from his efforts and experiences in occupational therapy. Lack of progress is frequently blamed on poor motivation of the child. The child might be highly motivated not to do what the occupational therapist directs. Keeping the treatment session pleasurable helps to align the therapist's and child's goals. Whenever possible the treatment goals should reflect the aspirations of the child as well as his parents. It is most important to know what the child feels about his treatments and what he expects from them. When the treatment goals have been set, the treatment can begin.

Occupational Therapy Goals

A sample of some initial treatment goals that reflect the developmental approach will be given. The specific techniques that might be used in implementation of the goals will not be described. The sample treatment plan is not meant as a treatment recipe, but an example of the initial thinking using a developmental approach that would be modified after treatment has commenced. An ongoing process of evaluation, treatment planning, treatment implementation modification, re-evaluation, etc., occurs.

Case Description   D. J., a female infant of twelve months, was born after prolonged labor and was delivered by forceps. During the first few weeks of her life she was irritable and had to be fed by tube. During the first year she cried frequently and was difficult to feed. After the general flexor pattern began to break up, the baby was "floppy." At twelve months of age she continues to be a slow weak feeder, has very poor head control, and cannot roll or sit.

A consultation with the parents should be arranged to initiate a home feeding program, suggest methods of handling and positioning the baby, suggest toys and activities to stimulate the baby, and to help solve any problems the parents may encounter handling the baby. Before the parent consultation a questionnaire is sent home. Following are questions selected from Western

Long Range Goals	Short Term Goals
Mastery of the basic ocular movements.	1. Ocular fixation on stationary objects. 2. Ocular pursuit (180°).
Develop head control.	1. Controlled rotation of head. 2. Controlled lateral head movements. 3. Supine head lifting.
Ingestion of solid foods.	1. Facilitate sucking, swallowing, and chewing. Inhibit tongue protrusion, gagging, choking, bite reflex.
Support on arms in prone position with the head and upper body raised off the surface.	1. Facilitate co-contraction of the shoulder girdle and trunk musculature. Facilitate the labyrinthine reaction on the head. 2. Facilitate the Landau reflex.
Voluntary grasp and release.	1. Encourage eye-hand regard. 2. Gross reaching movements in the side-lying and back-lying postures initially concentrating on shoulder movements. 3. Gross reaching movements which involve elbow extension and crude grasp.

QUESTIONS TO PARENTS

LOCOMOTION

Does your child attempt to move when placed on the floor? i.e. push himself around on his back? roll (to which side?), creep, crawl or shuffle along on his bottom? Describe.

WASHING

1. Do you have any difficulty with your child's balance in the bath? Does he need support? Does he fall over when you wash on leg? Does he sit or lie?

2. Does he cooperate when you wash or bathe him? How?

CARRYING

Do you have difficulties in controlling your child when you carry him? Describe.

DRESSING

1. In which position do you dress your child? On his tummy? On your lap? On his back? On the table? On his side? Or do you use different positions for various garments?

2. Are there any garments, including diapers, with which you have particular difficulties? (a) putting on? (b) taking off?

3. Does your child cooperate? i.e. lift his arms, put his head down? lift his leg, give his foot, etc.?

FEEDING

1. In what position do you feed your child? i.e. is he lying, sitting in your lap, on a special chair?

2. Does your child have difficulty in eating certain foods? Indicate those that are the hardest to manage and those that are impossible:
   Liquids: hot or cold, or ice cream?
   Crisp foods: cereals, raw vegetables, toast, biscuits?
   Slippery foods: eggs?
   Sticky foods: mashed potatoes, fish?
   Chewy foods: bacon, meat, chicken?
   Sipping and chewing: e.g. soup with vegetables, etc.?
   Large bites and chewing: e.g. apples?
   Are there any foods not listed that are especially difficult?

3. Are there any of the following difficulties when feeding? If so, describe:
   (a) Tongue thrust (b) Gagging (c) Continual sucking (d) Biting as soon as something is placed in his mouth (e) Inability to close mouth when feeding (f) Swallowing (g) Biting or chewing.

4. Are there difficulties when your child drinks? If so, what are they, and what do you do about them?

Does he drink from a bottle? through a plastic tube? from a cup? cup with spout? or a spoon?

Do you have to pour the liquid down his throat, head backward?

Does he try to hold cup or mug, and if so, with one hand, or both?

5. Do you have to help him with his feeding? How do you do this? Details please of help given to control him generally, and any specific help given to the jaw, lip, and tongue to enable him to chew and swallow.

BABY CARRIAGE OR CHAIR

1. Which type of baby carriage have you got? Is it satisfactory? If not, state why.

2. What type of chair do you have?

3. Describe difficulties, if any, when he sits on your lap or on the floor.

Are there difficulties when he sits on a chair? Does he fall to one side? Which? Does he slide forward? Does he push back? Can he place his feet on the support?

SLEEPING

1. Does he go to sleep in a preferred position? Which?

2. Does he move in his sleep? Or do you find him in the same position? Are his bedclothes undisturbed, and do you have to turn him?

PLAYING

1. In which position does he find it easiest to play? i.e. sitting on the floor or a chair? lying on his tummy or on his side? squatting? kneeling?

Is he always in the same position or does he move about?

2. If a baby, does he play "peek-a-boo," wave "bye-bye"? Join in nursery rhymes with actions? Describe. Take toys to his mouth?

3. What type of toy does your child prefer? How does he play with them? (e.g. move them, bang them, etc.). Does he use one (which?) or both hands? Can he build, bang together, screw, unscrew, etc.? Does he push and pull toys?

Acquisition of the Facilitation Techniques

The occupational therapist is committed to utilizing her mind and body as an instrument within her professional capabilities to aid the child and his parents. The therapist is limited by the scope of his knowledge and skills. Each theoretical school of treatment stresses the importance of correct application of its techniques. Indiscriminate and incorrect use of the treatment procedures may be detrimental to the child, to the occupational therapy profession, and to that specific theoretical school of treatment.

Many therapists live and work far from major medical facilities. The Bobaths reside in Great Britain. Brunnstrom and Delacato reside on the East Coast. Knott, Rood, Ayres and Semans reside on the West Coast. The optimal way of acquiring the specific treatment techniques is to take the formal courses offered, which may not be possible. Local workshops should be set up and attended whenever possible. Each area should seek people who have taken the courses and who have had direct experience with the techniques to demonstrate. As the systems of treatment are not static, but evolving, it is vital to stay abreast of the current trends. A primary source of information is the *American Journal of Occupational Therapy* and *Physical Therapy; Journal of the American Physical Therapy Association.* Another very useful journal is *Developmental Medicine and Child Neurology.* Each month current books are reviewed and abstracts presented in these journals. A periodic review of the pertinent subjects in *Index Medicus* at the local medical library is often rewarding and promotes a broader view of the subject. Other sources of professional publications and materials including films, audio tapes, reprints of journal articles, pamphlets, study course manuals, the subjects and sources of physical and occupational therapy theses and dissertations are available from the American Occupational Therapy Association Inc.[81] and the Physical Therapy Association Inc.[82] A primary source of information is through direct inquiries to the specific centers of treatment concerning their short term courses and the availability of materials and films.

> Strange how much you've got to know
> Before you know how little you know.
>
> *Anonymous*[83]

204

References

1. Gesell, A. L. "Behavior Has Shape." *Science* 134 July (1961), p. 266. Copyright 1961 by the American Association for the Advancement of Science.
2. Gesell, A. and Amatruda, C. S. *Developmental Diagnosis,* Second edition (New York: Paul B. Hoeber, 1947), p. 187, p. 194.
3. Ames, L. B. "Individuality of Motor Development." *Physical Therapy* 46 (1966), pp. 121-127.
4. Castner, B. M. "The Development of Finè Prehension in Infancy." *Genetic Psychology Monographs* XII (1932), pp. 105-193.
5. Schneirla, T. C. "The Concept of Development in Comparative Psychology." In *The Concept of Development* (Minneapolis: University of Minnesota Press, 1967, pp. 78-108.
6. Nelson, W. E. *Textbook of Pediatrics,* Eighth edition (Philadelphia: W. B. Saunders Company, 1964), pp. 36-41.
7. Nelson, W. E. *Textbook of Pediatrics,* p. 20.
8. Nelson, W. E. *Textbook of Pediatrics,* pp. 34-35.
9. Peiper, A. *Cerebral Function in Infancy and Childhood,* Translation of Third edition (New York: Consultants Bureau, 1963).
10. Hellebrandt, F. A. "Physiology of Motor Learning as Applied to the Treatment of the Cerebral Palsied." *Quarterly Review of Pediatrics* 4 (1952), pp. 5-14.
11. Twitchell, T. E. "Attitudinal Reflexes." *Physical Therapy* 45 (1965), pp. 411-423.
12. Magnus, R. *Lancet* 2 (1926), pp. 531-536, pp. 585-588.
13. Milani-Comparetti, A. and Gidoni, E. A. "Pattern Analysis of Motor Development and Its Disorders." *Developmental Medicine and Child Neurology* 9 (1965), pp. 625-630.
14. Zador, J. *Les Reactions d'Equilibre Chez l'Homme* (Paris: Masson et Cie, 1938).
15. Martin, J. P. "Tilting Reactions and Disorders of the Basal Ganglia." *Brain* 88 (1965), p. 855.
16. Twitchell, T. E. "Normal Motor Development." *Physical Therapy* 45 (1965), pp. 419-423.
17. Halverson, H. M. "An Experimental Study of Prehension in Infants by Means of Systematic Cinema Records." *Genetic Psychology Monographs* 10 (1931), pp. 212-215.
18. Halverson, H. M. "A Further Study of Grasping." *Journal of General Psychology* 7 (1932), p. 41, p. 44.
19. Castner, B. M. "The Development of Fine Prehension in Infancy."
20. Gesell, A. *The First Five Years of Life* (New York: Harper and Row, 1940).
21. Illingworth, R. S. *The Development of the Infant and Young Child, Normal and Abnormal,* Second edition (London: E. & S. Livingstone Ltd., 1963).
22. McGraw, M. B. *The Neuromuscular Maturation of the Human Infant* (New York: Hafner Publishing Company, 1969).
23. Gesell, A. and Amatruda, C. S. *Developmental Diagnosis.*

24. Gesell, A. and Ilg, F. L. *Child Development* (New York: Harper and Row, 1949).
25. Illingworth, R. S. *The Development of the Infant and Young Child, Normal and Abnormal.*
26. Moore, J. C. "A New Look at the Nervous System in Relation to Rehabilitation Techniques." *The American Journal of Occupational Therapy* XXII (1968), p. 489.
27. Dekaban, A. *Neurology of Infancy* (Baltimore: The Williams & Wilkins Co., 1970).
28. Gesell, A. and Amatruda, C. S. *Developmental Diagnosis.*
29. Knoblock, H. "Developmental Screening Instrument." (Columbus, Ohio: Child Developmental Service, The Children's Hospital, 1963).
30. Zdanska-Brincken, M. and Wolanski, N. "A Graphic Method for the Evaluation of Motor Development in Infants." *Developmental Medicine and Child Neurology* 11 (1969), pp. 228-241.
31. Jones, M. H. "Cerebral Palsy Diagnosis in Young Children." In Wolf, J. M. *The Results of Treatment in Cerebral Palsy* (Springfield, Illinois: Charles C Thomas, Publisher, 1969), pp. 255-266.
32. Ingram, A. J., Withers, E. and Speltz, E. "Role of Intensive Physical and Occupational Therapy in the Treatment of Cerebral Palsy: Testing and Results." *Archives of Physical Medicine and Rehabilitation* 40 (1959), pp. 429-438.
33. "Motor Development Test" developed at New York State Rehabilitation Hospital. *In* Wolf, J. M. *The Results of Treatment in Cerebral Palsy,* pp. 246-253.
34. Zausmer, E. and Tower, G. "A Quotient for the Evaluation of Motor Development." *In* Wolf, J. M. *The Results of Treatment in Cerebral Palsy,* pp. 312-317.
35. Footh, W. K. and Kogan, K. L. "Measuring the Effectiveness of Physical Therapy in Treatment of Cerebral Palsy." *Journal of the American Physical Therapy Association* 43 (1963), pp. 867-873.
36. Tyler, N. and Kogan, K. L. "Measuring Effectiveness of Occupational Therapy." *The American Journal of Occupational Therapy* XIX (1965), pp. 8-13.
37. Dehaven, G. E. and Mordock, J. B. "Coordination Exercises for Children with Minimal Cerebral Dysfunction." *Physical Therapy* 50 (1970), pp. 337-342.
38. Stott, D. H., Moyes, F. A. and Headridge, S. E. "Test of Motor Impairment." (Ontario, Canada: Centre for Educational Disabilities, University of Guelph, 1970).
39. Bobath, K. and Bobath, R. "An Assessment of the Motor Handicap of Children with Cerebral Palsy and of Their Response to Treatment." *American Journal of Occupational Therapy* 21 (1958), p. 19.
40. Semans, S. et al. "A Cerebral Palsy Assessment Chart." *Physical Therapy* 45 (1965), pp. 463-468.
41. Milani-Comparetti, A. and Gidoni, E. A. "Routine Developmental Examination in Normal and Retarded Children." *In* Wolf, J. M. *The Results of Treatment in Cerebral Palsy,* p. 292.

42. Daniels, L., Williams, M. and Worthingham, C. *Muscle Testing*, Second edition (Philadelphia: W. B. Saunders Company, 1969).
43. Brunnstrom, S. "Motor Testing Procedures in Hemiplegia." *Physical Therapy* 46 (1966), p. 360.
44. Brunnstrom, S. "Motor Testing Procedures in Hemiplegia." pp. 357-375.
45. Brunnstrom, S. *Movement Therapy in Hemiplegia* (New York: Harper and Row, 1971)
46. Defibaugh, J. J. "Measurement of Head Motion." *Physical Therapy* 44 (1964), pp. 157-168.
47. Werner, J. L. and Omer, G. E. "Evaluating Cutaneous Pressure Sensation of the Hand." *The American Journal of Occupational Therapy* XXIV (1970), pp. 347-356.
48. Kent, B. E. "Sensory-Motor Testing." *Physical Therapy* 45 (1965), pp. 550-561.
49. Von Prince, K. and Butler, B. "Measuring Sensory Function of the Hand in Peripheral Nerve Injuries." *The American Journal of Occupational Therapy* 21 (1967), pp. 385-395.
50. Fiorentino, M. R. *Reflex Testing Methods for Evaluating C.N.S. Development* (Springfield, Illinois: Charles C Thomas, Publisher, 1970).
51. Ayres, A. J. Perceptual Motor Test Battery. *In* Ayres Space Test (Los Angeles Western Psychological Services, 1962).
52. Johnson, M. K., Zuck, F. N., and Wingate, K. "The Motor Age Test: Measurements of Motor Handicap in Children With Neuromuscular Disorders Such as Cerebral Palsy." *Journal of Bone and Joint Surgery* 33 (1951), pp. 693-707.
53. The Dallas Motor Development Test (Dallas: Dallas Society for Crippled Children, 1963).
54. Anderson, R. Bargowski, E. and Blodgett, W. H. "A Code Method for Evaluating Function in Cerebral Palsy." (Detroit: Detroit Orthopedic Clinic, 1961).
55. Wolf, J. M. *The Results of Treatment in Cerebral Palsy* (Springfield, Illinois: Charles C Thomas, Publisher, 1969).
56. Harris, F. A. "Multiple-Loop Modulation of Motor Outflow: A Physiological Basis for Facilitation Techniques." *Physical Therapy* 51 (1971), pp. 391-397.
57. Fay, T. "Neuromuscular Reflex Therapy for Spastic Disorders." *Journal of the Florida Medical Association* 174 (1960), pp. 257-262.
58. Fay, T. "The Neurophysiological Aspects of Therapy in Cerebral Palsy." *The Archives of Physical Medicine* 29 (1948), pp. 327-334.
59. Fay, T. "Use of Pathological and Unlocking Reflexes." *American Journal of Physical Medicine* 33 (1954), pp. 347-352.
60. Doman, R. J. et al. "Children with Severe Brain Injuries." *Journal of the American Medical Association* 174 (1960), pp. 257-262.
61. Delacato, C. H. "Neurological Organization." *Human Potential* (Philadelphia: The Institutes for the Achievement of Human Potential, 1, 1967).

62. A Summary of Concepts, Procedures, and Organization (Philadelphia: The Institutes for the Achievement of Human Potential, 1967).

63. Doman, R. J. et al. "Brain Injury as a Diagnosis and the Results of Treatment in 335 Brain Injured Children." *In* Wolf, J. M. *The Results of Treatment in Cerebral Palsy*, p. 214.

64. Rood, M. A. "The Use of Sensory Receptors to Activate, Facilitate, and Inhibit Motor Response, Autonomic and Somatic, in Developmental Sequence." *In* Sattely, C.: Study Course VI, Third International Congress, World Federation of Occupational Therapists (Dubuque, Iowa: William C. Brown Co., 1964), pp. 26-37.

65. Stockmeyer, S. A. "An Interpretation of the Approach of Rood to the Treatment of Neuromuscular Dysfunction." *The American Journal of Physical Medicine* 46 (1967).

66. Bobath, B. "Treatment Principles and Planning in Cerebral Palsy." *Physiotherapy* 49 (1963), pp. 122-124.

67. Bobath, B. "The Very Early Treatment of Cerebral Palsy." *Developmental Medicine and Child Neurology* 9 (1967), pp. 373-390.

68. Bobath, K. and Bobath, B. "The Facilitation of Normal Postural Reactions and Movements in the Treatment of Cerebral Palsy." *Physiotherapy* (1964), pp. 3-19.

69. Bobath, K. *The Motor Deficit in Patients with Cerebral Palsy* (London: Wm. Heinemann Medical Books Limited, 1966). Clinics in Developmental Medicine No. 23.

70. Voss, D. E. "Proprioceptive Neuromuscular Facilitation: Demonstrations with Cerebral Palsied Child, Hemiplegic Adult, Arthritic Adult, Parkinsonian Adult." *In Exploratory and Analytical Survey of Therapeutic Exercise*, Northwestern University Medical School, July 25-August 19, 1966. *American Journal of Physical Medicine* 46 (1967), pp. 838-898.

71. Knott, M. "Neuromuscular Facilitation in the Child with Central Nervous System Deficit." *Journal of American Physical Therapy Association* 46 (1966), pp. 721-724.

72. Knott, M. "Specialized Neuromuscular Technics in the Treatment of Cerebral Palsy." *Physical Therapy Review* 32 (1952), pp. 73-75.

73. Knott, M. and Voss D. E. *Proprioceptive Neuromuscular Facilitation: Patterns and Techniques*, Second edition (New York: Hoeber Medical Division, Harper and Row, 1968), p. 4.

74. Knott, M. and Voss, D. E. *Proprioceptive Neuromuscular Facilitation: Patterns and Techniques*, preface xiii.

75. Knott, M. and Voss, D. E. *Proprioceptive Neuromuscular Facilitation: Patterns and Techniques*.

76. Ayres, J. "Integration of Information." *In* Sattely, C.: Study Course VI, Third International Congress, World Federation of Occupational Therapists (Dubuque, Iowa: William C. Brown Co., 1964) p. 49.

77. Brunnstrom, S. *Movement Therapy in Hemiplegia*.

78. Froebel, F. *In Maria Montessori: Her Life and Work* (New York: Mentor-Omega Book by Arrangement with Academy Guild Press 1962), pp. 324-325.
79. Curran, P. In Ayres, A. J. "Occupational Therapy for Motor Disorders Resulting from Impairment of Central Nervous System." *Rehabilitation Literature* 21 (1960), pp. 302-310.
80. Muller, P. *The Tasks of Childhood* (New York: McGraw-Hill Book Company, 1970).
81. The American Occupational Therapy Association, Inc., 251 Park Avenue South, New York, N. Y. 10010.
82. The American Physical Therapy Association, Inc., 1156 15th Street, N. W., Washington, D. C. 20005.
83. In Henry, L. C. *Five Thousand Quotations for all Occasions* (New York: Doubleday & Company, Inc., 1945).

Bibliography

"Exploration and Analytical Survey of Therapeutic Exercise." *American Journal of Physical Medicine* 46, Number 1 (1967).

Finnie, N. R. *Handling the Young Cerebral Palsied Child at Home* (New York: E. P. Dutton & Co., Inc., 1970).

Gillette, H. E. *Systems of Therapy In Cerebral Palsy* (Springfield, Illinois: Charles C Thomas, Publisher, 1969).

Ingram, T. S. *Pediatric Aspects of Cerebral Palsy* (Edinburgh and London: E. & S. Livingstone Ltd., 1964).

Mysak, E. D. *Neuroevolutional Approach to Cerebral Palsy and Speech* (Columbia University: Teachers College Press, Library of Congress Catalog Number 68-19524, 1968).

"The Child with Central Nervous System Deficit." *Physical Therapy.* Part I, May 1965, Volume 45 Number 5, February 1966; Part II, February 1966, Volume 46 Number 2; Part III, July 1966, Volume 46 Number 7.

NOTES

NOTES

Chapter Five

Psychosocial Development: Function and Dysfunction

Carolyn Abbe Kent, M.S., O.T.R.

(July 1970)

Psychosocial Development

Unlike perceptual-motor and neuromotor development, psychosocial development is a process which continues throughout the life cycle. Maturation is not acquired in the childhood or adolescent years, but is an ongoing process lasting from birth until death. The term *psychosocial* is used to group a number of concepts under a single heading, such as the development of object relations, ego development, the development of peer relationships, psychosexual development, and superego development.

Organizing the psychosocial area of normal development into a cohesive, sequential exposition is a difficult task because of the lack of an integrative theory. Theories have been developed about specific behaviors — Freud's theory of infantile sexuality and Spitz's theory of the development of object relations for instance. For this reason psychosocial development is approached by topics. Each topic will be followed from its inception through the childhood years; adolescent behavior will be presented only in order to complete the developmental sequence of certain topics. The order of topic presentation has been chosen in order to approximate chronology and to minimize repetition. For example, the first topic, ego development, is highlighted during the first year of life with the development of object relations, while the development of the self image is primarily a task of the second and third year. The development of ego identity, the last task of this topic, is an adolescent achievement.

213

I.

EGO DEVELOPMENT

(1) See child as separate from environments

Development of Object Relations

The development of object relations is the process of differentiating the self from the environment and forming relationships with objects in the environment. Objects may be human, nonhuman, or abstract concepts. The term *libidinal object* is often used to indicate that objects have the ability to satisfy primary needs and therefore come to be cherished (cathected) by the individual. The infant develops object relations through the mothering relationship, the mothering person being the primary libidinal object.

As it has been defined, the concept of object relations encompasses much of psychosocial development. The common use of the term, however, implies the mother-child unit and those aspects of development which are dependent upon this relationship.

A primary researcher in the development of object relations is Rene Spitz. His book, entitled *The First Year of Life: A Psychoanalytic Study of Deviant and Normal Development of Object Relations,* describes his work and the theory derived from his research. Spitz divides the development of object relations into three stages: the objectless stage, the precursor of the object stage, and the establishment of the libidinal object stage.

The objectless stage   Spitz maintains that the newborn is unable to distinguish himself from his environment; he experiences his body and surroundings as continuous. The source of food, whether breast or bottle, is experienced as coming from himself, much in the manner in which nutrition came to him prior to birth.

During this neonatal stage, Spitz feels that the infant is protected from the environment by a high threshold to stimuli, as shown by the newborn's lack of response to noise, pain (a pin prick), and bright lights. The threshold barrier serves to cushion the "trauma of birth" which has been emphasized by some psychoanalists such as Otto Rank. The trauma of birth is described as the stress felt by the neonate in the transition from the secure "nirvana" of the womb to the cold, insecure, external world.[1]

In the early days of life the mother protects the neonate further by shielding him from environmental stimuli. Such child-rearing practices as keeping infants in warm rooms, wearing proper clothing, and with suitable support are some examples. The mother also helps the infant deal with unpleasant stimuli by changing his soiled diapers, feeding him when hungry, and burping him to aid his newly functioning digestive system.

At about eight days, the neonate begins to reach out to his new environment by responding to some cues. One of the first cues to which the neonate responds is that of being held in the feeding position. The hungry infant will turn his head toward the chest of the person holding him and actively seek the nipple of the bottle or breast.

With repetition and reinforcement this response generalizes. At about eight weeks the hungry infant may begin to make sucking movements at the sight of an approaching human, and at about three and one-half months he will watch the human's movements while he prepares the feeding.

During these first months the infant is coming to learn about his environment. The mother is the vehicle for this learning since she is usually the one who provides pleasure and relieves discomfort. As the mother cares for the child, it is her face which is the constant stimulus and as such, it becomes associated with pleasant changes.

Precursor of the object stage — the smiling response   The infant's ability to recognize the human face in the environment of many stimuli and to associate it with pleasurable experiences is shown at about the end of the second month by the smiling response. This response has been studied extensively by Spitz, who feels that this response marks a definite milestone in the formation of object relations. The smiling response is the "first active, directed, and intentional behavioral manifestation, the first indicator of the infant's transition from complete passivity to the inception of active behavior..." [2]

Certain conditions must be met to elicit the smiling response. The full human face must be presented with the head in motion. A nodding mask or any headlike object containing two eyes will provoke the response. A profile will not cue a smiling response, nor will a nonmoving rigid face. No other stimuli, such as the baby's bottle, will evoke this smile, and unlike the visual following and positional responses, the infant need not be hungry in order for the configuration of the human face to elicit the smile.

The smiling response seems to be an age-specific response. Spitz found that the first smiling responses were observed toward the end of the second month. Spitz's subjects, however, tended to be institutionalized children from lower socioeconomic parentage. More recent research on a more cross-sectional population seems to indicate that the smiling response occurs somewhat earlier. Fifty percent of one infant population smiled at 1.9 months — with a range of from 1.4 to 5.0 months.[3] By age six months Spitz found that the smile could no longer be elicited by the configuration of the human face alone. Beyond this age, the face must be alive and familiar to the infant in order for the smiling to occur.

The smiling response of the infant also suggests the presence of a rudimentary ego, a sense of self. The baby is able to make a coordinated, intentional response to a perceived stimulus. The infant also shows a trace of memory in that the familiar stimulus of the human face has become associated with pleasure. It indicates that the infant is now able to act upon this environment and become a participant, rather than a passive object upon which the environment acts.

The smile of the infant must also be considered as a stimulus for the mother. It reinforces her interest in the infant by providing rewarding feedback for her efforts and a new form of communication with her child. A new stimulus-response cycle is established: the baby smiles and the mother is rewarded; she responds in a way to restimulate the smile; and the behavior is continued, strengthening the relationship within the dyad.

Spitz terms the stage of the smiling response "the precursor of the object stage" because the face is as yet undifferentiated. It is only the moving configuration of the eyes, forehead, and nose which triggers the smile, and not the true libidinal object, the mother's face. The infant is unable to differentiate between familiar and unfamiliar faces. In other words, the human face is a *preobject,* or a sign for the true object.

Establishment of the libidinal object — stranger anxiety   Spitz states that between the sixth and eighth month the child no longer smiles indiscriminately at all human faces. As with the smiling response, however, this cessation may actually occur earlier than demonstrated by Spitz's subjects. He begins to differentiate between familiar and unfamiliar faces and indicates this new ability by a new response that is called stranger anxiety. This response can range from a mild, indifferent nonsmile to violent screams and tears.

Spitz attributes this stranger-anxiety response to the establishment of the libidinal object. The mother is the object in the true sense of the term, having become the cathected love-object. When confronted with a stranger's face, Spitz believes that the child feels he has lost his true object and reacts to the situation in the manner he deems appropriate.

The appearance of the stranger-anxiety response suggests the acquisition of new skills by the child. His ego abilities have increased, as illustrated by his discriminatory powers and variety of action responses. His sense of *self versus nonself* (or environment) has expanded, while his memory traces have enlarged to include differentiating facial characteristics.

Following the establishment of the libidinal object there is a spurt in development. The child's development of object relations rapidly progresses once he has had the initial experience of establishing his first relationship with an object. New forms of social relations develop. Communication expands to include gestures. For example, the infant of nine months may make his wishes known by pointing and making a familiar sound. Some capacity for reciprocal play develops, such as handing toys to an adult. The amount of space the child can utilize expands. Objects which fall from his crib no longer cease to exist, but can be found in the space surrounding the crib. With increased ability to travel about, the child can begin to explore his surround and the objects in it. As his manipulative skills increase objects are touched, mouthed, pushed, pulled, lifted and dropped.

Erikson's trust versus mistrust   Erik Erikson describes the events of the first year of life in a slightly different manner, although like Spitz, he does it from a psychoanalytic viewpoint. Erikson's Chapter "Eight Stages of Man," in his *Childhood and Society* describes ego development as evolving from critical periods of development.

Erikson describes the first stage of ego development as *basic trust versus basic mistrust.*[4] The infant must successfully establish a sense of social trust in order for his ego development to continue. The development of basic trust is described in a manner similar to Spitz's description of the development of object relations. The infant, in his relationship with his mother, comes to trust and recognize the predictability and continuity of her maternal care and her power to relieve unpleasurable stimuli.

The development of basic mistrust is the negative outcome of the first crisis of development. The child cannot learn to trust his environment if there is discontinuous mothering, or poor child care. Erikson feels that the result is a basic weakness of the personality which interferes with more mature ego development.

The psychosexual stages of development originally formulated by Freud have been expanded by Erikson to include data from different cultural sources. The term *oral stage* is used to identify the observation that the infant experiences his environment through his mouth. The first stage, trust versus mistrust, incorporates Freud's oral stage of infantile sexuality.

At first the oral experience is incorporative or receptive; the infant learns through sucking and taking in, and his first experience is with that object which provides him stimulation and nourishment, the nipple of the breast or bottle. This stimulus is gradually generalized to the adult which provides the nipple. The mouth or oral area is the source of pleasure for the infant, the center of trust and warmth.

Toward the end of the first year the incorporative behavior of the oral stage shifts to a more aggressive mode. With teething the pleasure of oral stimulation comes to include pleasure with biting and holding on. Conflicts arise at this time, particularly with the breastfed baby, when the pleasure of biting interferes with the pleasure of incorporating. In Western culture this conflict is heightened by the practice of weaning at about the time of teething. Without the basis of a strong trust relationship the effects can alter the personality. Erikson's study of the feeding patterns of other cultures illustrates this point.

Development of the Self Image

The development of the self image is the task of establishing a concept of the self as an autonomous, complete being. In a sense it is the natural continuation of the development of object relations, but with a slightly different focus. The inner child is the focus of this task, rather than the process of the child differentiating himself from his environment.

Locomotion in the development of the self image   The primary stage in establishing a self image is closely linked with the development of object relations. Just as locomotion is important for the child in learning about his environment, it is important for the child in learning about himself. The tremendous drive to move and explore is aptly described by Selma Fraiberg in her book, *The Magic Years*. The attraction of the environment and the compulsion to be active are expressions of the needs to explore the environment and to gain mastery of the body.

The ability of the child to get around by himself is a tremendous step toward independence and autonomy. He is no longer at the mercy of an adult as to where he will be placed and what objects will be available to explore. A new element of free will has entered his life — as well as a whole new world of experiences. He can learn that the family dog is not so big when you are standing rather than sitting; he can learn how tall he is by hitting his head while trying to stand under the kitchen table; he learns the abilities of his hands by the manipulation of the myriad objects he finds about the house.

The process of developing autonomy is seen also in the changing relationship with the mother. The process of individuation is beginning to occur. With locomotion the child can test his ability to separate from his mother. He can voluntarily leave her presence and return, rather than always be a victim of her departures.

The mother's approach to the child is also changing. In addition to being the agent of care and support, she must begin limiting the child to protect him from the environment he is so recklessly exploring. The word "no" comes to be used more frequently in the relationship, and certain social behaviors come to be expected of the child.

Bowel control in the development of the self image   The mother's and family's expectations for the child to control his behavior are usually brought to a climax over the issue of toilet training. The child is encouraged to conform to the more mature standards of cleanliness and pleasant odor.

These expectations usually begin shortly after the child has gained physical control of his bowel functions. He gains a great deal of pleasure in being able to autonomously control his bowel movement, an act which, like locomotion, contributes to the development of his self image. The pleasure of evacuating the bowels with the resultant feelings of well-being and release of tension and discomfort is described as the *anal stage* of psychosexual development. Extreme demands made upon the child to comply in using the toilet can destroy the sense of autonomy and pleasure he gains from this act of voluntary control.

Erikson[5] describes this crisis of development as *autonomy versus shame and doubt.* The positive attitude resulting from this stage, autonomy, is analogous to the development of a positive self image. The child develops an image of himself as a wholesome, independent being. He is able to stand on his own two feet and exhibit his ability to make free choice, as illustrated by his oppositional behavior and liberal use of the word *no.*

The negative outcome of shame and doubt is similar to a negative self image. It is a feeling of self-consciousness and a lack of assurance. The child feels ashamed and small.

The development of a sense of autonomy is the primary task of the toddler stage in development. Erikson feels that this task is universal for all cultures, but that toilet training need not be the focus of the development of autonomy. Our Western culture seems to increase the stress of this period of development by expecting early toilet training. The development of the self image continues throughout the childhood years, culminating in adolescence with the development of ego identity.

Development of the Sexual Image

The next major task in the ego development of the child is the development of a sexual image. The child has developed a sense of autonomy or a self image through locomotion and bowel control. He understands the capacities of his body and the power he has to exercise a degree of free will. At about the age of three, the child discovers that he is more than an autonomous being, but that he is a being of a definite sex. The development of a sexual image is the process of gaining an appreciation and acceptance of himself as a boy or girl, male or female. In a sense, the development of a sexual image is a refinement of the development of a self image.

The development of a sexual image does not suddenly begin at about the age of three. From birth on the sex of the child has had a powerful influence on his development, primarily because of the approach and expectations the mother and the rest of the family have had for the child. However, it is not until this stage that the child becomes aware of sexual differences.

Awareness of sexual differences   Children may begin to view sexual differences as a matter of clothing and only later discover anatomical differences. The realization that the sex organs of boys and girls are different may be particularly difficult for the girl, who may feel that she has lost a vital organ. This fear is termed *penis envy;* many psychoanalysts feel that many sexual problems in women are due to an unresolved feeling of having been deprived of the penis. Boys, on the other hand, may have *castration anxiety;* that is, the fear that they may lose their penis or that it may be removed.

Concomitant with an awareness of sexual differences is the growing awareness of the child's own genital area. Erotic feelings are now focused in the genitals, and thus the term, *infantile genitality.*

Oedipal behavior   Oedipal behavior received its name from Freud, who found Sophocles' tragic hero to be a classic illustration of the sexual predicament of early childhood. In the Greek myth, Oedipus killed his father and married his mother. The term *Oedipal conflict* is used to designate the tendency of children from about three to five years to develop a sexual attraction for the parent of the opposite sex. The problem tends to be more intense in a mother-son relationship, for it is the mother who cares for the bodily needs of her son. The father-daughter relationship tends not be as physically intimate.

The child seeks erotic gratification from the parent who is the love object and desires eventually to marry this parent. The parent of the same sex is considered an intruder — the child wishes to be rid of the rival parent and may imagine killing him or driving him away. At the same time, the child fears retribution for these fantasies and develops anxiety for his own well-being. Moreover, he feels ambivalent because he also loves the parent of the same sex and wishes no harm to befall him.

Behavior characteristic of the Oedipal stage may or may not be clear-cut expressions of love or hate, but may take the form of seemingly irrational fears and odd behavior. Nightmares, fear of the dark, and behavior which can be extremely frustrating for the parents may be manifestations of Oedipal feelings. It is also difficult for parents to understand their child at this crisis in development for their own Oedipal feelings have been repressed to the point where they can no longer empathize with the child's feelings. For this reason the detection of Oedipal behavior is often difficult.

Initiative versus guilt is the crisis of this stage, according to Erikson. Initiative refers to a vigorous, self-confident mode of behavior with the new freedom of autonomy. Initiative is an enhancement of autonomy expressed in planning and attacking a task for the sake of the activity, rather than engaging in a task to assert one's independence. There is pleasure in accomplishment. Men express initiative in pleasure over attack and conquest, while women tend toward modes of catching and snaring. The guilt of this stage is over the goals and tasks contemplated and actual acts engaged in during the exuberant expression of one's activity.

Erikson emphasizes that this is the point in the child's life when be begins to separate himself from the pregenital relationship with his parents and begins the process of becoming a parent himself.

> Infantile sexuality and incest taboo, castration complex and superego all unite here to bring about that specifically human crisis during which the child must turn from an exclusive, pregenital attachment to his parents to the slow process of becoming a parent, a carrier of tradition.[6]

Establishment of the sexual image   The establishment of the sexual image is closely related to the resolution of the Oedipal stage. The process is a gradual one. The mother-child relationship begins to weaken. The mother gradually frustrates the child's attachment to her, since the need for her care diminishes as the child is able to care for himself. The child comes to learn that the father also is a focus on the mother's love and attention, a fact which until this time he has been unable to recognize. He comes to realize that his mother loves not only him, but his father and siblings as well.

The child begins to renounce his love for the parent of the opposite sex. He becomes struck by the positive ties to the parent of the same sex, ties which are strengthened by the normal sharing of interests. Boys, for example, find that by being like their fathers, they can gain a new form of recognition from both of their parents. As Selma Fraiberg states, "It's as if the child says, 'Since I cannot take my father's place, be my father, I will be like him,' and now begins to model himself after his father."[7]

Through this process of identification the child develops his sense of his sexual role, and comes to view himself as male or female. As Erikson points out, however, this is only the beginning of the process of sexual identification. The individual cannot truly develop a sense of his sexual role until late adolescence and adulthood.

The period of late childhood, from about six to eleven years, is a relatively quiescent period in ego development. For this reason it is often referred to as the *latency stage*. The child utilizes this period to consolidate his ego development and to practice and master other childhood tasks. Late childhood is a relatively stable period prior to the abrupt changes which occur at puberty.

Development of Ego Identity

The onset of puberty marks the beginning of a new challenge to the ego of a child. The self image and sexual image which the child worked so hard to establish are in a state of upheaval. The body that he once mastered is rapidly changing and a new sexual urgency is felt within him. The adolescent must rework his ego development to accommodate these changes and must in turn meet the challenge of a new step in his development, the establishment of his identity.

Ego identity is more than the sum of the integration taking place during childhood. The problem of establishing ego identity can be likened to the adolescent answering the question, "Who am I?" It's a problem of preparing for the future by establishing what to do with his life. It is the transition from dependent childhood to independent adulthood.

Adolescent sexual identity   Puberty brings physical sexual maturity and with it a changing body and a new inner drive toward sexual gratification. Genital sensations cause restlessness and thoughts and dreams of sexual behavior and objects. There is a reactivation of Oedipal feelings as the parent of the opposite sex once again becomes the focus of sexual fantasies.

The adolescent must learn new modes of behavior to accommodate these changes and gain relief from sexual tension.

Sexual feelings tend to be sublimated or drained off through activity; an increase in masturbatory behavior also occurs. There tends to be a turning away from the parents in order for the adolescent to protect himself from the guilt of his Oedipal feelings and seek sexual objects outside the family. The family remains important to the adolescent as a source of support and identification, but not as a source of sexual expression.

The adolescent turns to his peer group as the source of sexual outlet and support. He gains their approval through conformity to certain patterns of behavior — modes of dressing and special interests.

In early adolescence the members of the peer group are of the same sex. This helps the adolescent integrate his sexual changes by exchanging information and experiences. As the ego learns control over sexual feelings, the peer group tends to become heterosexual. At first there is a teasing relationship between groups of boys and girls which tends to occur at public events or "hangouts." Certain members of the opposite sex are singled out as objects of sexual fantasies, although overt behavior would rarely indicate anything more than casual interest. Gradually the youth group grows smaller, offering the opportunity for couples to pair off, but continuing to have the protection of peers close at hand. Necking and petting behavior seem to be an opportunity for the adolescent to explore his own feelings and learn control over his impulses, rather than provide the adolescent a release of sexual tensions or a sharing of an intimate relationship. Erikson states that the self-abandonment necessary for serious lovemaking is felt as threatening to the adolescent who has not yet established his identity.

In mid- or late adolescence the youth is likely to fall in love. These early love relationships are important in establishing the sexual identity. Once a love object outside the family has been established, there comes relief from many tensions within the family. The adolescent in becoming a love object secures his sexual or gender identity. The girl finds herself attractive and capable of ensnaring, while the boy insures his masculine prowess.

Establishment of ego identity   The establishment of gender identity is part of the adolescent process of answering the question, "Who am I?" As the beginnings of sexual identity are being made, the adolescent focuses on his total being and on the responsibility for his future.

A major decision which helps to establish the identity is the choice of an occupation. The basis of this decision is largely a result of the previous experience of the adolescent: his skills and interests, his socioeconomic background, the types of occupations with which he has had contact, the occupations of influential people in his life, and so forth.

Once this choice has been made, many of the questions concerning "Who am I?" will have been answered. Who the adolescent is becomes largely a statement of the life for which he is preparing. By making an occupational choice the adolescent has to some extent picked a life style and has more or less determined much of his future ego development. As Erikson points out, without the establishment of ego identity, there is role confusion. In large part the turmoil of late adolescence can be measured by the length of time necessary for the adolescent to reach his decision, for it seems that once introspection is forfeited for the establishment of a goal, his life becomes less complicated.

The establishment of ego identity is marked by a homeostasis of the self. The individual seems to have an inner resistance to radical change; his behavior and approach to life become predictable.

Ego development is by no means complete with the establishment of the identity. Each period of crisis in the life cycle must be met with ego change and development. It is, however, during the childhood years that the development of the ego is most marked.

II. SOCIAL DEVELOPMENT

Social development may be considered to be the development of the ability to function within a group and to accept the demands of the culture and society in which one lives. Inherent in social development is the development of the superego. The *superego* is the internal control of the individual which promotes behavior in accordance with the norms of his society and his culture. A discussion of social behavior emphasizes the manner in which the child learns to conform to group standards and traditions, and comes to be a cooperative, contributing member of society, in other words, the process of socialization.

Early Social Behavior

The neonate is an asocial or presocial being. He does not show interest in people and in no way does he desire the company of others. He is egocentric. Behavior that could be considered social in nature, such as crying, has nothing to do with human contact or the lack of it, but with some internal discomfort.

As the baby learns to associate pleasure and the alleviation of discomfort with adults, he begins to show contentment with the presence of others. At about two months he begins to respond to human stimuli, such as a human voice or face. The smiling response, in addition to being an indicator of the development of object relations, is also a sign of early social behavior.

The baby at about nine months tries to initiate playful behavior with adults by imitating gestures, such as "peek-a-boo" and "bye-bye."

Development of the Superego

Locomotion and language in superego development With the development of locomotion there is more need to limit the child's behavior. He is exposed to more potentially harmful stimuli, such as electric outlets and stairs, and has more access to damageable items, such as record collections, books, and potted plants. The parents, usually the mother, must take the responsibility for providing these limits, in essence acting as the child's superego. It is through this process of setting limits for the child that the child comes to incorporate them into his own functioning.

Through his mother's "no, no, no" and stern facial expression — as well as physical prevention from engaging in certain activities —he learns that certain impulsive behaviors are not in accordance with the wishes of others. Behavior such as throwing food on the floor, pulling the dog's ears, and playing with daddy's books are not pleasing to the members of his family and they express this in varying ways. Prior to the development of language, however, it is difficult for the child to forego these behaviors. His instinctual needs to explore and manipulate far outweigh his capacity for control.

The development of language greatly facilitates the task of superego development. Words can come to substitute for an act or object. The mental experience of using the words allows the child control over his behavior. The words, "Dad's books, no, no," can help the child inhibit his urge to explore the bookcase. Postponement of gratification becomes possible by language.

Of course the child's ability to control his own behavior does not occur overnight. Parental intervention is required for some time after language develops. Gradually, however, the prohibitions become more a part of the child himself.

The child is also learning social behavior by imitation. Such activities as feeding himself, becoming toilet trained, and dressing and undressing himself are all modes of behavior which tend to make the child a more social being. Other social behaviors, such as waving "bye-bye" and giving bedtime kisses, help the child to accept daily periods of stress in his relationships with others.

The establishment of the superego The Oedipal stage offers opportunity for further superego development. Through the resolution of the Oedipal conflict, the child comes to grasp some of the social and cultural restrictions of sexual expression. Through the attitudes and behavior of his parents and others, he comes to incorporate appropriate behavior and acquire some moral responsibility. Erikson's emphasis upon the guilt which can be felt at this age is testament to the fact that superego development has begun.

> ...the 'Oedipal' stage results not only in the oppressive establishment of a moral sense restricting the horizon of the permissible; it also sets the direction toward the possible and the tangible which permits the dreams of early childhood to be attached to the goals of an active adult life.[8]

Through resolution of the Oedipal stage and identification with the parent of the same sex, the child's self-control is strengthened. The child now accepts a model of behavior to follow.

Through the acquisition of language and the identification process, the superego emerges. The child begins to gain inner controls over his behavior and establishes a sense of social responsibility. He continues to be dependent upon parental standards of right and wrong and adult authority in enforcing these standards. Superego development only begins in the childhood years. It continues to develop throughout the life cycle.

Erikson's Industry Versus Inferiority

Later childhood produces new shifts of behavior which indicate social development. Erikson characterizes the stage as *industry versus inferiority*[9] and emphasizes the process of the child's learning to become a contributing member of society.

The emphasis upon industry at this age indicates that the child is beginning to be judged by his works. The child is preparing to become a worker and provider. He feels that he must earn the love and esteem of others by producing things. He comes to feel gratification at "a job well done." School becomes important as a place to accomplish and produce; he learns skills that will help him function as an adult. The child's own sense of worth comes to be reflected in his work — if his work is judged as inferior, he comes to feel that he is inferior.

Preparing to become a contributing member of society includes many skills. Learning to use tools, becoming proficient with language acquiring specialized knowledge and skills, and learning to work effectively with others are all important in taking one's place in society.

Development of Peer Relationships

Until now, this chapter has emphasized the relationship between the adult and the child. In order to prepare to function within a group, the child must develop the ability of relating to his peers.

Early peer relationships Babies first become aware of other babies at about the age of four months. They smile and are attentive to the cries of another child. Later in the first year, they like to touch and explore other children, in a manner similar to their exploring other objects in the environment.

During the second year children like to follow one another about and imitate each other's behavior. Toys may be used as a means of establishing social contact and may be extended as a gesture of friendliness. Looking-on play is apt to occur — especially between an older and younger child: the younger child looking on while the older demonstrates his skills. Parallel play consists of two children engaged in solitary play while in close physical proximity. The interaction of toddlers may consist of friendly or unfriendly exchange of toys, and gross motor behavior of following, imitating, and chasing.

The play group In early childhood (about three and one-half to five) cooperative play develops; the children work together to accomplish a specific task. There is an amount of conscious cooperation and a relationship may exist for the duration of the task.

With increased maturity the size of the play group expands and the complexity of the task increases. There is increased verbal communication. In the process of cooperative behavior there are many displays of aggression and verbal fights, but these are short-lived, and quickly forgotten. Rules and laws are developed by the play group to regulate the behavior of the members, and roles are assigned to insure the accomplishment of the task. The rules and roles are constantly being modified to meet the needs of the individual members.

Although peer interaction has been initiated, there continues to be a great deal of solitary play. The play group is a flexible social group. Membership is largely determined by physical availability. There is no sense of group loyalty, nor is there unity once the task has been completed. If the neighborhood does not provide natural peer contacts, the initiation of the play group may come from outside forces, such as a nursery school or parental planning.

The gang   The gang is spontaneously formed by the children themselves. It exists independently from activities and seems to form as a result of the needs of older children (about six to twelve) to gain what an adult society cannot give them. They find increasing pleasure in being with small groups of their own sex. A sense of worth is achieved by being a member of a gang, as well as providing the vehicles for companionship and fun. Devices such as passwords, nicknames, initiation ceremonies, and secret meeting places help to form gang solidarity.

The gang engages in numerous types of activity, some of which is constructive and worthwhile, some destructive and mischievous. The member of a gang is susceptible to the approval and disapproval of the other members. He conforms to the norms of his gang by behaving in the manner in which the gang approves. When there is a discrepancy between the norms of the gang and the norms of the parents, the child is faced with a difficult dilemma. Chastisement from either source can be extremely unpleasant.

Competitive and rivalrous behavior are also experimented with by the gang. The competition may be within the gang for the leadership position. This type of behavior tends to undermine the stability of the gang and weaken the group. Rivalry between gangs, however, strengthens the group and increases the loyalty. Competition between peer group members may lead to physical aggression or more subtle means of vying for power, such as teasing, bullying, and "ganging-up" on another member.

Gang behavior favors development of both desirable and undesirable behavior in the child. It teaches the child group cooperation, social consciousness, and to be sensitive to the needs and wishes of others. Courage, loyalty, and sportsmanship are other positive behaviors learned in the gang. Negative qualities that may result from gang life are lying, snobbishness, discriminations of minority groups, and contempt for parental ideals. These negative factors tend to be eliminated in later development and do not provide a serious threat to the personality of the child. In fact, membership in a gang is a very important aspect of a child's development. Without its socializing influence the child is handicapped.

Summary

Rather than attempting to summarize normal psychosocial development, a chart is provided (Figure 5-1). This method of presentation has been chosen in order to illustrate the interrelationship between the various aspects of psychosocial development, and their critical periods of development.

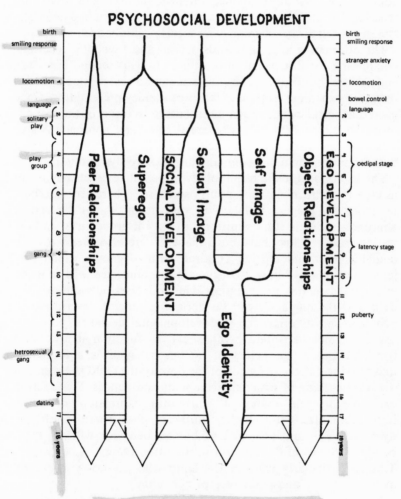

FIG. 5-1. Psychosocial development.

Psychosocial Dysfunction

Two approaches are feasible in organizing a discussion of psychosocial dysfunction. One approach tends to reinforce the chronological sequence of development. This approach begins by presenting those syndromes which result from deviations in early development, and proceeds in chronological order to those conditions which are a result of deviations in later childhood and adolescence. As an example, infantile autism and psychotic reactions of childhood appear first in this approach, since their genesis is felt to be in infancy and early childhood.

The alternative approach finds autism and psychotic reactions completing the discussion of dysfunction. This second approach emphasizes the continuum from normalcy to severe illness, and is the more expedient method in terms of literary presentation, since each diagnostic category can be discussed in terms of the manner in which it compares to less severe illness. This approach is also more in line with rates of incidence; less severe psychosocial dysfunction is far more common than severe dysfunction.

The use of diagnostic terminology in pediatric psychiatry is not as clearly defined as it is in adult psychiatry. There seems to be a tendency for diagnostic labels to vary according to theoretical approaches, diagnostic definitions, treatment procedures, and the setting in which they have been made. There also seems to be a tendency to avoid tagging children with diagnoses which may jeopardize their future. Diagnostic terminology will not be emphasized in this presentation. General classifications will be used and the emphasis will be upon the general description of behavior and its relevance to developmental deviance.

The attempt to isolate psychosocial dysfunction in the child from the other parameters of human behavior is a foolhardy undertaking, for the behavior of the developing child is a result of the intermeshing of many environmental influences. Dysfunction exclusive to one realm of behavioral expression is nearly impossible. It seems highly unlikely that there could be dysfunction in any one area of human behavior without there being overtones of dysfunction in the other realms of behavior.[10] This is particularly true for the child who has not yet reached maturity in any one parameter of behavior.

The problem of establishing the cause of psychosocial dysfunction is another difficult task for the clinician working with children. Unlike neuromotor—and to some extent perceptual-motor dysfunction — there are no clearcut signs, symptoms, and diagnostic procedures which can be used to confirm or dispel a diagnosis and establish the cause. The signs and symptoms of psychosocial dysfunction are nefarious, attributable to either psychological or physiological causes.

Many assumptions are made in regard to etiology, each based upon the theoretical framework of its proponent. Many clinicians regard the environment as the primary cause; they feel that the child's behavioral manifestations are made in response to the environment. The environment includes the mother-child relationship, the family relationship, as well as the environment external to the home, such as the school and neighborhood. This assumption seems to explain a great many cases of psychosocial dysfunction.

Some clinicians, however, have begun to see the danger in the assumption that the parents, and more particularly the mother, are the cause of psychopathology in their children. To place the blame on the parents serves no useful purpose when it comes to treating the child, and, in fact, it often complicates the treatment process. "Momism," as Erikson terms the syndrome, is a product of our culture, and must be understood as such, if parents are to be relieved of the tremendous burden they presently feel in rearing their children.

Although most clinicians agree that in some cases the environment may be the cause of psychosocial dysfunction, more and more questions are being raised as to the role of the child in the etiology of the disorder. Children from similar environments do not all develop dysfunction. What is it about any one particular child which causes a neurotic or psychotic reaction, when children from very similar backgrounds have made normal adjustments? Is there a genetic predisposition to psychosocial dysfunction? Can it be possible that the child who develops a psychosocial disorder has some organic illness and/or damage which is undetectable?

There has been some research which seems to indicate brain dysfunction in some cases of psychosocial dysfunction. Behavioral disturbances have long been known as symptoms of identifiable brain injury and disease (see *Psychosocial Dysfunction Due to Brain Damage*). The more recent research into diagnostic tools which are used to identify minimal brain dysfunction seems to indicate that behavioral manifestations correlate with positive findings of brain damage. The question, then, becomes: are the behavioral manifestations primary or secondary to the minimal disturbance? In other words, are the behavioral problems a means of compensating for the organic handicap, or are they caused by the organic impairment?

At this time very little is known about the manner in which the environment and the child react to create pathology. An interesting study by Thomas, Chess, and Birch attempted to record the beginnings of psychosocial disorders by longitudinally studying the temperament of children and the influence of and reaction to the environment. Temperament was defined as "the behavioral style" of the child, and was explained in such terms as adaptability, persistence, activity level, distractability and rhythmicity. The results were inconclusive, since they were not able to predict the situations in which pathology would occur, but their study, along with others, indicates some methods by which research can begin to solve the etiological dilemma of psychosocial dysfunction in children.

The Normal Child

Stella Chess, in her text, *An Introduction to Child Psychiatry,* proposed the following description of the child functioning normally in the psychosocial realm of behavior.

> ...he [the normal child] gets along reasonably well with parents, siblings, and friends, has few overt manifestations of behavioral disturbance, is using his apparent intellectual potential to a degree close to its estimate, and is contented for a reasonable proportion of the time.[11]

The ability to play at a level expected for the child's chronological age is also a good index of mental health.

Many behavioral manifestations, such as thumbsucking, selfishness, aggressive or negative behavior, nightmares and so forth, are expressions that normal development is occurring. They indicate that the child has not yet found effective, social methods of coping with the situation. It is only the excessive, compulsive continuance of these patterns of behavior beyond their normal range that should cause concern. As Anna Freud states, "Many of the inhibitions, symptoms, and anxieties of children are produced not by processes which are truly pathological but. . . by the strains and stresses inherent in development itself."[12]

Other normal behavioral reactions may occur as the result of specific experiences. For example, a child may have a fear of dogs for several weeks or months after having been bitten by a dog in the neighborhood, or a child may develop a sleep disorder after having a nightmare about a recent television program. These reactions are only transitory in nature, and are easily considered to be within the realm of normal development.

The occupational therapist must be cognizant of the fact that these normal developmental problems are more likely to occur — during — or may be intensified by — illness, and unfamiliar environment, or separation from parents. Ill and/or hospitalized children face increased amounts of environmental stress. Their usual patterns of behavior may be inadequate to deal with the situation and they may need to utilize less mature patterns of behavior or employ less effective methods of handling the situation.

Reactive Behavior Disorders

Reactive behavior disorders are behavioral expressions in response to external circumstances. The behavioral expressions may be developed as a defense to inappropriate handling, physical illness, and traumatic occurrences.[13] The severity of the reactive disorder is a matter of the rigidity of the response. The more pervasive the response in the total functioning of the child, the more severe is the reaction. As Anna Freud states,

> ...there is only one factor in childhood the impairment of which can be considered of sufficient importance..., namely, the child's capacity to move forward in progressive steps until maturation, development in all areas of personality, and adaptation to the social community have been completed. Mental upsets can be taken as a matter of course so long as these vital processes are left intact.[14]

Children with reactive disorders are likely to be patients of occupational therapists. Severely ill or hospitalized children, or children who are the victims of accidents are likely to develop reactive disorders if not properly managed. Children from home environments which are unable to manage them appropriately are also likely candidates for reactive disorders. The occupational therapist must be able to modify his approach to the child in order to prevent these reversible reactions from becoming fixed, neurotic patterns of behavior.

Certain symptoms are common to reactive disorders. The pervasiveness of the symptoms vary from those which can be considered a part of normal development to those which severely hamper the functioning of the child. There are many behavioral symptoms which might be discussed; however, there are many similarities among them. A discussion of a few symptoms will serve as a model for the remaining ones.

Enuresis Urinary incontinence is normal behavior for all children until they have mastered full control of their bladders. A child is usually not considered fully toilet trained until he is able to go through the night without wetting his bed. At about the age of three the child usually ceases wetting himself at night or he is able to wake himself to use the toilet.

Enuresis beyond the age of three may result from many normal situations. Wetting often occurs during periods of stress. Starting nursery school or kindergarten, or being away from home at summer camp or in the hospital may cause "accidents." Wetting may also be preferable to certain environmental problems. The child may prefer the social repercussions of his act, rather than tread through the darkness of the house or venture outdoors in homes that have no indoor toilets.

Enuresis which persists into later childhood may also result from incomplete toilet training. The parents may never have taken the steps necessary to prevent bedwetting. It may have been more convenient for them to diaper the child at night, than to change soiled beds and/or toilet the child at night.

There may be physiological causes of frequent enuresis beyond the age of three. Wetting may be a secondary symptom to convulsive disorders, brain damage, infections of the urinary tract, and systemic illnesses. Organic causes for enuresis must be checked before a psychogenic cause can be assumed.

Despite the previous exceptions, enuresis often is psychogenic in origin. It can be a behavioral expression of many problems. It may represent an inability to achieve the autonomy normally mastered at the toddler or anal stage of development. There may be hostility toward the parents in not allowing the child to experience independence and the wetting may be an expression of this feeling. Enuresis may also be an indicator of stress. For example, the child who feels anxiety at school may wet his bed on each school night, but not on the weekends.

Enuresis must also be considered a source of further problems. The child who wets himself is often the target of teasing and rebuke from his peers. Nocturnal enuresis may prevent a child from going to summer camp or staying overnight with friends. He may come to feel the "shame and doubt" described by Erikson which prevents him from developing a positive self image.

In general, enuresis is not indicative of a severe mental problem unless it is one of a number of behavioral symptoms. Deep-rooted neurotic disorders generally are expressed by more than one such symptom. Enuresis may be the symptom, however, which brings the parents to seek help for their child.

Negative behavior Negative behavior, like enuresis, is normal behavior for children two to three years of age. In the process of developing a sense of self, negativism of oppositional behavior is practically a prerequisite. In developing their own egos, children of this age assert their independence by making decisions in opposition to their parents.

Negative reactions in children may result from several normal developmental situations. Unreasonable requests of parents for their children to comply with modes of behavior inappropriate for their age is one major cause. For example, parents who expect their three-and-a-half year old to sit quietly at the dinner table for an hour or more while the adults discuss politics, are asking for a glass of spilled milk, or a handful of food to be thrown on the floor.

Another source of negative behavior is seen when adults consistently give a child attention for "bad" behavior. The attention may not be favorable, but it is preferred to no attention at all. Many cases of sibling jealousy can be attributed to a situation similar to the following. A family birthday party is arranged for Johnny. He receives presents from his parents, his grandparents, and his older brother, and it takes him nearly half an hour to open them all. During this time everyone's attention is focused on Johnny. Suddenly there is a loud crash from the other room. Everyone rushes in to find mother's antique dish in pieces on the floor with Johnny's older brother standing over it with a guilty look on his face. The brother is reprimanded in front of everyone and is dragged screaming to his room, quite delighted at stealing the spotlight from his brother.

The negativism illustrated in the previous two situations are normal reactions to stress. When these patterns of behavior become fixed so that the child reacts in this manner despite the situation, negative behavior is becoming more of a neurotic symptom. As an example the case of Bob is presented. Bob rarely received any positive attention from his parents. His mother expected him to play in his room a great deal of the day while she studied for her master's degree. He received attention from his mother when he did something negative, such as breaking the furniture in his room, and tearing up his bedclothes. This type of negative behavior spread to other periods of the day. At mealtime he became picky about what he would eat, never accepting the first dish offered to him. He made elaborate demands at bedtime, extending the going-to-bed process for several hours. When Bob began school he carried this behavioral pattern to the new situation. His teacher could not understand, nor could she cope with Bob's behavior, and she consulted the occupational therapist working in the school.

School phobia   The term *school phobia* must not be considered a disease entity, as the term might imply, but as a behavioral reaction or symptom.

Slight cases of school phobia are normal for some children during the beginning of their school career; they fear they will not be successful or that they will be unable to function in the unfamiliar situation away from the home. They cope with the situation by refusing to leave home or by refusing to leave their mothers. School phobia may be masked by physical complaints of stomach ache, headaches or nausea, either prior to having to go to school or while actually in attendance. After a few days and a few successful experiences, the anxiety disappears.

Phobic reactions may be considered normal after certain experiences in school. A harsh, punitive teacher, or a failure in a spelling test may cause anxiety about attending school. A physical handicap, or behavioral pattern due to organic brain damage, such as hyperactivity, may make adjustment to school difficult, and cause an anxiety reaction.

Psychopathic school phobia is often a symptom of more encompassing behavior dysfunction. It is merely one expression of a general dysfunction. The stress eliciting the school phobic reaction may be centered around fear of separation from the parents, fear of failure, fear of peer-group rejection and so forth. It may also be symptomatic of a general, diffuse anxiety as severe as schizophrenia.

Neurotic Reactions of Childhood

Neurotic reactions are more fixed patterns of behavior than are reactive disorders. The original environmental situation which triggered the behavioral response is no longer a direct cause of the behavior. The response has been generalized to situations which no longer justify the reaction. Neurotic reactions can be considered pathological extensions of reactive behavior. They are more severe behavioral disorders since the presence of neurotic symptoms may interfere with the process of development and lead to developmental lag.

Neurotic behavior patterns can be described as self-fulfilling prophesies. For example, a child who through some environmental situation has come to feel that everyone is hostile, is apt to react in a defensive manner. A slight brush in the school hallway, or a muffled laugh in class when the child is reciting is interpreted as an intentional, hostile act. Intentional acts or not, the child reacts as if they were, and flies into physical or verbal defense of himself. The offending child then reacts to this response by defending himself and the original prophesy is affirmed — the world is hostile. This constant reinforcement of the assessment of the environment strengthens the child's behavioral reaction pattern and makes it more fixed and rigid.

Organized neurotic behavior commonly found in adults is relatively rare in childhood.[15] Neurotic symptoms in adults are incorporated in their personality structure. This is not so in children; symptoms often occur in isolation. For example, compulsive, ritualistic behavior exhibited around the bedtime hour may be the only evidence of this symptom, while other symptoms are found in connection with other situations. This characteristic is probably due to the immaturity of the child's personality. There has not been adequate time for the child's neurotic reactions to have become a part of his personality. For this reason the incidence of neurosis increases with later childhood and adolescence.

Childhood neurosis differs from adult neurosis in another way. The neurotic symptoms of the child seem to be an effective method of alleviating the precipitating anxiety. Unlike adults, neurotic children do not suffer with their symptoms.[16] It is not the children who seek relief from their symptoms, it is their distressed families.

Neurotic children may develop phobias about such things as animals, heights, and insects, and may exhibit compulsive or obsessional behavior such as counting toys, touching certain objects, or asking repetitious questions. (Less exaggerated forms of these behaviors are normal for children of certain ages. The two- to four-year-old is likely to be very fearful of many things: animals, the dark, or strange grotesque people. Compulsive talking and counting are common when a child has just mastered these tasks.) Hysterical symptoms, such as paralysis, sensory loss, or abdominal complaints are found in later childhood and adolescence.

Children with neuroses may be treated by occupational therapists working in a community setting, such as a school or community mental health agency. Adolescents exhibiting hysterical symptoms might be seen in a general medical setting. In situations where the family is unable to cope with the child's symptoms, residential care may be recommended.

Psychosomatic Illness

Psychosomatic illnesses are those diseases or conditions which are affected by psychological variables. It is questionable as to whether the illness is actually caused by psychological stress or whether it is precipitated by it. Of course all disease has psychological components, but those termed *psychosomatic* are triggered in large part by psychological factors.

Psychosomatic illnesses can be distinguished from hysterical reactions in that they are not purely psychological in origin; physiological changes do occur within the body. Common illnesses in children that may be psychosomatic are asthma, hayfever, colitis, convulsive disorders, rheumatoid arthritis, obesity, and skin reactions such as hives, eczema and acne — although virtually any illness has the potential for being psychosomatic. A common factor in these disorders seems to be the phasic quality of the illness. There seem to be periods of remission followed by "outbreaks" or attacks. The exacerbation period can be triggered by psychological as well as by physiological stress. For example a child's asthma attack could be triggered by a high pollen count in the air — or by the child's parents planning to spend the weekend in the next city.

Occupational therapists in most pediatric settings must be aware of the possibility of illness triggered by psychological stress. Keen observations to assess the cause-effect relationships and to ascertain the stress producing situation are necessary in order to help these children find more gratifying methods of dealing with stress.

Infantile eczema   Infantile eczema was studied by Spitz in the same institution in which he researched the development of object relations. He found that the infants who developed eczema in the second half of their first year had two variables in common. First they seemed to have congenital predisposition for skin reactions, since from birth they had exaggerated responses to touch triggered reflexes, such as the rooting reflex. It seemed as if the skin of these infants was more receptive in some way.

The second common variable seemed to be the personality of the mothers of the children who developed eczema. The mothers seemed to have an attitude of anxiety about their children, with large amounts of repressed hostility toward them. These mothers did not like to touch their children and avoided doing so as much as possible. They expressed concern about the fragility of infants, yet their children seemed to be the ones most often exposed to risk and danger.

Spitz theorizes that the babies' development of eczema was brought about by the interplay of these two variables. The child who somehow seemed to require extra tactile stimulation was denied it because of his mother's personality. Eczema seemed to be the result. The children with eczema also seemed to be functioning at a lower level in terms of social functioning and learning. For example they tended not to exhibit stranger anxiety at eight months. These symptoms Spitz feels are indications of impairment in the development of object relations. The eczema might help the child by (1) providing tactile stimulation through the itching of the eczema or (2) forcing the mother to provide more tactile stimulation in caring for the eczema, or a combination of the two.

Most of the eczema was spontaneously cured near the end of the first year. Spitz feels this was due to the child's development of locomotion. The development of his object relations was no longer dependent solely upon the mother. The child now had access to the environment and the many objects in it.

It would be interesting to have follow up data which would show whether or not the child developed eczema later in life in response to environmental stress. Spitz states, "It is to be expected that the interlude of eczema, during the first year of life, will leave permanent traces on the psychic development of the child; what they are we can only surmise."[17]

Sociopathic Reactions

The types of psychosocial dysfunction which have been discussed until now have largely been concerned with psychological dysfunction. *Sociopathic reactions,* as the name implies, are disorders of social functioning. They are disorders of superego, as well as ego development. Several terms are used to denote this group of behavioral reactions: sociopathic reaction, psychopathic personality, character disorder and antisocial personality. "Sociopathic reactions" was chosen from among these terms as it seems the most descriptive and the least offensive.

Sociopathic reactions are characterized by impulsive behavior, an inability to plan ahead, a lack of empathy and concern about the feelings of others, and a lack of guilt about engaging in antisocial acts.[18] The sociopathic child tends to be intelligent, yet there seems to be a lack of consideration for the past and future, as well as a lack of consideration for the welfare of others. This child may actually exploit others to obtain his own goals. Sadistic behavior is not uncommon. The sociopathic child seems to lack insight into his own behavior and is considered incorrigible by those around him; he often becomes involved in criminal acts as the result of his impulsive behavior and need for immediate gratification.

There is some evidence to indicate that sociopathic reactions result from maternal deprivation in the first two years of life.

Children raised in orphanages, foster homes, or in their own homes with a number of mother substitutes; who received inconsistent, unstable, or rejecting care seem to have a greater tendency toward sociopathic reactions.[19] It is theorized that the child fails to develop the very early object relationships necessary for later social development to occur.

A sociopathic reaction must be differentiated from purely antisocial acts. Children who have been raised in an environment where antisocial acts are not uncommon do not develop a sense of "right and wrong" that is compatible with society at large. For example some disadvantaged ghetto adolescents may consider stealing a parked car for a "joy ride" as normal entertainment for a Saturday night. In their environment the act is not deviant. The child feels no remorse in having taken the car; he cannot, therefore, be termed a sociopathic personality because an examination of his relationships with his parents and peers shows normal ability to relate and an adequate sense of social responsibility. In contrast, a sociopathic personality would present additional indications of a poorly integrated personality, particularly in his relationships with others.

Occupational therapists employed in community mental centers, and other facilities supported by society, such as psychiatric hospitals, detention centers, and residential schools or care facilities are especially likely to come into contact with children with sociopathic reactions.

Psychosocial Dysfunction Due to Brain Damage

Damage or disease of the brain may cause behavioral dysfunction, as well as neuromotor or perceptual-motor dysfunction. It has long been known that cases of clearcut brain damage or injury also include behavioral symptoms. Disease or conditions such as epilepsy, brain tumors, severe burns, encephalitis, and meningitis are often accompanied by behavioral changes. A post-encephalitic syndrome, in a child for example, might include hyperactivity, aggressiveness, a short attention span, and sleep disturbances. [20]

What is not known, however, is the effect of less clearly defined or undetected brain damage. The effects of mild brain dysfunction due to anoxia at birth or some less severe childhood illness or injury are not well studied. The incidence of this type of etiology for behavioral symptoms may actually be on the increase with the development of greater skill in obstetrics and pediatrics. The lives of infants and children with a greater potential for minimal brain damage are being saved.

It is often difficult to distinguish between behavior problems that are the result of primary brain damage or that are secondary to organic deficit. In other words, the behavioral manifestations may be the direct result of the portion of the brain that is injured, or they may be caused by the stress of brain injury in other areas of functioning. In the latter case, treatment to improve the functioning of the child should also alleviate the reactive behavior disorder.

Symptoms of clear cut cerebral dysfunction include muscular weakness, sensory impairments, paralysis, and tremors (see neuromotor chapter). Less severe brain dysfunction may be indicated by perceptual problems, clumsiness, poor reading ability, and distractability (see perceptual-motor chapter). Behavioral symptoms which may result from brain damage are negativism, temper tantrums, withdrawal, clowning, running away, and overt signs of anxiety. These symptoms may either be the direct result of the brain damage or may be a secondary reaction to stress. Behavior reactions due to brain damage are not unlike those previously discussed. The child may present psychosomatic, sociopathic, neurotic or psychotic symptoms to the clinician.

Occupational therapists working with children must remain cognizant of the fact that behavioral symptoms may result from brain injury. In cases of severe brain damage, such as cerebral palsy, it is well to bear in mind that there may be behavioral, as well as neuromotor and perceptual dysfunction. In cases where brain damage can only be assumed, it is well to keep in mind that behavioral manifestations may be debilitating.

Psychotic Reactions of Childhood

The characteristic symptoms of psychotic children have been outlined by Creak and her associates. The symptoms are not intended as diagnostic criteria for childhood psychosis in that any or all of the symptoms must be present for the child to be considered psychotic.

1. Gross and sustained impairment of emotional relationships with people. This includes the more usual aloofness and empty clinging...; also abnormal behavior toward other people or persons, such as using them or parts of them, impersonally. Difficulty in mixing and playing with other children is often outstanding and long-lasting.
2. Apparent unawareness of his own personal identity to a degree inappropriate for his age. This may be seen in

abnormal behavior toward himself such as posturing or exploration and scrutiny of parts of his body. Repeated self-directed aggression, sometimes resulting in actual damage, may be another aspect of his lack of integration (see also point 5), as also the confusion of personal pronouns (see point 7).

3. Pathological preoccupation with particular objects or certain characteristics of them, without regard to their accepted functions.

4. Sustained resistance to change in the environment and a striving to maintain or restore sameness. In some instances behavior appears to aim at producing a state of perceptual monotony.

5. Abnormal perceptual experience (in the absence of discernible organic abnormality) is implied by excessive, diminished, or unpredictable response to sensory stimuli — for example, visual and auditory avoidance (see also points 2 and 4), and insensitivity to pain and temperature.

6. Acute, excessive, and seemingly illogical anxiety is a frequent phenomenon. This tends to be precipitated by change, whether in material environment or in routine, as well as by temporary interruption of a symbiotic attachment to persons or things (compare points 3 and 4, and also 1 and 2).

7. Speech may have been lost, or never acquired, or may have failed to develop beyond a level appropriate to an earlier stage. There may be confusion of personal pronouns (see point 2), echolalia, or other mannerisms of use and diction. Though words or phrases may be uttered, they may convey no sense of ordinary communication.

8. Distortion of motility patterns — e.g. (a.) excess as in hyperkinesis, (b.) immobility as in catatonia, (c.) bizarre postures, or ritualistic mannerisms, such as rocking and spinning (themselves or objects).

9. A background of serious retardation in which islets of normal, near normal, or exceptional intellectual function or skill may appear.[21]

The above symptoms cannot be considered exclusive to childhood psychosis. For example, Symptom 3, "pathological preoccupation with objects," is also common to mentally retarded and brain-injured children. Symptom 5, "abnormal perceptual experience," more or less defines the child with perceptual-motor dysfunction. The last symptom, "a background of serious retardation in which islets of normal, near normal or exceptional intellectual function may appear," is perhaps the single, best criteria for differential diagnosis.

Psychosis in children may be psychogenic or organic in origin. Psychotic episodes resulting from acute illness with high temperature and white blood count are not considered serious since the etiology is understood and the symptoms follow the course of the precipitating disease. Organic psychosis may also be chronic in nature as the result of degenerative disease, or as the remaining symptoms of brain injury.

Many theorists have looked to deviations in normal development in an attempt to explain psychogenic psychotic reactions. Margaret Mahler describes one theory leading to psychosis in children. She feels that the normal symbiotic relationship between the mother and child is either gravely distorted or missing in the child who develops psychosis. This may be due to a deficiency or defect in the child or to inadequate mothering. As Erikson might state, the child is unable to gain autonomy from the first primary relationship with his mother. He is not able to achieve a self image.

Bruno Bettelheim [22] offers a theory which differs only slightly from Mahler. He feels that psychosis in children develops as a result of the infant's experience at any one of several critical periods in development. Some children may develop a psychotic reaction as the result of experiences prior to the period of stranger anxiety. These are children who probably have been deprived in their early lives and have failed to develop early object relations. A second critical period in the development of psychosis parallels the development of stranger anxiety, age five to nine months. If the child in his attempts to relate to the newly differentiated object (the mother) is met with unresponsiveness, he may give up and his development of object relations will be impeded at this immature stage. The period from eighteen months to two years is the third period when psychosis may develop, according to Bettelheim. This is the age when the child can avoid contact with the world, not only on a psychological or emotional level, but also on a physical level. He can walk away and isolate himself from people and objects.

Spitz theorizes that psychotic reactions in children may be caused by disturbed development and integration of perceptual modalities. The information originating from the various senses is not correlated, for some reason, giving a distorted picture of the environment. These children appear to Spitz to be slow or unable to make the transitions from contact perceptions, such as touch and pressure, to distance perceptions, such as vision and hearing. There is research evidence to support this view; it is not known, however, whether the perceptual dysfunction of a psychotic child is a cause of the mental illness, or whether somehow the severe mental illness may cause the perceptual abnormality.[23]

Psychotic reactions of childhood are divided into several syndromes based upon a set of characteristic symptoms. The symptoms are not exclusive to the syndrome and may be seen in other psychotic reactions. For this reason, the use of these categories is not altogether justified, and many clinicians prefer to use only the more general classification of childhood psychosis. Brief descriptions of three of the more commonly used categories will be utilized as a method of describing childhood psychotic reactions in general.

Symbiotic syndrome   Mahler describes the symbiotic child as being unable to separate or individuate himself from the caring person. There does not appear to be any clear distinction between the child and the mother, and the child panics with any separation from the mother. The symbiotic child appears overly sensitive to his environment and extremely dependent upon others.

The earliest symptoms of the symbiotic syndrome may be a difficult baby who does not sleep well, cannot adjust to change, and in general is oversensitive. Severe reactions do not usually occur until early childhood when in normal development the child begins to become independent from the mother. Mahler feels that the maturational acquisition of locomotor abilities, and the challenge to self by the Oedipal conflict during the third and fourth year are the precipitating factors. The world is interpreted as threatening because it must be met as a separate being. Separations caused by enrollment in nursery school, birth of a sibling, or by illness may trigger the psychotic reaction.

The resultant anxiety is overwhelming and incapacitating. Delusions and hallucinations may serve to restore the symbiotic relationship. The boundaries of the self and the nonself become blurred and the child maintains closeness to the mother at every opportunity to protect himself.

The symbiotic child is prey to many traumas. Every small incident is enough to cause regression for a number of weeks. A normal bump or bruise may be enough to keep the child from walking. Excessive autoerotic activities, such as rocking, masturbation, and the "twiddling" of small objects between the fingers are behaviors the symbiotic child may use to relieve anxiety during periods of stress.

The symbiotic reaction is very trying for the parents. In the symbiotic syndrome the parents, and particularly the mother, become involved in the illness. The symbiotic child is also difficult in that he appeared to be normal until about three to four years of age, at which time his behavior deteriorated and regressed.

Infantile autism   Infantile autism is perhaps the most severe form of psychosis in childhood and one that is commonly seen as a unique form of childhood psychosis. Bettelheim calls these children "strangers to life."[24] He theorizes that they never develop the initial forms of object relations and, therefore, they have no means of knowing life.

The most typical symptom of autistic children is their noncommitment to the world. They show no perceivable response to their environment of humans and objects. Everything in the environment, from a sonic boom to their parents, is disregarded equally. Bettelheim feels that this mode of behavior is adopted as a defense against extreme anxiety and panic.

> Autistic children ... not only fear constantly for their lives, they seem convinced that death is imminent; that possibly it can be postponed just for moments through their not taking cognizance of life.[25]

Bettelheim feels that the anxiety is a result of the child's correct interpretation of the negative emotions which the significant figures in his environment have for him. He develops the state of mind that life is without hope. The child at such an early age has no counterbalance for such a force, and his defense is to adopt the autistic position.

Kanner outlined the traditional symptoms of autism as an inability to relate to other people, a delay in the acquisition of speech along with abnormalities of language, an exceptional rote memory, and a desire to prevent changes in the environment.

Language is never used or is characteristically given up in the autistic child. Echolalic speech, the use of neologisms or the continuous repetition of songs and television commercials may remain as uncommunicative speech. In children who do retain their language, there usually is a marked developmental lag in its use and consequently a lag in intellectual processes. Bruno Bettleheim has found that autistic children who do retain the use of language have a much better prognosis than those who do not. Pronouns tend not to be used, especially *I*. The child seems unable to make reference to himself as "I," and instead refers to himself as "you" or by his own name.

Autistic children also seem insensitive to pain. Bettelheim reports the case of an autistic girl who was obviously quite ill, having a high temperature and white blood count. It was suspected that she had appendicitis but there was no reaction to abdominal palpatation and she showed no signs of abdominal pain. Eventually she became comatose and exploratory surgery revealed a ruptured appendix. This insensitivity to pain seems to indicate that autistic children are as alienated from the inner world of their body as they are from the world external to them. Despite the seeming lack of response to pain within the body, these children characteristically fight any intrusion into their body from the outside world. Injections or dental repair are two intrusions which they struggle valiantly, and often successfully, to avoid.

In the clinical setting it is often difficult to observe children who present a clearcut picture of either the autistic or symbiotic position. As Bettelheim illustrates in his case histories, the autistic child may present many symbiotic behaviors in the process of giving up his autistic position. Bettelheim considers this a step toward more mature functioning.

Childhood schizophrenia   The term *childhood schizophrenia* is used by most clinicians instead of, or synonomous with, childhood psychosis. Childhood schizophrenia is not defined by a set of symptoms or a "position" as is autism or symbiosis. Some clinicians use it as a more general term, including infantile autism and symbiotic syndromes as subcategories of childhood schizophrenia.[26]

Other clinicians prefer not to use the term in diagnosing children, since there are few parallels to adult schizophrenia.[27] Anna Freud feels that the child's illness is unlike the adult's, much as childhood neurosis differs from adult neurosis. This is not meant to imply that the origins of adult schizophrenia do not lie in childhood. Anna Freud suggests that the origins of adult schizophrenia may be reactive disorders, neurosis, or psychosis of childhood, or that the basic personality defect resulting in adult schizophrenia may have been undetected in childhood, and seen only in retrospect.

Adult-like schizophrenia may develop in adolescence with the characteristic indifference to the events of reality, and the splitting of thought from its normal affect.[28] The stress of adolescence together with the capacity for a more organized type of illness due to further ego development make a schizophrenic reaction possible. Virtually any type of schizophrenic reaction is possible in adolescence. Acute reactions and catatonia are two of the more common adolescent responses.

The child with a psychotic reaction is often placed in a residential care situation, particularly once he is of an age when he may be difficult to manage in the home. A residential treatment center can offer the protection of confined play areas and the specially adapted living quarters necessary for many of these children. Some, particularly the younger children, may remain at home and be treated in day-care centers or on an outpatient basis. These children may also turn up in unlikely places, such as special classes for aphasic children, and institutions for the retarded.

Summary

Childhood psychosocial dysfunction has been traced from so-called normal functioning to the most severe psychosocial disorder, childhood psychosis. Normal functioning was shown to include behavioral problems resulting from the stress of the maturational process. Reactive behavior disorders included those behavioral manifestations which were reactions to environmental stress. Neurotic behavior was identified as pervading most of the functioning of the child and as being a fixed response no longer attributable to environmental stress. Childhood psychosis was defined in terms of nine characteristic symptoms and of its origins in the deviation of early development. The diagnostic categories of symbiotic syndrome, infantile autism, and childhood schizophrenia were discussed. Psychosomatic illness, sociopathic disorders, and behavior problems due to brain damage were also presented (see Figure 5-2).

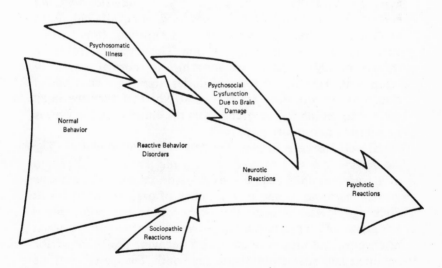

FIG. 5-2. Continuum of psychosocial functioning.

The occupational therapist working with children in any setting will be confronted by behavior problems. The purpose of this section has been to aid the therapist in making an assessment of the severity of the problem and its probable cause. The purpose of the next section will be to aid the therapist in managing and treating the problem.

Evaluation and Treatment of Psychosocial Dysfunction

UNDERSTANDING AND MANAGING NORMAL CHILDREN

Several manuals designed to aid parents in managing their children are equally useful to the occupational therapist working with children. They are helpful when actually working with normal children as in a general medical setting, and are equally helpful when working with children with psychosocial dysfunction.

Dr. Benjamin Spock's best seller, *Baby and Child Care,* is one such manual. He outlines possible solutions to many physical as well as emotional problems encountered in childhood. Such problems as colic, weaning, thumbsucking, toilet training, feeding problems, stuttering, sex education, and so forth are discussed from a pediatrician's point of view.

Selma Fraiberg's book, *The Magic Years: Understanding and Handling the Problems of Early Childhood,* is equally helpful to the occupational therapist working with children. It is written from more of a psychoanalytic viewpoint. The author discusses the problems of childhood in relationship to normal stages of development. Her discussions of toilet training, the Oedipal period, and sex education are particularly helpful. Her approach of presenting childhood problems from the child's point of view is both amusing and informative.

The Gesell Institute Books, *The First Five Years of Life, The Child From Five to Ten,* and *Youth, the Years From Ten to Sixteen,* are helpful because they provide data on the average child's functioning in any of a number of areas of behavior at various age levels. Growth gradients follow the sequence of development of such behaviors as personal hygiene, interpersonal relationships, and ethical sense, while behavior profiles describe the child at each year of childhood and youth. The Gesell Institute books are useful in outlining the types of problems typical of children at any given age.

A fourth source recommended for its usefulness in working with children is Haim Ginott's *Between Parent and Child.* Ginott recommends a method he calls *talking childrenese.* This approach is particularly useful in working with children with psychosocial dysfunction.

Childrenese is a method of verbal communication used with children. It is based upon respect and skill. Ginott developed this method in his work with group play therapy. He presents several principles of conversing with children. He illustrates each principle with examples of how to implement his method.

1. When a child tells of, or asks about, an event, it is frequently best to respond, not to the event, but to the relationship implied.
2. When a child tells of an event, it is sometimes helpful to respond, not to the event itself, but to the feelings around it.
3. When a child makes a statement about himself, it is often desirable to respond, not with agreement or disagreement, but with details that convey to the child an understanding beyond expectation.[29]

Dr. Ginott also recommends helping the child to know his feelings by mirroring his emotions for him. Statements like, "I know you must hate to have to share your room with your brother," help the child to acknowledge his feelings and provide him with the opportunity for examining them.

Guidelines to help the adult deal with his feelings when working with children are also provided by Dr. Ginott. Adults should be able to express their emotions to the child in a manner which will help the child to understand what he has done to provoke these feelings. He provides adults with "three steps to survival":

1. We (adults) accept the fact that children will make us angry.
2. We are entitled to our anger without guilt or shame.
3. Except for one safeguard, we are entitled to express what we feel. We can express our angry feelings *provided* we do not attack the child's personality or character.[30]

Statements such as "I feel angry" and "I'm greatly annoyed" expressed with the proper affect help the child to know how the adult is feeling. Sometimes it is necessary for the adult to add to the statement of feeling the reason for the anger and the inner reaction it is causing, for example, "When you leave your things lying around I get furious. I feel like gathering them up and tossing them out the door."

INTRODUCTION TO THE EVALUATION
AND TREATMENT OF
CHILDHOOD PSYCHOSOCIAL DYSFUNCTION

A rationale for the treatment of psychosocial dysfunction in children will be proposed followed by a method of evaluation and treatment based upon this rationale. Other approaches to treatment and evaluation will then be presented. Each approach will be discussed in terms of its advantages, its disadvantages, the role of the occupational therapist using its methods, and the required evaluation. Examples of treatment will then be presented as a method of acquainting the reader with the treatment procedure.

Each of the approaches to treatment are presented in their "pure form"; that is, they are presented as proposed by the theorists or clinicians who developed the approach. In some cases the approaches are not original to occupational therapy, but come from other clinical professions, such as pediatric psychiatry and psychology.

The approaches to treatment were chosen based upon their current or suggested use in pediatric occupational therapy. They are approaches not unknown to occupational therapists, nor are they antithetical to the occupational therapy approach.

The treatment examples are not all from the occupational therapy literature. The reason for the choice is that in attempting to present the "pure form" of a treatment approach, it was felt most expedient to present a treatment example which clearly illustrates the approach. Most occupational therapy treatment is not "pure" in this sense. Occupational therapists usually create treatment plans based upon a number of approaches which, therefore, do not serve as good illustrations of any single approach. (References to occupational therapy literature which have not been utilized in this chapter are provided in the reading list.)

The purpose of this approach to the presentation of the treatment of childhood psychosocial dysfunction is to provide the reader with a firm understanding of the various treatment rationales. It is intended that with this background, the reader will then be able to formulate the treatment plan most appropriate for his patient.

Proposed rationale for the evaluation and treatment of psychosocial dysfunction in children   In the course of the development of normal psychosocial behavior, development proceeds in approximately the same sequence for each child. To state this another way, each child recapitulates the same sequence of development as have children before him. This principle is basic to most theories of development, although it is frequently left unstated. Each theorist describes the developmental process from a slightly different point of view or in slightly different terms, but basically what he is describing is the sequence in which development occurs.

Children who present some form of psychosocial dysfunction are exhibiting a deviation in the sequence of normal development or normal functioning. The deviation may be an exaggeration of normal development, as with reactive behavior disorders, psychosomatic illnesses, and neurotic reactions, or they may be due to faulty development — as is suspected in psychotic reactions of childhood, brain-damaged children with behavioral manifestations, and sociopathic children.

To correct or treat the child exhibiting psychosocial dysfunction, it would seem rational that the approach would be to facilitate the sequence of normal development. The person treating the child would help him adopt normal patterns of behavior. Lela Llorens expressed this view succinctly in her 1969 Eleanor Clarke Slagle Lecture, although her remarks were not confined to psychosocial dysfunction in children. They were intended as a conceptual model for treatment in all of occupational therapy.

> ... occupational therapy is a facilitation process which assists the individual in achieving mastery of life tasks and the ability to cope as efficiently as possible with the life expectations made of him.... The occupational therapist serves as the enculturation agent for the conditions of physical, social and psychological health in which the developmental level being experienced by the individual in any one of a number of parameters of development is unequal to the age-related demands of that organism as a result of natural or traumatic incident.[31]

Mastery of Developmental Tasks Approach (MDTA)

The MDTA can be described as a direct application of the theoretical approach outlined above. It is characterized by helping the child master tasks appropriate to his age level by recapitulating the sequence of normal development until parity is achieved between the child's chronological age and his level of functioning.

The advantages of the MDTA are many. First, it is applicable to all areas of dysfunction in children — indeed, to dysfunction of all individuals, according to Llorens. This general applicability of the

MDTA has advantages when the total field of pediatrics is considered. Children, unlike adults, are changing quickly. The maturation process does not stop if there is a slow down dysfunction in one area of development. For this reason, dysfunction in one carries over to the other areas. The MDTA is effective because it can ameliorate dysfunctions simultaneously in many different areas.

This approach is also appropriate when the problem of differential diagnosis is considered. Because of the difficulty in determining etiology and, therefore, making an accurate diagnosis, treatment appropriate for only a specific disease may miss its mark. For example, the distinction between infantile autism and mental retardation may be impossible to make. If the child is treated on the basis of his deviation from normal development, however, the MDTA will be appropriate no matter what the diagnostic label; if the child were treated with psychotherapy, the approach may be appropriate if the child is autistic, but not if he is mentally retarded.

The MDTA is flexible in its application. It is appropriate for children with dysfunction of varying severity. It can be applied in nearly any treatment setting. It is equally applicable to a residential treatment center as it is to a community mental health program. It is applicable to both group and individual treatment sessions. It can be a formal, well-planned treatment approach, or an adjunct to another treatment method.

The disadvantage of this approach lies in the lack of knowledge of how the normal recapitulation sequence is modified by faulty development in one parameter of behavior. For example, an autistic child seems to have gross motor abilities nearly commensurate with his chronological age. His fine motor and perceptual-motor abilities are perhaps further behind his age level. In the parameter of psychosocial behavior, however, he continues to function at the level of an infant or toddler. How does the fact that this child's motor ability far exceeds his psychosocial ability affect the sequence in which his psychosocial development will occur? To carry this example further, it is known that locomotion is an important contributor to the development of the self image in the toddler; yet the autistic child has not successfully developed his first object relations. How does the fact that he has developed locomotion modify the manner in which he will develop his self image? This issue is one that deserves much research and investigation. Perhaps as more clinicians use this MDTA to treatment, the more will be learned.

The role of the occupational therapist utilizing a MDTA is that of a developmental therapist. His goal is to facilitate mastery of developmental tasks. Anne Mosey sees the relationship between the therapist and child in the MDTA as a teaching-learning one. She describes the occupational therapist as a teacher who is "oriented to 'assisting the individual to develop those skills which will permit him to function more adequately in his environment...' "[32]

Evaluation To evaluate a child in preparation for treatment using the MDTA, it is necessary to ascertain his present level of functioning in several parameters of psychosocial behavior. Anne Mosey's manual, *Occupational Therapy: Theory and Practice,* or her text, *Three Frames of Reference for Mental Health,* can be helpful in providing some guidelines. Mosey organizes development into several learned patterns of behavior which she terms "adaptive skills." She then traces the usual sequence of development of each adaptive skill from its inception to its maturity. For example, one such skill is the Primary Group Interaction Skill which she defines as "the ability to participate productively in a variety of primary groups." [33] She outlines five sequential stages in the development of this skill, the first four of which apply to the childhood years.

1. The ability to attend to individual tasks in the presence of others.
2. The ability to interact in a short-term task with others, the duration of the relationship being determined by the task.
3. The ability to interact cooperatively and competitively in a long-term task, the interaction of the self being characterized by enlightened self interest.
4. The ability to satisfy social-emotional needs of others in a same sex group.[34]

Havighurst's developmental tasks, the work of the Gesell Institute, and Erikson's "Eight Stages of Man" offer other sources of guidelines in evaluating the psychosocial functioning of the child.

Once the guidelines have been set the method of obtaining the evaluation data are determined. An interview with the child's parents is one method of obtaining data (Chapter Two). For example, an inquiry such as "How does Johnny participate when there are other children present for him to play with?" may elicit information pertinent to establishing Johnny's level of functioning in the Primary Group Interaction Skill described earlier.

An alternate method, and perhaps a preferable one, would be to place Johnny in a group situation and observe his participation. It would then be possible to make a direct assessment of his functioning in this area of development.

Unfortunately, not all aspects of psychosocial functioning are as simple to evaluate. Direct observation may not provide the needed data to make an assessment about the status of the self image, for example. Less direct indicators may need to be interpreted in order to make the evaluation. This is a dangerous practice because it lends subjectivity to the evaluation. This problem is one that both plagues and provides the challenge of the behavioral sciences.

Using the self image parameter of behavior as an example, what methods of investigating its status are possible? Verbal information provides the most obvious source of data. Does the child seem to convey a positive picture of himself or does he speak of himself in deprecatory terms? Nonverbal clues of posture, facial expression and gait are also helpful.

Another source of information might come through an interpretation of a child's human figure drawings. Several sources suggest the correlation between the child's sense of self and his drawing, and have developed criteria of normal drawings of children at various ages.[35]

The close proximity between the psychosocial concept of self image and the more perceptual-motor concept of body concept have led to the use of diagnostic tools designed for assessing body concept as fairly accurate indicators of self image. Some of the assessment techniques designed by Jean Ayres, such as body visualization, crossing the mid-line of the body, and gross and fine motor planning, are one source of body concept data which may shed light upon the status of the self image.

The occupational therapist working in a pediatric psychiatric setting may wish to evaluate a child in other areas of functioning — in addition to the psychosocial area. Some clinicians recommend that the occupational therapist assess neuromotor and perceptual-motor functioning, as well as psychosocial, as an aid to diagnosis and in preparation for treatment.[36] In this situation the occupational therapist would be conducting a developmental evaluation (Chapter Seven).

Special problems exist in evaluating children with psychosocial dysfunction. The problems are inherent in the nature of their dysfunction. One problem may be gaining the cooperation of the child. It may be difficult to assess the potential of a child who consistently responds in a negative or withdrawn manner — or that of the child who responds to new situations as stressful. His use of ritualistic or autoerotic behavior to reduce the stress may make evaluation impossible until such time as the situation is no longer stress producing.

Various methods can be utilized to reduce stress for these children. They may be evaluated in the presence of their mothers or in a familiar environment, such as the home. Evaluation may need to be preceded or accompanied by time to adjust to the therapist and the situation.

In addition to assessing the child's level of functioning in several behavioral parameters, it is also important to gain other information to aid in the treatment planning process. Data about the specific interests of the child can be useful. Is the child particularly interested in drawing and painting, cooking or playing outdoors? It is also useful to know what methods of management have been successful or have failed with the child. Does he respond to a structured approach rather than an informal one? Does he respond to a verbal or nonverbal approach?

Occupational therapy evaluation techniques have some advantages over the more formal methods of psychological testing of children with psychosocial dysfunction, particularly those children whose illness is quite severe. By its very nature the occupational therapy evaluation can be less formal or structured and can easily be adapted to the needs and wishes of the child. Psychological tests, however, must be administered in a systematic and formal manner in order for the results to be valid. These characteristics often make it impossible for the child with psychosocial dysfunction to tolerate formal testing. Another advantage of an occupational therapy evaluation is that it is not dependent upon verbal responses. Nonverbal behavior is equally received. The occupational evaluation has the third advantage of using materials familiar and interesting to the child. The toys, equipment, art materials, games and food available in the occupational therapist's repertoire of evaluation materials makes the occupational therapy evaluation more appealing to the child.

Once the evaluation data has been gathered it should be studied to designate the primary areas of developmental deficit in the child. Treatment goals should be established and the priorities of treatment worked out. Plans for treatment are then made utilizing all the data, and taking into account the "givens" of the setting in which treatment is to occur (see section on treatment planning, Chapter Three).

Treatment   The goal of treatment in the MDTA is to help the child develop psychosocial patterns of behavior more closely in line with what is expected for his chronological age. The exact techniques employed vary widely — depending upon the child, the therapist, and the setting in which treatment is to occur.

The first example of treatment using the MDTA comes from a paper which discusses methods of achieving mastery of problems involving separation-individuation.[37] Occupational therapy was used in a residential treatment center to help children of varying ages and with varying degrees of psychosocial dysfunction to master tasks of separation-individuation.

Separation anxiety was illustrated by behaviors such as refusal to leave the ward for occupational therapy — and then refusal to leave therapy to return to the ward. Individuation problems were seen as the inability to make decisions, requiring the help of the therapist to draw or paint, and a need for the close physical presence of the therapist.

In each case, the use of activities that were meaningful to the child were employed. These activities included making a scrapbook, cooking, reading to the child, painting, and making a garden fence. Along with the activity as the basis for treatment, several methods of helping the child master the tasks of separation-individuation were used. "Leaving rehearsals" were used to give the child practice in the difficult process of separation. Teaching the child to tell time was used as a method of helping the child to anticipate and prepare for separation at the end of the session. Transitional objects, such as a painting the child had done, or a paper airplane he had folded, were used to make returning to the ward easier, since he could take along a small reminder of the occupational session. Sometimes games were utilized to help the child master the task of separation-individuation.

Sandra Watanabe presents another example of MDTA to treatment in a completely different setting and utilizing different techniques. Her patients were treated in the home with the treatment modalities found in the home and community. She describes her treatment goal as "helping the individual to master his life tasks." She presents her treatment of Robert, a nineteen-year-old schizophrenic. She helped him master his life tasks utilizing such activities as learning how to use public transportation, buying birthday presents for his family, and learning the carpentry trade. With this help Robert was better able to function at a level more nearly commensurate with his age.

A third example of the MDTA comes not from an occupational therapist, but from a child psychiatrist. Stella Chess sees mastery of an activity as one approach to the treatment of psychotic children. Her rationale for this treatment approach is based upon her observations that psychotic children have prolonged and intensified problems in mastering their environment, as evidenced by their repetitious and perseverative behavior. Echolalic speech, compulsive and ritualistic behavior, exaggerated reaction to certain stimuli and primitive patterns of thought are all indications of mastery problems.

She describes her treatment of a psychotic child using this approach. She utilized the child's interest in balloons as the vehicle of her treatment. She began by getting the child to differentiate between the "long skinny" balloons and the "round fat" ones. Matching and picking out differently colored balloons was then learned. Further along in treatment the child was taught some of the physical laws of nature using the balloons. For example, the child was shown that a balloon filled with water falls faster than a balloon filled with air. Activities of daily living were incorporated into this lesson when the inevitable occurred: the water-filled balloon broke.

Gradually other toys were introduced as the patient demonstrated a willingness to master other objects. More and more verbal communication took place — with the patient asking questions of the therapist. Questions were asked about the relationships between people and the wishes and desires of others. More and more social behavior was discussed with an emphasis upon teaching the child the rules of behavior, such as how to share, what it means to be polite, and in contrast, what it means to hurt others.

Chess reports a feeling of warm attachment growing between herself and the patient, an attachment which Chess describes as similar to that which children frequently form with certain teachers. The relationship she feels stems from the satisfaction and success the child feels over developing mastery of his environment.

Milieu Therapy

The term *milieu* is used in two similar but slightly different contexts in relationship to treating children with psychosocial dysfunction. The term *milieu therapy* is used to designate a plan for residential treatment of children in which the everyday environment is arranged to help the child learn more appropriate methods of behavior. The second use of the term, *therapeutic milieu,* is a more general concept. Its goal is to establish an atmosphere conducive to recovery and in which the basic needs of the child are met. The two terms, milieu therapy and therapeutic milieu, are not clearly separated in the literature and are often used interchangeably.

Milieu therapy is appropriate for nearly all diagnostic categories when removal from the home is either necessary for treatment or required because of the behavioral symptoms of the child. The milieu therapy approach usually can be modified to work in nearly any setting which provides some degree of residential care. Many of the principles used in creating a therapeutic milieu for the child with psychosocial dysfunction are applicable to all areas of pediatrics. In any situation in which an environment must be created for the child away from home, consideration must be given to planning the environment to be conducive to recovery.

Milieu therapy may be difficult to provide because of personnel limitations and to limitations in the physical setting. It is often difficult to find personnel willing to become ward staff for mentally ill children. It can be a threatening, taxing, thankless responsibility, with long hours and poor working conditions. Many times the physical setting is unable to be adapted to accommodate a therapeutic milieu. Residential care centers built to accommodate many children in a dormitory fashion do little to meet the individual needs of children for privacy and a place of their own.

Anne Mosey and Gail Fidler describe the role of the occupational therapist in providing a therapeutic milieu as a mental health worker. A mental health worker works with others to provide an environment in which the basic psychological needs of the child may be satisfied. The occupational therapist who works as a mental health worker may act as a consultant to non-professional ward staff in helping to provide a therapeutic milieu — or may actually provide an environment in occupational therapy treatment — which helps to meet the needs of children. The therapist may also be meeting treatment goals specific to each patient at the same time.

Evaluation   Much of what was discussed about the evaluation procedure in the MDTA is appropriate to an evaluation in a milieu approach. It is important to assess the area of psychosocial development in which the child is not functioning at the expected level for his age.

Data about the home environment is often useful in knowing how to create a successful therapeutic milieu. Information — such as the child's daily schedule, his food and eating habits, his sleeping patterns, his favorite activities, his usual playmates, and household responsibilities — can help in creating an environment conducive to treatment and aid the child in adjusting to new living conditions.

Once the assessment has been made of the child's present level of functioning, the treatment goals are established. The occupational therapist and other mental health workers determine how to plan the milieu to meet the treatment goals. For example, for a child with a bedwetting problem, the milieu therapy team may decide that the best approach would be to have the ward staff get the child up twice a night for toileting.

Treatment   Two examples of a milieu approach to treatment will be presented. The first describes the role of the occupational therapist in helping to provide a therapeutic milieu. Llorens and Rubin describe a therapeutic milieu appropriate for emotionally disturbed children in their book, *Developing Ego Functions in Disturbed Children: Occupational Therapy in Milieu.* The occupational therapist is a member of a mental health team, each member of which is responsible for a certain aspect of the therapeutic milieu. Occupational therapy

> ...provides a setting, activities, and interpersonal relationships through which the child can increase his mastery of objects and management of his body as well as acquire appropriate social skills and behavioral control.[38]

The authors provide some guidelines for helping emotionally disturbed children change their behavior, and some techniques that can be used effectively by the occupational therapist in providing a therapeutic milieu. They make the following recommendations for managing aggressive behavior:

1. Define the boundaries of the limits to the child, delineating what behavior will be permitted, what behavior will be tolerated, and what behavior will be controlled.
2. Define the purpose for the boundary and explain why certain kinds of behavior will be controlled — it will hurt him or someone else.
3. Keep limits consistent, clear, and reasonable.
4. Avoid seducing children into behavior which is unacceptable by suggestion, such as "I know you won't be able to listen," or by introducing forbidden objects into the child's environment.
5. Restate and enforce the limits as often as necessary.[39]

The following are techniques which can be useful in helping the child control his behavior:

1. Planned ignoring: ignoring unacceptable behavior which may be tolerated but not approved, in such a way that the

behavior is discontinued from lack of attention paid to it.

2. Proximity or touch control: sitting next to the child or touching him on the shoulder or arm may be enough to control certain kinds of behavior.
3. Extra attention and affection: giving reassurance, attention, and affection before the child finds it necessary to behave unacceptably to receive the attention and affection he desires.
4. Extra help over a difficult situation: clarifying the situation for the child, using the situation to help the child to develop insight and realize why things went wrong and what might be done to avoid a recurrence.
5. Restructuring the activity or situation: removing gadgets and other objects which seduce the child into unacceptable behavior; changing the activity for the child if it is too stimulating, too difficult, or too boring; and removing the child from situations contributing to unacceptable behavior.
6. Direct appeal: appealing to the child's sense of fairness and his responsibility as a member of a group.[40]

Useful methods of managing the environment for withdrawn, fearful or inhibited children are also presented.

1. Provide the child with a benign setting and easily available protective adults.
2. Reduce stress of competition and expectation beyond the child's level of competence.
3. Provide structure and routine initially. A gradual decrease of such structure may be introduced as the child is able to tolerate it.
4. React in a nonjudgmental manner to behavior and attitudes displayed by the child.
5. Avoid a too-close affectional relationship by personnel initially.[41]

An example of a more intense use of milieu therapy with psychotic children has been provided by Bruno Bettelheim in his book *Love Is Not Enough*. This book outlines the milieu of the Orthogenic School for psychotic children. He describes many aspects of a child's life, waking in the morning, eating, learning, playing, bathing, toileting and bedtime, and how the successful management of each can help the child learn new behavior. "Love is not enough" to treat these children; it is also necessary to provide a certain milieu which will foster normal behavior.

The staff of the Orthogenic School is the provider of this milieu. The staff members come from varied backgrounds and training. Each comes with special skills, as well as his own unique personality, which present a set of characteristics which will appeal to the needs of some particular child.

The role of the occupational therapist working in this setting would differ somewhat from the role described by Llorens and Rubin. The therapist's work would be limited to a few children for whom he would provide a primary relationship and environment. The therapist would not be working as a representative of his profession, but as an individual with a unique personality and set of skills for working with mentally ill children. In some ways this role might be more fulfilling for the therapist who would be the primary treatment agent for a small number of children. It would also have its drawbacks, since the therapist would also have the primary responsibility for the child's mental health.

The intensive milieu approach outlined by Bettelheim is quite effective in treating some psychotic children. It is, however, a long treatment process and one that is very expensive. For these reasons, it is difficult to implement in many residential treatment centers to the extent which Bettelheim and his staff utilize it. A team approach similar to the one described by Llorens and Rubin is perhaps more feasible for treating larger numbers of children.

Behavior Therapy

Behavior therapy, or conditioning therapy, is a set of therapeutic methods based upon principles of learning. The methods of experimental psychology have been applied to the clinical setting as a method of changing behavior. Inappropriate behavior is felt to be the result of faulty learning. In order to change behavior, the environment of the child is manipulated so that the child will be able to learn appropriate behavioral responses. Appropriate behavior is positively reinforced, whereas inappropriate behavior is either not reinforced or is reinforced negatively.

Behavior therapy is gaining increasing recognition as an effective treatment method in psychiatry. It is particularly effective with children for whom many "things" and events can act as positive reinforcement. Adults, it seems, are not as easily pleased. Behavior modification has been effective in changing the behavior of many types of clinical dysfunction, but perhaps it is best known for its results in changing neurotic reactions, particularly phobic reactions.[42] The effectiveness of the treatment varies, of course, with the pervasiveness of the dysfunction. More success is to be expected with children with limited inappropriate behavior, such as phobic reactions, than children with pervasive psychotic reactions. The effectiveness of behavior therapy is also dependent upon the strength of the reinforcers used to shape behavior and the manner in which they are utilized. A formal treatment program in which many variables can be controlled and in which a strong reinforcement can be applied will be more effective than a loosely applied treatment program in which there is no strong reinforcement. Despite a seemingly loose program, however, the effectiveness can still be dramatic. Such natural reinforcement as positive attention from a therapist, in the form of a "good" or "uh-huh" or a smile, have been shown to produce dramatic changes in behavior.

Behavior modification techniques are particularly useful in treatment planning. Unlike psychoanalytically oriented techniques, which are based upon theoretical assumptions, behavior therapy deals directly with the behavior that is inappropriate. For example, phobic reactions are assumed to be the result of a faulty learning process, whereas the psychoanalytic interpretation of the behavior might assume that the phobic reaction is due to unresolved castration anxiety. In the behavioral approach, the treatment procedure follows the assumption quite clearly; some method must be utilized which will help the child unlearn the inappropriate behavior and learn a more appropriate mode of response. Behavior therapy offers several concrete methods of approach; the psychoanalytic assumption, in contrast, leaves the treatment approach unclear.

Perhaps the most positive aspect of behavior therapy is its promise for the future. As more skill is obtained in evaluating psychosocial dysfunction from a behavioral point of view and planning treatment to change behavior, behavior therapy will become increasingly useful.

Objections to using a behavior therapy approach to treatment arise from several sources. Some clinicians seem to be apprehensive about the responsibility of modifying behavior, feeling that unintended behavior may be propagated as well as intended behavior. They are frightened by both the desirable and undesirable behavioral changes which have been made with animals. They also question their right to manipulate the existence of another human and to be the determinant of what behavior is to be considered desirable. If it were not for the effectiveness of this approach these fears would not be founded. Discussion fostered by such fears are healthy and useful in controlling the ethical uses of behavior modification techniques.[43]

Several clinicians have recommended occupational therapy as providing an environment which can be utilized to modify behavior."⁴⁴ Occupational therapy is also recommended as providing a setting in which an assessment can be made of possible positive reinforcers for a child. Food, specific playthings, positive attention, or other things attractive to the child can be used as rewards, and then evaluated in terms of their potential for changing behavior.

Behavior modification principles can be used in an informal way in conjunction with other approaches to treatment. For example, an occupational therapist who employs the MDTA in treatment may incorporate behavior therapy techniques in helping the child to develop mastery of certain tasks. The procedure may also be occurring in a setting in which the occupational therapist is helping to provide a therapeutic milieu for the child.

Evaluation The evaluation of the child with psychosocial dysfunction in preparation for treatment with behavior therapy techniques is designed to assess the child's behavior. Kanfer and Saslow offer some helpful suggestions on approaches to this task. They suggest assessing the behavior of the child that is both problematic and nonproblematic, by answering such questions as: Under what conditions does the problematic behavior occur? What satisfactions continue for the child if such problematic behavior were to continue? Who objects to the problematic behavior? What reinforces nonproblematic behavior?

The answer to these questions may be ascertained by direct observation of the child in his daily activities, by interview with the child and/or parents, and by observation of the child in a controlled setting such as occupational therapy. It takes skill and practice, however, to become astute in answering the questions. It is difficult to be able to react to the child and at the same time assess the factors that are influencing his behavior.

Example of treatment   There are many techniques of behavior therapy which have been employed to change the behavior of children. Shaping, systematic desensitization, and aversion therapy are three commonly employed methods. It is not within the scope of this presentation to outline the techniques of each type of behavior modification method, rather an example of behavior therapy will be discussed to provide a model.

Loovas et al. present a method of initiating imitative speech in mute autistic children, which is the discrimination-training procedure they utilized with two six-year-old boys whom they describe as being "profoundly schizophrenic."

The training was intensive. It was conducted six days a week for seven hours each day with a fifteen-minute rest during each hour.

The child sat facing the therapist and the therapist prevented the child from leaving the training session. Single spoonfuls of the child's meal were used as positive reinforcement, while spanking or yelling at the child was used to punish inattentive, self-destructive, or negative behavior.

The training program consisted of four steps. In the first step the child was rewarded for all vocal responses and for visually focusing on the therapist's mouth. The first step was continued until the child was making at least one verbal response during every five seconds, and was visually attending to the therapist's mouth at least fifty percent of the time.

Step two involved getting the child's verbal response to follow the therapist's verbal stimuli. The adult would emit a vocal stimuli about every ten seconds, and the child would be positively reinforced if he responded vocally within six seconds.

Step three differed slightly in that the child's response must approximate the vocal stimuli. The therapist chose the stimuli from a number of possible choices. The words and sounds were selected for several reasons. First, sounds were chosen that were easily visible (the sound of *b* as in "baby" and "bottle" is a good example). Sounds frequently used by the child in step one were also employed.

Step four was similar to three except that different stimuli were added to the words and sounds presented for the child to imitate. The child actually had to discriminate between new and old words and sounds. This was true imitative speech. Additional sounds, words and phrases were then added as quickly as the child could correctly imitate ten consecutive stimuli. After twenty-six days of training, starting with the introduction of step three, both children had learned to imitate new words with rapidity and ease. They were then introduced to a new program, wherein they were taught to use language for communication rather than just to imitate language.

Play Therapy

Play therapy is characterized by allowing the child to "play-through" his conflicts, tensions, frustrations, insecurities, and fears. The responsibility for changing behavior is the child's. The therapist acts as an accepting, understanding adult who provides security in the play situation. The therapist's role is to reflect back to the child in a nondirect manner that which he is expressing either in his play or verbally. The therapist's goal is to provide the environment from which the child can change his behavior.

Play therapy is particularly effective with children with reactive behavior disorders, psychosomatic illnesses, and with some neurotic reactions. It also has the advantage of being applicable to either group or individual therapy sessions. Group therapy sessions have the advantage of helping the child change his behavior in peer group relationships, as well as adult relationships.

The disadvantages of play therapy are the length of time necessary for treatment to continue and the lack of effectiveness with some children. In order for play therapy to be effective, the child must have the ability to express his "problem" in a symbolic manner. For this reason play therapy cannot be used with a young child or with a child with limited intellectual capacity.

The concept of play therapy is readily amenable to occupational therapy. An occupational therapist's familiarity with children's activities makes the play therapy treatment model a natural for occupational therapy. The possible problem might be the reluctance of the occupational therapist to act as a feedback system for the child. Several therapists have felt that this is an appropriate role for the occupational therapist and have recommended the practice in other contexts. Diasio sees the occupational therapist helping the patient to understand the implications and consequences of his behavior. She suggests that the occupational therapist can function as a feedback system for the patient by clarifying his behavior for him.

Evaluation   Evaluation of a child in preparation for treatment with a play therapy approach is geared to determining whether the child could utilize such an experience. As Ginott points out, in *Group Psychotherapy with Children,* not all children are appropriate candidates for play therapy. A determination must also be made as to whether a group or individual therapy session would be indicated.

Axline suggests that individual therapy is appropriate for children with deep-seated emotional problems, whereas group therapy is more helpful in problems centered about social adjustments. She does not, however, define any criteria for selecting children appropriate for play therapy.

Ginott outlines the criteria he feels a child should meet in order for group play therapy to be effective. The first criteria for acceptance into a play group is the need for acceptance and status by peers. Given the opportunity, the child will be motivated to change his behavior in order to gain peer acceptance. This need presupposes a considerable amount of ego development; the child must have had a satisfactory primary relationship with his mother and have been able to mature to the point where he also needs acceptance from others. Children who have not had a satisfactory primary relationship are not good candidates for group play therapy. Ginott recommends investigating the problematic behavior of the child and determining its possible sources, such as the school or home, the child's level of maturity, and his reaction to frustration.

Ginott recommends play groups for the following types of children: withdrawn children, immature children, children with phobic reactions, effeminate boys, children with habit disorders such as thumb-sucking and temper tantrums, and children with conduct disorders such as negative behavior, fighting, and destructiveness. The following types of children, he feels, are not suited to treatment by group play therapy: sociopathic children, intensely jealous children, children with abnormal sexual needs, and extremely aggressive children.

The evaluation of the child must also extend to the assessment of what the child can offer to a play group, as well as what he needs from a play group. Children must be carefully grouped in order to obtain maximum results. Ginott suggests grouping children so that they have a corrective influence on each other. The child should be able to associate with children who have problems both complementary with and different from his own. The group must not produce fear in any of its members. The child must be free of overwhelming anxiety in order to utilize the group experience. Considerations of age, sex, and group size must also be worked out to maximize the therapeutic effects of the group.

Suggested toys and media for play therapy are doll houses with family member dolls, water play, climbing equipment, toy animals, transportation toys, media allowing creative expression such as paints, clay, fingerpaint and blackboards, puppets, housekeeping equipment, sand box and aggressive toys.

Treatment example   In the appendix to her book, *Play Therapy,* Virginia Axline presents excerpts from some of her play therapy sessions as illustrations of how closely the child's problem is related to his free play. She presents the case of Dickie:

Dickie, age seven, was living in a private children's home, having been placed there four months previously when his divorced mother remarried. The stepfather wanted nothing to do with Dickie and, as a result, his mother rarely visited him. His natural father, whom Dickie had not seen in several years, lived in a distant city. Before her marriage, the mother had worked, leaving Dickie in the care of an older woman. He was allowed to do as he pleased as long as he played quietly and did not disturb the woman.

Dickie seemed unable to adjust to his new environment. He had never played with his peers or led a regimented life. He felt rejected by his mother, lonely and hostile. He was a problem in the home because of his immature behavior. He cried easily, was withdrawn and enuretic.

Much of what Dickie was feeling was expressed clearly in his first play therapy session. He accepted the permissiveness of the play session and seemed to utilize it as an opportunity to be in control of his environment. He told the therapist exactly what he wanted her to do. They were playing with clay and he told her to make a cat and hide it behind a rock. He made a rabbit which proceeded to smash the cat. This was repeated several times, each time the therapist's animal succumbing to Dickie's. Finally he asked the therapist to see if her animal could smash his. When it did, Dickie demanded that the therapist fix his animal and left the table to explore the other toys. He returned with a nursing bottle and asked the therapist for permission to drink from it. When permission was given, he spent the remainder of the session lying on the floor with his eyes closed, drinking from the bottle.

Reality Therapy

Reality therapy is an approach to the treatment of psychosocial disorders which places the responsibility for behavior change with the patient. William Glasser, the proponent and introducer of reality therapy, feels that all individuals with psychosocial disorders have one basic inadequacy; they were unable to fill their basic needs; the two basic needs being "the need to love and be loved and the need to feel that we are worthwhile to ourselves and others."[45] Unable to fill their needs realistically, individuals with psychosocial dysfunction choose some unrealistic method of attempting to do so. Glasser describes these unsuccessful methods as irresponsible behavior.

The first step in reality therapy is involvement. The therapist and child must become involved so that the patient can begin to face reality and learn how his behavior is unrealistic. The second step involves rejecting the irresponsible behavior of the child while continuing to maintain involvement. Thirdly, the therapist must teach the child responsible behavior, that is, more successful methods of fulfilling his needs.

The advantages of reality therapy, as outlined by Glasser, are its widespread applicability and its relatively straightforward approach. Glasser recommends his approach with children, delinquents, institutionalized psychotics, neurotics and people with psychosomatic illnesses. He also suggests that his approach can be helpful to persons such as parents, teachers, good neighbors, friends, and clergymen, who must deal with slight behavior problems.

The disadvantage of reality therapy is the difficulty of establishing an involved relationship with the dysfunctioning child. This relationship may be very difficult with a severely ill person, and Glasser suggests that not all therapists have the personality which would allow them to develop such an involvement. However, once an involved relationship is established, the techniques of reality therapy are quite easily employed. The therapist's ability to accept, understand, and not be frightened of irresponsible behavior usually facilitates the development of involvement.

The occupational therapist can utilize the method of reality therapy in the occupational therapy setting if he is able to establish an involved relationship with the child. This involvement may take time to establish; but once it is established, the techniques of reality therapy can be effective. Reality therapy can be employed in conjunction with other treatment techniques.

Example of treatment   Glasser presents illustrations of how reality therapy can be applied to several types of psychiatric settings: hospital treatment of psychotic patients, office treatment of private patients, and treatment of delinquent girls. He also proposes the application of reality therapy to public schools.

Glasser presents his treatment of Jeri, an adolescent girl, committed to the Ventura School of the California Youth Authority. Jeri had been confined to the school for a series of arrests for shoplifting. The most difficult aspect of Dr. Glasser's treatment with Jeri was to establish an involved relationship with her. Once she had exhausted the usual repertory of behaviors trying to secure her release from the Ventura School, she settled down to an adequate but unenthusiastic adjustment to the school's program, marking time until her parole was to be discussed. During her treatment sessions, up until this time, she was friendly and ingratiating with her therapist and anxious to know what he could do for her. Dr. Glasser's approach met with little success until she was denied parole. She couldn't understand why her referral had been denied and became very upset; she stated that her therapist had let her down and had been unfair to her. In retaliation she began spreading stories that Dr. Glasser was doing special favors for her, in particular mailing letters which had not been censored.

The turning point in Jeri's relationship with Dr. Glasser seemed to come when he disciplined her for the tall tales. He confined her to the disciplinary unit but stated that he would see her at their regular treatment time. When next he saw Jeri their involvement had apparently been strengthened by this encounter. Dr. Glasser's refusal to accept Jeri's irresponsible behavior while continuing to accept her seemed to make the difference in their relationship. During that session Jeri related her life story to her therapist and stated that she was worried about her future. She said she felt guilty about her behavior and that she wished to change. In the treatment which followed, Jeri and her therapist carefully worked out her plans for the future and how she would behave once she was paroled.

The Psychodynamics of Activities Approach (PDAA)

Several occupational therapists recommend treatment in occupational therapy based upon the psychodynamics of activities. They suggest that certain activities are symbolic of early relationships and that by using regressive or symbolic activity the occupational therapist can help the child to communicate his feelings and thus deal with them.[46]

Amelioration of symptoms may result from this approach, as the basic needs of the child may be filled. In some ways the PDAA is similar to play therapy, in that during play therapy the child expresses himself through his play, while in the PDAA it is his expression through creative activities. The PDAA has the advantage of being less dependent upon verbal communication; the child can express himself exclusively through his activity if he wishes. The PDAA is a useful method of initiating treatment and establishing a relationship with a child.

The disadvantage of the PDAA is the amount of time that may be required before behavior change occurs. It may be that the PDAA is more effective in relieving symptoms than it is in initiating change in psychosocial behavior.

The role of the therapist in a PDAA is to be an accepting, need-filling adjunct to activity. The therapist must be able to provide the appropriate activity, present it to the child in a manner in which he can use it, and in an environment which allows him to do so. The therapist must be prepared to accept the feeling which the activity elicits and to understand the nonverbal clues the child presents.

Evaluation   The PDAA can be particularly useful as a method of evaluating a child's status in treatment. His well being can more or less be recorded through his work. Llorens [47] describes this clearly in her case illustration of children treated with

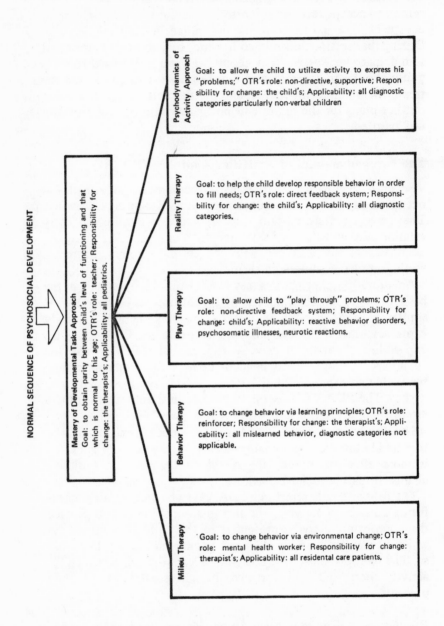

NORMAL SEQUENCE OF PSYCHOSOCIAL DEVELOPMENT

Mastery of Developmental Tasks Approach
Goal: to obtain parity between child's level of functioning and that which is normal for his age; OTR's role: teacher; Responsibility for change: the therapist's; Applicability: all pediatrics.

Psychodynamics of Activity Approach
Goal: to allow the child to utilize activity to express his "problems;" OTR's role: non-directive, supportive; Responsibility for change: the child's; Applicability: all diagnostic categories particularly non-verbal children

Reality Therapy
Goal: to help the child develop responsible behavior in order to fill needs; OTR's role: direct feedback system; Responsibility for change: the child's; Applicability: all diagnostic categories.

Play Therapy
Goal: to allow child to "play through" problems; OTR's role: non-directive feedback system; Responsibility for change: child's; Applicability: reactive behavior disorders, psychosomatic illnesses, neurotic reactions.

Behavior Therapy
Goal: to change behavior via learning principles; OTR's role: reinforcer; Responsibility for change: the therapist's; Applicability: all mislearned behavior, diagnostic categories not applicable.

Milieu Therapy
Goal: to change behavior via environmental change; OTR's role: mental health worker; Responsibility for change: therapist's; Applicability: all residental care patients.

FIG. 5-3. Comparison of treatment approaches.

fingerpainting sessions. The goal was to have the children express their feeling through their paintings. She presents pictures that children have done which illustrate different levels of emotional expression.

Example of treatment   Llorens' treatment of emotionally disturbed children with fingerpainting is illustrated by her description of a neurotic boy, Bobby. Bobby suffered from severe obsessive-compulsive, ritualistic behavior which was interpreted as his method of controlling his impulsive behavior. Fingerpainting was initiated as a method of having Bobby express his fantasy material and as an outlet for his aggressive feelings. His first paintings characterized his compulsiveness. The colors were separated into stripes and he washed his hands between applications of different colors. In a later session he asked if he could mix the colors and he was assured that this was acceptable. He began to mix the colors and to refrain from washing his hands as frequently. Gradually he expressed his enjoyment in fingerpainting, and he and the therapist discussed how his paintings differed from his original ones. He began to relate some of his fingerpainting behavior to his relationships with people and was able to make some changes in his behavior.

Summary

The previous chart is presented both to summarize this section of the chapter and to compare and contrast the various approaches utilized by the occupational therapist in treating children with psychosocial dysfunction. (See Figure 5-3.)

References

1. Brown, J.A.C. *Freud and the Post-Freudians,* Revised edition (Baltimore: Penguin Books, 1964).
2. Spitz, R. *The First Year of Life: A Psychoanalytic Study of Normal and Deviant Development of Object Relations* (New York: International Universities Press, 1965), p. 85.
3. Frankenburg, W. and Dodds, J. "The Denver Developmental Screening Test." *Journal of Pediatrics* 71(1967), pp. 181-191.
4. Erikson, E. *Childhood and Society,* Second edition (New York: W. W. Norton, 1963), pp. 247-251.
5. Erikson, E., pp. 251-254.
6. Erikson, E., p. 256.

7. Fraiberg, S. *The Magic Years: Understanding and Handling the Problems of Early Childhood* (New York: Charles Scribner's Sons, 1959), p. 205.

8. Erikson, E., p. 258.

9. Erikson, E., pp. 258-261.

10. Kent, C. "Perceptual Functioning of Emotionally Disturbed Children: Figure-Ground Perception." (Unpublished Master's thesis, Boston University, 1968).

11. Chess, S. *An Introduction to Child Psychiatry* (New York: Grune and Stratton, 1959), p. 87.

12. Freud, Anna. *Normality and Pathology in Childhood* (New York: International Universities Press, 1965), p. 119.

13. Chess, Stella. *An Introduction to Child Psychology.*

14. Freud, Anna, p. 123.

15. Freud, Anna. *Normality and Pathology in Childhood;* Chess, S. *An Introduction to Child Psychiatry.*

16. Freud, Anna. *Normality and Pathology in Childhood.*

17. Spitz, Rene, p. 241.

18. Coleman, J. *Abnormal Psychology and Modern Life,* Second edition (Oakland, N.J.: Scott, Foresman and Company, 1956); Chess, S. *An Introduction to Child Psychiatry.*

19. Bowlby, J. *Child Care and the Growth of Love* (Baltimore: Penguin Books, 1953).

20. Brain, R. *Diseases of the Nervous System* (London: Oxford University Press, 1956); Elizur, A. and Wijenbeck, H. "A Case of Psychiatric Complications after Encephalitis." *Psychiatria, Neurologia, Neurochirurgia* 69(1966), pp. 169-174.

21. Creak, M. "Schizophrenic Syndrome in Childhood." *Lancet* 2(1961), p. 818.

22. Bettelheim, B. *The Empty Fortress: Infantile Autism and the Birth of Self* (New York: The Free Press, 1967).

23. Hermelin, B. and O'Conner, N. "Perceptual and Motor Discrimination in Psychotic and Normal Children." *Journal of Genetic Psychology* 110(1967), pp. 117-125; "Visual Imperception in Psychotic Children." *British Journal of Psychology* 56(1965), pp. 455-460.

24. Bettelheim, B. p. 63.

25. Bettelheim, B.

26. Kanner, L. "Autistic Disturbances of Affective Contact." *Nervous Child* 2(1943), pp. 217-250; Meyer, R., Levitt, M., Falick, M., and Rubenstein, B. *The Essentials of Pediatric Psychiatry* (New York: Appleton-Century-Crofts, 1962); Bettelheim, B., *The Empty Fortress.*

27. Rutter, M. "Concepts of Autism." In Mittler, P.J. *Aspects of Autism* (London: British Psychological Society, 1968), pp. 1-29; Freud, Anna. *Normality and Pathology in Childhood.*

28. Coleman, J. *Abnormal Psychology and Modern Life.*

29. Ginott, H. *Between Parent and Child* (New York: Avon Books, 1969), pp. 30-32.

30. Ginott, H. pp. 57-58.
31. Llorens, L. "Facilitating Growth and Development: The Promise of Occupational Therapy." *American Journal of Occupational Therapy* 24(1970), p. 93.
32. Mosey, Anne. *Occupational Therapy: Theory and Practice* (Medford, Mass.: Pothier Brothers, 1968), p. 1-2.
33. Mosey, Anne, p. 29.
34. Mosey, Anne, pp. 30-32.
35. Koppitz, E. *Psychological Evaluation of Children's Human Figure Drawings* (New York: Grune and Stratton, 1968); Goodenough, F. *Measurement of Intelligence by Drawings* (New York: World Book, 1926).
36. Llorens, L. and Rubin, E. *Developing Ego Functions in Disturbed Children: Occupational Therapy in Milieu* (Detroit: Wayne State University Press, 1967); Barker, P. and Muir, A. "The Role of Occupational Therapy in a Children's Inpatient Psychiatric Unit." *American Journal of Occupational Therapy* 23(1969, pp. 431-436.
37. Buskirk, M., Cunningham, J. and Kent, C. "Disturbed Children: Therapeutic Approaches to Separation and Individuation." *American Journal of Occupational Therapy* 22(1968), p. 289-293.
38. Llorens, L. and Rubin, E., p. 18.
39. Llorens, L. and Rubin, E., p. 20.
40. Llorens, L. and Rubin, E., pp. 21-22.
41. Llorens, L. and Rubin, E., p. 22.
42. Paul, G. "Outline of Systematic Desensitization: I." In Franks, C. (ed.) *Behavior Therapy, Appraisal and Status* (New York: McGraw-Hill, 1969), pp. 63-104.
43. Krasner, L. "Behavior Modification — Values and Training: The Perspective of a Psychologist." In Franks, C. (ed.) *Behavior Therapy, Appraisal and Status* (New York: McGraw-Hill, 1969), pp. 537-568.
44. Diasio, K. "Psychiatric Occupational Therapy: Search for a Conceptual Framework in Light of Psychoanalytic Ego Psychology and Learning Theory." *American Journal of Occupational Therapy* 22(1968), pp. 400-407; Smith, A. and Tempone, V. "Psychiatric Occupational Therapy within a Learning Theory Context." *American Journal of Occupational Therapy* 22(1968), pp. 415-420.
45. Glasser, W. *Reality Therapy* (New York: Harper and Row, 1965, p. 9.
46. Azima, H. and Azima, F. "A Theory of Dynamic Occupational Therapy." *American Journal of Occupational Therapy* 13(1959), pp. 215-221; Fidler, G. and Fidler, J. *A Communication Process in Psychiatry: Occupational Therapy* (New York: Macmillan, 1963); Linn, L., Weinroth, L., and Samah, R. *Occupational Therapy in Dynamic Psychiatry* (Washington, D. C.: American Psychiatric Association, 1962); Llorens, L. "Projective Technique in Occupational Therapy." *American Journal of Occupational Therapy* 21(1967), pp. 226-229.
47. Llorens, L., "Projective Technique in Occupational Therapy."

Bibliography

Axline, V. *Play Therapy,* Revised edition (New York: Ballantine Books, 1969).

Ayres, A.J. "Patterns of Perceptual-Motor Dysfunction in Children: A Factor Analytic Study." *Perceptual and Motor Skills, 20* (Monograph Supplements 1-V20, 1965).

Barker, L. "An Emotionally Disturbed Child." In *Perceptual-Motor Dysfunction, Evaluation and Training.* Proceedings of Occupational Therapy Seminar (Madison, Wisconsin, 1966), pp. 292-306.

Bettelheim, B. *Love Is Not Enough* (New York: Collier Books, 1965).

Doyle, P. "The Treatment of Psychotic Children: A Multiple Therapist Approach." In West, W. (ed.) *Occupational Therapy for the Multiply Handicapped Child* (Proceedings of Conference, Chicago, Illinois, 1965), pp. 211-227.

Fahl, M. "Emotionally Disturbed Children: Effects of Cooperative and Competitive Activity on Peer Interaction." *American Journal of Occupational Therapy* 24(1970), pp. 31-33.

Forward, G. "Observation and Treatment of Psychotic Children, Part 1." *Occupational Therapy* (March 1958), pp. 23-34.

Forward, G. "Observation and Treatment of Psychotic Children, Part 2." *Occupational Therapy* (April 1958), pp. 22-31.

Gesell, A. and Ilg, F. *The Child from Five to Ten* (New York: Harper and Row, 1946).

Gesell, A. et al. *The First Five Years of Life* (New York: Harper and Row, 1940).

Gesell, A., Ilg, F. and Ames, L. *Youth: The Years from Ten to Sixteen* (New York: Harper and Row, 1956).

Ginott, H. *Group Psychotherapy with Children: The Theory and Practice of Play Therapy* (New York: McGraw-Hill, 1961).

Havighurst, R. *Developmental Tasks and Education,* Second edition (New York: David McKay, 1952).

Kanfer, F. and Saslow, G. "Behavioral Diagnosis." In Franks, C. (ed.) *Behavior Therapy, Appraisal and Status* (New York: McGraw-Hill, 1969), pp. 417-444.

Llorens, L., Rubin, E., Braun, J., Beck, G. and Beall, C. "The Effects of a Cognitive-Perceptual-Motor Training Approach on Children with Behavior Maladjustment." *American Journal of Occupational Therapy* 23(1969), pp. 502-512.

Loovas, O.I., Berberich, J., Perloff, B. and Schaeffer, B. "Acquisition of Imitative Speech by Schizophrenic Children." *Science* 151(1966), pp. 705-707.

Mahler, M. *On Human Symbiosis and the Vicissitudes of Individuation; Volume I: Infantile Psychosis* (New York: International Universities Press, 1968).

Mosey, A. *Three Frames of Reference for Mental Health* (Thorofare, N.J.: Charles B. Slack, Inc., 1970).

Mosey, A. "Treatment of Pathological Distortion of Body Image." *American Journal of Occupational Therapy* 23 (1969), pp. 413-416.

Spock, B. *Baby and Child Care,* Revised edition (New York: Cardinal Pocket Books, 1957).

Thomas, A., Chess, S. and Birch, H. *Temperament and Behavior Disorders in Children* (New York: International Universities Press, 1968).

Watanabe, S. "The Developing Role of Occupational Therapy in Psychiatric Home Service." *American Journal of Occupational Therapy* 21(1967), pp. 353-356.

Watanabe, S. "Four Concepts Basic to the Occupational Therapy Process." *American Journal of Occupational Therapy* 22(1968), pp. 439-445.

NOTES

Chapter Six

The Development of Visual-Perceptual-Motor Function

Maureen Hayes, O.T.R.
M. Patricia Komick, O.T.R.

(July 1970)

The Development of
Visual-Perceptual-Motor Function*

Visual-perceptual-motor development begins shortly after the child is born and reaches a peak about age seven. Perceptual-motor development is primarily based in neurological development and dependent upon it. In turn, the experience gained through visual and auditory perception during what Piaget terms the "sensorimotor period" forms the basis for cognitive development.

Definition of Perception

The term perception has different meanings within different contexts. Of the five definitions offered by Webster's Dictionary the following one is most applicable to this discussion: Perception — the awareness of objects or other data through the medium of the senses. This chapter will be concerned only with visual perception (the development of auditory perception and speech are similar to visual perception but will not be included here). It is important to note that one's awareness of his environment is determined by his ability to receive stimuli and the amount and quality of his experience. Therefore, for this discussion the definition of visual perception shall be modified to: *visual perception is the awareness of meaningful objects or symbols gained through visual experience.*

*Portions of this chapter have been adapted from section three of *Curriculum Guide for Psychoneurologically Inefficient Preschool Children,* developed at the Meeting Street School, Providence, R.I., under Grant B89-4596 from the Office of Economic Opportunity, 1968-1969.

Visual-Perceptual-Motor Development

There are two other systems which directly affect visual awareness: the motor (or muscular) system which serves to bring objects within the view of the infant or child; and the tactile-kinesthetic system through which the sensations of touch and movement are gained. A child who sees and feels a round ball becomes aware of roundness from two complementary sources, visual and tactile-kinesthetic.

To understand perceptual motor functioning, one must first understand normal visual-perceptual-motor development. In studying this area of development, three elements or systems are examined: visual intake, sensory intake and motor function. These may be viewed separately as a medium of study; however, it is the integration of these three systems which causes further development and facilitates function.

Through the many apparently meaningless activities of infancy, these three systems develop into a repertoire of experiences which becomes integrated into new skills and causes the phenomenon that we know as *development.* It is the integration of the systems that causes development and development which facilitates further integration. Visual-perceptual-motor development, then, is the integrated development of visual and tactile-kinesthetic experience; the motor skills used to enhance that experience facilitate new development and express the individual's awareness of the experience through function.

Visual-Perceptual-Motor Functioning

There are several areas basic to efficient visual-perceptual-motor functioning. Difficulty or inefficiency in any one or a combination of these areas will affect performance. Although these areas do not follow each other successively, but develop simultaneously, it is beneficial to separate them in an attempt to pinpoint the area in which inefficiency exists. Furthermore, by outlining a logical order of skill development in these areas, it will then be possible to modify a particular inefficiency before allowing a child to attempt integration of this skill into higher and more complex levels of functioning.

The framework for looking at visual-motor functioning is divided into three main sections: (I) Basic Sensory Awareness and Discrimination; (II) Basic Visual-Motor Activity; and (III) Advanced Perceptual-Motor Functioning.[1] While skills in all

[1] Model adapted by M.P. Komick from: A. Jean Ayres: "Perceptual-Motor Training for Children, in a monograph edited by C. Sattely, OTR, *Approaches to the Treatment of Patients with Neuromuscular Dysfunction* (Third International Congress World Federation of Occupational Therapists, 1962. Wm. C. Brown Book Co.; Dubuque, Iowa).

areas continue to develop throughout the child's growing years, we feel that those areas mentioned as basic are the foundations for performance at the advanced levels. Difficulty at the advanced level, however, may not always be due to inadequacies on a basic level, but rather to problems of integrating the basic skills. At times visual skills may advance and be integrated on a higher level than motor skills and vice versa. Development of visual motor functioning is spiral in nature. There is a continuous progression toward more complex tasks with emphasis at one point in the motor area, and a constant interweaving or blending of these areas throughout the developmental growth of the individual. This interweaving also occurs in the overall development and integration of visual, gross and fine motor and language skills.

The first two sections of this framework are understood to be most basic to general visual-motor functioning and are developed during the early preschool years. They will be discussed in the first section in order to provide the background for the third section where more integration between visual-perceptual and visual-motor skills is important.

BASIC SENSORY AWARENESS
AND DISCRIMINATION

Visual

The term *visual attention and motility* refers to the individual's ability to attend, follow, and localize stimuli for efficient processing of visual information. This area begins to develop at birth and becomes increasingly more efficient as the individual successfully experiences and learns to control his attention and motor apparatus. The young infant, in the first few months of life, is able to achieve gross head movement and only a minimum of independent eye movement. As head control and eye motility improve, a child directs his gaze at specific objects — a rattle or the face of an adult — and is able to hold that visual attention for longer periods. He is then able to follow a moving target from one side of the crib to the other, as his mother walks around or moves an object at close range. Soon thereafter, he learns to gaze upward and downward. These patterns are closely associated with his total head movements and ability to control head position. As the child develops, he becomes increasingly more able to separate eye movements from head movements. This allows him to attend to any target for longer periods of time and to follow this target in its general movement until it disappears from his visual field. As visual stimuli become more familiar to the child, scanning becomes more selective and random eye movements begin to fixate upon objects of interest to him. The child gradually becomes efficient in pursuing visual stimuli with a maximum of eye movement and a minimum of head movement.

This early experimental training and development of efficient eye movement (eye motility) in the young child is essential to the use of the eyes as a tool for directing hand movements. A child of kindergarten age should be able to attend to an object for at least twenty seconds, pursue a moving target in all directions with a minimum of head movement, and localize different visual stimuli within the environment (both at far and near distances). If a child demonstrates difficulty in this area, one may provide specific guidance and exercises for the child as described below.

Evaluation   In order to evaluate the child's ability to localize, track and scan, the therapist holds an object such as a puppet or a small toy in his hand within the child's range of vision saying, "See the puppet." He then notes whether the child locates it with efficiency and attends for at least twenty seconds. If the child is able to attend to the puppet the evaluator says, "Let's play a game. I want you to follow the puppet with your eyes, but don't move your head." (Evaluator may need to demonstrate.) If the child cannot follow immediately without head movements, the evaluator may place the tips of his middle three fingers gently under the child's chin to remind him to stabilize his head. The puppet is moved slowly back and forth in front of the child's line of vision. After this has been done about six times, it is moved in an oblique line from upper left to lower right a few times and then from upper right to lower left. The child with a very short attention span may not be able to complete this test; this sort of difficulty should be noted, but it is not to be considered an indication that he cannot perform the task. Children with certain neurological and ophthalmological problems will not be able to follow the stimulus object with a smooth motion. One should refer to the child's medical records, if available, to determine the presence or absence of such problems. If he simply loses track of the object and cannot follow in smooth pursuit, then the exercises mentioned later in the book are appropriate and should be used.

This evaluation should be done very carefully. One should not trust his testing procedure until he has gained a great deal of practice and can be reasonably sure of moving the object with a steady, slow speed at the appropriate height for the child's eye level.

Suggestions for Stimulating the Development of Visual Attention and Motility   One may begin training the very young or deficient child by placing visual stimuli at close range in different positions in relation to his head: first, directly in front of the child; then, a few inches to the right side and to the left. As the child demonstrates response to these visual targets, one can move them to different locations further from him in both directions, so that he must attempt to relocalize. If the child is extremely young, the nature of the visual target is probably of great importance. It should be colorful, with some pattern. It should also possess some element of movement or sound, as multisensory stimulation may encourage visual attention. Such objects include rattles, mobiles, music boxes that move, as well as people in his environment who take the time to stand in front of him and talk to him and play peek-a-boo with a small blanket or some other similar size shield. As a child is able to sit up, crawl, and move about, one can increase visual attention and motility by providing toys such as a ball or truck that can be moved at a slow rate of speed past his field of vision, encouraging him to follow these as they come toward him or go away.

While seated, the child can be asked to look at a visual target as it is moved by the therapist in different directions or at wind-up toys, such as those which run on a track, or clowns which tumble down a ladder, and so forth. A variation found to be enjoyable is to flash a strong flashlight on the table surface or on a blackboard in a slightly darkened room. When the light goes on, the child points to the lighted spot. The child can be asked to follow the light with his eyes as it moves in vertical, horizontal, circular, and finally complex irregular paths. Other activities which achieve the same end include the visual tracking of bubbles blown from a wand or two children blowing a balloon back and forth across a table top. To help a child improve his ability to scan or search his environment for a specific object, one might play games of "where is the ball" (truck, dog). The object sought is kept within the child's field of vision; he need not move, therefore, but only look carefully around the area. The same type of game may be used with an older child by changing the stimuli to objects which are more appropriate to his interest level (including articles of clothing and household objects). One must remember to begin training with activities that require a maximum of visual attention and motility and a minimum of fine visual discrimination such as size and color.

One may occasionally find a child with an obvious strabismus (crossed eyes) or other physical eye problem for which he may be wearing corrective glasses or an eye patch. This should not limit the use of these activities, since the child is not asked to use one particular eye but rather to coordinate both eyes. Even the child who has difficulty with vision or with control of one eye can still benefit from these activities. One should never attempt to control or restrict the use of one eye unless it has been medically prescribed.

Thus, even with normal acuity, a child may be inefficient in visual processing. If he is so distractable that he cannot choose or localize a certain stimulus and attend to it for at least ten to twenty seconds he certainly will be unable to compare, discriminate or retain sets of symbols adequately enough to function in an academic situation. If he cannot follow a target smoothly with his eyes or with a minimum of head movement, he will probably have a great deal of difficulty in reading and spelling; for without smooth eye movement he is likely to lose his place and waste time and energy in retracing or reread that which he has already gone over. If he does not have sufficient ability to scan, which is a discriminatory process in which one must discard irrelevant stimuli in favor of the visual cues, he will encounter many obstacles to learning. Another factor in this selection process is the ability to discriminate between different forms and objects in order to choose the one which is desirable.

Development of Visual Discrimination and Constancy of Form   Another visual consideration is the development of discrimination and constancy of form position, and size, and the recognition of primary and secondary colors.

It is believed that the child first recognizes three-dimensional forms as "wholes," being unaware of the size, color, position, or geometric aspects. Therefore, one's first concern should be with the recognition of three-dimensional forms (such as a rattle, spoon, cup, ball) that are familiar to the child. Generally, it is those objects which are functional or have special meaning for him that are recognized first. It is through the manipulation of these objects that awareness of the properties of form begin to develop. The child must also learn that objects which are removed from his immediate visual field continue to exist. It is during the first year that the child begins to search for objects that have been temporarily or partially hidden from view, as he develops a visual memory or image of these objects and the realization that they continue to exist. Memory of form is the basis of visual recognition.

Visual exposure, manipulation, and verbal labeling help to reinforce the visual constancy of form. As the child broadens his experience and his ability to recognize a variety of forms, he begins to develop some method of generalization or categorization. He also begins to develop specific discriminative abilities within classes of objects. For example, he recognizes cups, both those used by the family and his own cup; he can discriminate between his old toys and new ones, between things which are edible and those which are not.

As familiarity with three-dimensional objects increases, he begins to transfer the recognition to pictorial representations of these objects. He enjoys finding and pointing to pictures of objects with which he is familiar. He will probably recognize realistic photograph-type pictures in magazines and books first. A little later, he will develop the ability to recognize black and white and stylized line drawings of these same objects. Recognition of objects and the association with verbal labels usually develop concurrently and thus enhance the development of each other. In addition, as the sensory-tactile area develops, the attributes of objects discriminated by this mode can be added or blended with the information the child obtains visually, for example, a soft ball or a heavy truck. Thereafter, he will not only be able to recognize the form visually but may add knowledge of the properties of texture and weight from his past experience.

After recognition of three-dimensional and pictorial representations has been established, the child begins to recognize the basic geometric shapes. The first shape generally recognized is the circle; then the square, triangle, cross, and later the oval, rectangle and trapezoid. It is this progression from three-dimensional to geometric form discrimination that is important to academic readiness.

As the child refines recognition of both three- and two-dimensional forms, he begins to become aware of a "natural orientation" of objects. He begins to realize that cups, trucks, dolls, and other toys can be turned upside-down and then re-oriented to their "correct" position. In doing such, he sees a visual difference between an object in an upright position and the same object turned upside-down. This awareness is an important point in the child's development. It is the beginning of directional concepts and spatial orientation and will eventually play an important part in his ability to follow directions — as to the position to place his name on a page and to discriminate between letters and words which, except for positional aspects, look the same. It is through manipulation of objects that the child is best able to appreciate positional variations. Thus he learns that the form remains constant. It is only his viewpoint of it that changes. This, for example, can be noted when a child wants to fill a cup or container — finding it upside-down, he quickly reorients it to the proper position for filling. The upside-down-ness of objects is more dramatically or visually obvious than the tilting of them to one side or the other. The young child who is still unable to identify many pictures looks at a picture book as comfortably in an upside-down position as he does when holding it right-side-up. As the child visually recognizes more details of forms, he begins to reposition the book toward a right-side-up position in order to "read" the pictures. But, for a time, the slight diagonal slant of a form on a page goes unnoticed. Development of left-right and diagonal orientation of objects should evolve during the fifth year.

Size recognition also proceeds from the three-dimensional to pictorial representations. The child initially recognizes extreme differences between things that are very large and very small; then he is able to discriminate the bigger and smaller of two objects more nearly the same size, until finally, he progresses to recognition of intermediate sizes or graduations. This is easily observable in play with nesting cups. At first the child makes only gross discriminations, and his random trial-and-error efforts diminish as more purposeful selection can be made by visual discrimination alone. In a similar way he learns to arrange graduated rings in order on the ring-stack. He also becomes aware of differences in size between familiar objects, such as his shoes in comparison to his father's. Development of size recognition also is enhanced by motor movements and kinesthetic feedback obtained as the child moves himself in relation to objects in space. The awareness of size and the discrimination of intermediate size graduations of three dimensional objects is then transferred to pictorial forms. This exists on a somewhat concrete level at first (for example, recognition that one picture is larger than another). By five years, he should be able to function on a more abstract or cognitive level, where he is able to project the concept of size, for example, that an automobile is bigger than a dish, regardless of the physical size of the picture on the page.

In respect to the development of color recognition, it is felt that although color may attract the infant's attention initially, this distinction is due not to his recognition of specific colors but to the variation given to forms by colors and their tone qualities. Form and pattern seem to be stronger attention-getting factors than color. However, as the child becomes familiar with form and size, he begins to be more interested in color recognition and identification. First, he is able to match the basic colors, then to find colors given the verbal label, and lastly, to give the verbal labels himself.

One must remember that early discrimination and constancy of forms, position, size, and color are developing, to some degree, simultaneously, and that the elaboration or refinement of each area continues for an extensive period. They have been separated in this presentation to focus more upon the development of each; however, development of one area may enhance development in other areas. The child's interest will fluctuate. At times he will be more concerned with the form or size of objects than in the relative position or color of them. It is, however, only when the child is capable of assessing and integrating all these aspects regarding any one object that he has established a sound basis for more detailed visual discriminative skills.

Evaluation   In order to determine whether the child can distinguish shapes the therapist may give him an empty formboard of three basic shapes. The therapist will present the child with one of the forms and ask the child to place it in the proper space. It is best to demonstrate the test first to maximize the chances for the child to understand the directions. The therapist will continue to give the child the forms until he has completed the formboard. One may then progress to more difficult formboards containing shapes which are more complex or more similar to each other.

A slightly more difficult task which is often used to determine the child's ability to distinguish form, size, position, or color is *sorting*. The therapist places two objects before the child (for example, a circle and a triangle). Another circle is held in the therapist's hand and he says, "Which one is like this?" or "Put this one on top of the one like it." The language and concepts involved (alike, different, on top of, next to and so forth) will vary according to the child's ability to understand.

Matching and sorting activities are highly variable. One may use familiar three-dimensional objects for children of a developmental level up to three years, two-dimensional objects such as formboards and cardboard cut-outs for four-year-olds, and children five and older may match and sort pictures, using a paper and pencil technique, crossing out the one that does not belong. The differences in the objects matched should be great when dealing with three-year-olds, but may be quite minimal with those who are developmentally at the fifth year.

One may, with little difficulty, devise matching and sorting games for the evaluation of constancy of position, size and color; therefore the exact procedure will not be described. Some brief suggestions of sources of materials follow under each category heading.

1. Constancy of position

    a. Use toy trucks. Place two going in one direction and one in another and ask, "Which one is going the wrong way?"
    b. Dolls with movable parts may be placed in different positions.
    c. Familiar objects, spoons, socks, and cups with handles may be especially helpful if the child is unfamiliar with the therapist or the objects she uses.

2. Constancy of Size

    a. Stacking cones are a standard. Ask the child to build with them or place one inside the other. This will quickly illustrate the child's ability to discriminate differences in size. Vary the number according to the level of ability of the child.
    b. Blocks of various sizes are useful and can be adapted many ways.
    c. Sharpen several pencils to various lengths and ask which is longer and which is smaller.

3. Constancy of Color

    a. Crayons may be matched to each other.
    b. Some toys have pieces which fit only when the colors match. These are quite helpful.

Suggestions for Stimulating Visual Discrimination and Constancy of Form, Position, Size and Color   If a child demonstrates particular delay or distortion of skill development in any one of the aforementioned areas, extra training may be necessary. One should first determine that the language component of the discriminatory skill is not the primary factor hindering the child. It is possible that the language symbol may not have meaning for the child. Thus when one asks a child to point to specific objects, he may fail, not because he doesn't have the ability to visually discriminate size and color, but because he does not recognize the verbal label or properly decipher the command. The problem is likely not one of visual perception if he can match two objects which are the same. Difficulty with position orientation is probably less likely to be influenced by labeling problems, as such an exercise is less often directed verbally at this level. Poor motor coordination may hinder a child's ability to perform these tasks, but this will be recognizable to the therapist through careful observation while the child is performing.

Methods of remediation in visual discrimination and form constancy follow the previously outlined stages of development. For example, when a child has difficulty identifying two-dimentional pictures, the therapist should revert to discrimination of three-dimensional objects with which the child may be familiar. In exposing the child to these objects, the therapist should talk about them and let the child handle them. When he has become familiar with a variety of objects in this manner, he may be asked to sort them or to match the ones which are the same. It is important to begin with objects that are familiar to the child functionally — such as a spoon or a shoe. As he becomes able to discriminate same and different with three-dimensional objects, the therapist may proceed to realistically colored pictures of the same objects, while simultaneously presenting the sample three-dimensional forms. Next, the child should be given the opportunity to match similar pictures, following which, objects with *two* variables may be presented to match (for example, select a large red ball from a choice of a large blue ball, a small red ball, and a large red ball). Gradually elaborate the number and type of discriminations to include form, size and color. In order to enhance recognition of geometric shapes, a simple formboard with deep insets of the basic shapes can be used. Have the child place each piece (circle first) into the holes. This exercise should be used in conjunction with verbal labeling by the therapist, and will provide him with auditory, visual and tactile feedback regarding the correct match. Once this is accomplished, one can use two-dimensional material such as flannelboard shapes or pictures of shapes for matching.

To develop concepts of position orientation, one might begin by reviewing orientations of the body. Can the child follow directions to lie on his back, on his side, turn over, stand up, turn upside-down, look to one side and now to the other? The therapist can present objects which have an obvious "right-side-up." Show the child three cups, one being turned open-side down, and ask him which one is different. Ask him to turn it in order to make it look just the same as the others. Again, manipulation in conjunction with verbalization should enhance development and visual recognition. The "sidedness" should be introduced, demonstrating that a difference exists between one toy animal facing left and one facing right (although these specific labels would not be used). This procedure can be followed, using felt picture pieces and the pictures in the same fashion.

In developing color discrimination, one must present one color at a time. One might start concretely by naming a color for the child and asking him to find objects in his environment that are of the same color. As he is able to identify one particular color from verbal command, add others, one at a time until finally he is able to discriminate all the primary and secondary colors easily. A good game to play is, "I see something red," and see if the child can find something of the particular color named. Once the child has developed recognition of these aspects singly, commence combining discrimination of two properties together, until the child can make discriminations involving all four aspects of form, position, size and color at once.

Tactile-Kinesthetic

Tactile Sensitivity   The term *tactile sensitivity* or *awareness* refers to the ability to receive and interpret stimuli through contact with the skin and exploration with the hands. Through the manipulation of objects, a child develops discriminations of temperature, texture, hardness or contour. When such tactile contact is meaningful, it can be integrated with information he gains visually and by audition, giving a richer and more pleasurable experience. When tactile contact is disturbing or not meaningful, there is a tendency to withdraw from or avoid such contact with the environment.

Initially, as the sensory system is beginning to develop, the child's overall physical contact with his environment is either pleasurable or irritating — and usually alternates between the two. The young child will react by crying or startling to unpleasurable stimuli — extreme heat, or cold, pain, sudden shift in body position or hunger. This early startle or altering response is the child's innate reaction to potential danger and is a protective reflex. At first, his only means of coping with the situation is to rely on adults to remedy the problem. Once the child becomes accustomed to certain positional changes or pressures, he no longer responds with such dramatic and undifferentiated reactions. He becomes discriminative and begins to control his more primitive protective patterns. As he becomes more comfortable with being touched, moved, and manipulated, he begins to understand that physical contact is happening not only to him as a total unit but is happening to a particular part of his body. He begins to experiment purposefully by reaching out and grasping his own body and his environment. His hands explore his mouth or feet, the blanket or rattle, and tactile exploration becomes an important means of gaining information. There are some children, however, who remain oversensitive to body contact. This rejection or disorganization at such a gross level inhibits the reinforcement and refinement of tactile exploration. These are the children who are often irritable and avoid passive or active contact with their environment. On the other hand, there are some children who from the beginning seem to have a diminished alerting system and do not respond to their environment unless contact is intense. They also tend to lag behind in tactile investigation, and therefore will frequently have difficulties in sensory-motor development. It is important that the child's sensitivity lie somewhere between these two extremes in order for sensory exploration to be a pleasurable and meaningful experience.

Evaluation techniques in this area are very unsophisticated at this time. A child with oversensitive tactile systems is usually referred to as "tactile defensive." This can be observed by watching and feeling the child's reaction (often physical withdrawal) to touch. If he withdraws with unusual speed or intensity or becomes exceptionally agitated, one may guess that he falls into this category. If the child does not respond at all (or only minimally) to the tactile stimulation he may be suffering from sensory deprivation. In either case the child usually needs more tactile experience.

Suggestions for Enriching Tactile Experience   Activities in this area should provide a variety of contact experiences which will lead toward purposeful exploration without the need for a high degree of manipulative skill. The materials used can be varied in terms of texture, resistance to movement and temperature, as well as the degree of manipulative skill necessary. To overcome a child's resistance to exploration and experimentation, one might hope to divert his attention from contact by interesting him visually in small boats, squeeze toys, plastic cups, bottles or other familiar objects to be played with in a basin of water. Because water is quite nonresistant, the child need only poke objects or pat the surface to produce some effect. A bubble agent added to the water will enable the child to produce and destroy bubbles, further encouraging contact with materials. He then can be asked to retrieve colored stones, shells, or other objects from the bottom of the basin. As an additional means of increasing tactile awareness, the temperature of the water can be varied. As the child finds waterplay to be an increasingly pleasurable experience, one can introduce ice cubes into lukewarm water, and have the child reach for these. This is a particularly good example of an activity at the introductory level, which encourages tactile exploration with a minimum of visual cues. The next step in removing visual cues and increasing tactile exploration is to have a child reach into a basin of ice cubes, held so that he cannot see into it and fish out one at a time. All these activities should be conducted on a voluntary basis, because the inability to see what he is touching can be very frightening to some children.

The next stage of tactile exploration might be to increase the resistance of the material presented. A container of sand in which articles (small trucks and marbles) are buried may be given to the child; ask him to find these objects with his fingers. Emphasis at this point is not on identification of the objects, but on the tactile discrimination between sand and objects without visual cues. Next a sequence of slightly more resistive objects such as mud, soft dough and then clay can be introduced for manipulation. Here the child is encouraged to push, pull, roll, squeeze and poke the material. Emphasis is not on producing some specific finished product, but on experimental manipulation.

Kinesthesia is the awareness of movement of the body and particularly of the position and direction of the extremities. This awareness is made possible through an internal mechanism that registers the direction and degree of muscle and ligament movement over joints. The individual knows when his arm is up or down, bent or extended, by feeling these positional changes without any visual clues. It is this internal process of feeling motor movements, in combination with visual feedback, that allows a child to monitor or refine patterns of movement. In other words, as the child purposefully reaches for an object, he can not only check visually whether he is reaching in the right direction, but he can also match this visual message with the sensory awareness of the movement he is making — establishing and refining coordinate eye-hand skill. This is important in being able to reach in correct directional patterns, position the hand for fine manipulation, and grasp and handle objects according to their weight. Kinesthetic awareness helps not only in gross movement but apparently has much to do with the speed and accuracy that a child must attain in fine motor skills. When there is inaccuracy or error in fine movement, such as falling short of a mark or losing grasp momentarily, it is kinesthetic awareness along with visual attention which allows for rapid adjustment and, therefore, successful completion of the act. As with all development, kinesthetic awareness proceeds in stages from gross to refined. A child first becomes aware of extreme and sudden adjustment, he is then able to detect more sensitive clues — and finally becomes able to produce smooth and continuous motor movements.

Evaluation   One may begin by asking the child to name his body parts as they are touched by the therapist. This will indicate his naming skill so that the therapist can evaluate his answers on the next part of the evaluation. A modified game of Simon Says may be played, with the therapist asking the child to keep his eyes closed and touch his nose, put his hands over his head, put elbows out to his side and so on. The A. J. Ayres tests, *Imitation of Postures* and *Crossing Midline of the Body,* are useful in determining the child's kinesthetic awareness and development. They may be found in a booklet entitled *Southern California Perceptual-Motor Tests,* by A. Jean Ayres.

Suggestions for Enrichment of Kinesthetic Awareness   To help the child become more acutely aware of kinesthetic sensation (especially the awareness of position and movement of his arms and hands) one may first apply resistance to his movements. Have the child push a heavy object (such as a two-pound sandbag) across the table as far as he can with two hands and then pull it back. The therapist should discuss the effort required to push and pull. Repeat the same procedure with a lighter object, discussing the difference in strength required as compared with the first object. Next he should pull a light object with one hand and a heavy one with the other in the same fashion. Again the difference in effort required to move each should be discussed. Another activity, emphasizing the same principle, would be to have the child simultaneously lift pails of identical size but different weights. A further exploration of both these activities would be to have the child push or pick up these objects in reciprocal or alternating pattern. Both objects should be moving at the same speed, at the same time but in opposite directions. This activity requires the child to accommodate his movements — by being aware of the effort required — to the difference in weight. This should enhance his awareness of movement and his ability to shift quickly and adjust movements as necessary. As awareness of movement is established, one may focus on the direction and position attained by moving the arm. Have the child stand with his eyes closed and his arms at his sides. Place one extremity in a certain position, extended over his head, out to the side, forward, back, or with elbow fixed, forearm up or down and so on. Tell the child to hold his arm in that position when you let go, and to place his other arm in a similar position — keeping his eyes closed. Then have him open his eyes to check whether the arms are exactly in the same position. If they are not, have him correct his error with his eyes open. Then repeat the attempt to match with his eyes closed.

Body Concept   As the child develops and refines his ability to localize and discriminate general stimulation of his body and awareness of movements of his body parts he develops a body concept. He becomes aware of the individual part of his body —

legs, fingers, head and nose — on the sensory as well as visual basis. He first discriminates his body parts as individual "things," and then begins to see their relationship to other parts of his body. For example, the baby suddenly becomes aware of his fingers as he waves them in front of his face, sucks them or manipulates a toy. Later he begins to realize the relationship of his hand to his whole arm (as an extension of his arm) and that the two combine to make an effective unit for manipulation. Thus, the child who derives pleasure from tactile exploration and who receives sensory feedback from his motor movements develops increased awareness and control of his body parts.

Evaluation   The child's knowledge of the arrangement of his body parts, his body concept, can be determined to some extent by asking him to put together a puzzle of a person. For a three-year-old, a two-part puzzle divided at the waist would be useful. A four-year-old may be given a puzzle with a head, a torso with arms and two legs. By age four and one-half to five years a child should be able to complete a five- or six-piece puzzle. The therapist should carefully observe the child while he is piecing the puzzle together in order to help determine whether any difficulty encountered is in lack of body concept or in general lack of ability to do puzzles (usually caused by a visual perceptual problem, which will be discussed in the next section). The therapist may wish to ask the child to do other puzzles or use a take-apart three-dimensional doll to further differentiate the possible problems.

The therapist may ask the child of four or more years to draw a picture of himself to give an indication of the child's concept of his own body. The therapist must be aware that a visual-perceptual problem or difficulty in motor control may prevent the child from drawing a person as he wishes.

Suggestions for Developing Body Concept   The child can be made readily aware of his own individual body parts through the use of singing games, ("I Touch my Nose" and others), but can also be emphasized sensorily through the application of various powders, handcreams, and spray perfumes to his knee, elbow, nose and finger, and so on. At first, the body part is pointed out and labeled for him, and he is instructed to apply the material to it. (He should be questioned whether he has two of these parts, or only one.) Next he should be asked to find the parts by himself on verbal command — and finally he can be asked to name these while he applies the lotion. Awareness is developed not only through visual localization, therefore, but is reinforced by the tactile stimulation of rubbing. The important factor is that he rub his own part rather than have the agent applied by someone else; he thus stimulates his own skin and receives feedback from tactile endings in his hand — as well as from the skin over the part being rubbed. Next, he must become cognizant of the relationship of these parts. This can be achieved by developing increased control of different body parts; first separately, and then in combination with other parts (for example, wiggle one finger, tap your knee with one finger, wiggle all your fingers above your head, and so forth). The use of a large mirror is also helpful in developing total body concept, since he can see as well as feel the different movements he makes. The therapist may have the child lie down on a large piece of brown paper while he traces around the child's body — the child can then draw in his body parts. The child will then have a copy of himself, and will be able to see all the separate parts as they are connected.

Steriognosis is the identification of forms through tactile manipulation with vision occluded. Initially the child begins to develop steriognostic ability in conjunction with visual recognition. Through increased manipulation of objects, he enhances not only his ability to visually discriminate objects — but also his ability to recognize them by tactile sense alone. Eventually he will be able to deduce something about an object's weight, softness or hardness, roundness or smoothness through visual observation alone — or vice versa — by simple feeling the object he will be able to recall a visual image of the form. It is this integration of the senses rather than the development of one exclusively that we are primarily concerned about, as they all are part of a basis for later development in transferring visual stimuli into motor patterns, such as seeing a circle and then drawing it.

Evaluation   A common test of steriognosis is to ask a child to guess what is in his hand while he is holding it behind his back. The therapist asks the child to stand in front of him with the child's back close to the seated therapist's knees. The child is asked to place his hands behind his back. The therapist places objects, one at a time, in one of the child's hands; and the child is to name the object. The therapist then repeats the process with the other hand. Familiar objects such as a key, a penny, a safety pin, a small ball and a small sponge are often used. For children with speech or language problems, or those who speak a foreign language, the therapist may place a duplicate set of objects on the table to which the child can point in order to indicate what is in his hand.

Suggestions for Stimulating Steriognostic Ability   Information concerning the world is developed initially through the combination and coordination of cues received visually and tactually (as well as by audition). Generally, an object can be identified visually before it can be identified by the tactile sense alone. Thus, when trying to enhance this latter means of obtaining information in isolation, one should be sure to use only those objects the child is familiar with visually and those he can name In establishing recognition of form tactually, one should proceed from three-dimensional to two-dimensional objects to geometric shapes. As specific forms are identified tactually, size variations may be introduced. Textural properties of hard, soft, rough and smooth should be included last.

Of primary importance when introducing these is that each element be presented in isolation. For example, do not ask the child to identify the object which is soft by having him feel a big round soft ball and a little round hard ball for he may get confused as to which is the element of softness. Verbal identification of textures is probably the last concept obtained, but the child should be able to make comparisons (same/different) between two objects — one in each hand — and indicate which one is soft or rough when the therapist uses the labels. Some pretraining on the meaning of "same" and "different" may be necessary to do this. In regard to the tactile discrimination of geometric shapes, these should not be attempted until the child can discriminate visually between shapes; have him match a heavy cardboard or plastic shape placed in his hand to one of several pieces placed in front of him. He can then be given two shapes, one in each hand, and asked if they are the same or different. Finally, he can be asked to name them as they are placed in his hand.

The following procedures may prove helpful in developing the child's ability to integrate tactile with visual and auditory cues. First, to eliminate the need for language, have the child match what he feels tactually with the visual stimuli. Place a single object in a bag or behind a screen and ask the child to feel the object. Then have him point to one of three objects which matches the one he is holding. The next stage is to place a variety of objects in the bag and ask the child to find a specific one from verbal command or visual stimulus. This step is more difficult since he must make a tactile discrimination between two or more objects; whereas before he had to choose the correct visual stimulus to match one tactile stimulus. Next he can be asked to find two objects which are the same by feeling in two different bags, thus matching tactile to tactile.

This establishment of a match between tactile-kinesthetic and visual recognition lays a foundation for future integrative processes, such as the translation of visual symbols into a motor pattern, necessary in copying or writing.

BASIC VISUAL-MOTOR ACTIVITY OR EYE-HAND COORDINATION

The second level within this developmental framework is that of basic visual-motor skills. Here there is a purposeful integration of visual-motor (eye-hand coordination) and sensory functions toward the development of skilled performance. This area is divided into two aspects: (1) motor planning, and (2) motor accuracy. The ability to plan motor movements seems to be of greater importance than the more often stressed aspect of accuracy of movement, since accuracy of incorrectly planned movements is of limited value. It must be remembered, however, that these aspects develop concomitantly, and that it is the successful interplay between the two that provides the foundation for advanced visual-perceptual-motor activity.

Motor Planning

Until a motor activity becomes a skilled pattern, there is a period when a child must consciously plan required movements. This motor planning involves recalling the movements and a sequence necessary for any specific action. Once the child has the correct movements and sequence in mind, smoothness and efficiency evolve through visual and kinesthetic feedback. For instance, the child who is learning to tie his shoes must concentrate and memorize the pattern and sequence of movements to be executed with each hand. He uses visual attention to check his performance, as well as tactile and kinesthetic awareness to monitor tension and control of the lace. Once this becomes a learned skill, a conscious motor plan is no longer required. The task soon can be accomplished easily without even looking; the tactile and kinesthetic feedback alone becomes sufficient.

The major factors related to efficiency in motor planning include directional concepts and imitative and self-initiated movement patterns.

Directional Concepts   Developing concepts and motor control of position orientations (up, down, front, back, side, over, under, in and out) are basic to motor planning. The child can both feel and observe his body movements; and therefore he learns these concepts first in relation to his own body and its movements. He then becomes aware of the movements of his body in relation to the environment (space) and then, finally, he is able to perceive the relationship of objects to each other. The child learns to control placement of his arms in front, to the side, in back, or above in his attempts to shift position or reach a specific object. As the child achieves accuracy in reaching for or placing objects in different positions in relation to his own body, he then begins to observe their relationship to each other. He begins by taking objects in or out of containers and placing blocks one on top, beside or in back of one another. The sequence of development proceeds from isolated movement, such as that produced in direct placement of an object, to a combination or pattern of movements, such as are required in assembling more complex construction toys, buttoning or tying shoe laces. At this point, he need not have established concepts of left and right, but he must be aware that he has two sides of his body, for it is this awareness that is the basis of later development of directional concepts of left and right. In addition to being aware of the two sides, the ability to cross over the midline of his body should also be established. For example, when picking up objects scattered on a table, a child should be able to hold a container in one hand while he picks up the pieces on either side of him with the other hand. This successful crossing of the midline can also be noted when a child draws a line across a piece of paper which is placed directly in front of him without switching the crayon to the other hand at the midpoint.

He must not only comprehend the basic directional movements, but realize that these have to occur in a correct sequence in order to complete any one motor activity. An example of planning separate motor patterns and then arranging them in the proper sequence is when the young child is learning to drink from a cup independently. At first he learns to drink from a cup which is held for him. Next, he learns to hold the cup and bring it to his mouth. Then, he learns to control how far he must tilt a full or partially filled cup. Still later, he learns to pick up the cup independently and, finally, to return it to the table without spilling. He has then learned to combine separate motor-planning units into one continuous and sequential operation. This process is established by an interweaving of both imitative and self-initiated movement.

Imitation of Motor Patterns   Through experimentation, the child produces movement. Those movements which are efficient are stored for future use in specific acts. Those movements which do not help him attain his goal are corrected or adjusted through visual and tactile-kinesthetic feedback; and, once successful, are memorized so that they may be recalled whenever necessary. Imitation is not only associated with attempts to repeat one's own random movements, but is often an attempt to copy another person's movements. It is through such trial-and-error, accompanied by a meaningful correcting process, that the child begins to attain command of his movements and, hence, develop efficient motor planning ability. This trial-and-error process is noted in the young child's spontaneous manipulation of objects, attempts at simple construction toys, dressing, drawing and scribbling. (Purposeful imitation of patterns is noticed when the child attempts to copy gestures (clapping hands or waving bye-bye) or daily activities (washing dishes, cooking or mowing the lawn) of his siblings or parents.)

Initiation of Motor Patterns   As imitated patterns become well established, the child develops a repertoire of motor patterns which he can recall and initiate at will. Once he can initiate these at will or on command, he can begin to elaborate and combine them to handle a variety of new situations. He learns to use these motor patterns in appropriate situations or at appropriate times in relation to external visual or verbal cues. For example, as soon as he hears or sees his mother preparing supper he runs to the high chair, when he sees his father getting the keys to the car he may get his jacket.

Evaluation of motor planning ability is usually achieved on the basis of clinical judgment, simply because there is no standardized test available. Therefore, all data gained in order to determine the child's ability is gained through observation. Diagnosis is made on the basis of the evaluation of observed behavior and by relating that behavior to other behavior reported by the mother, teacher, or other person who has had extensive contact with the child. In designing a diagnostic task the therapist must consider many aspects: the child's chronological age and estimated developmental age, his interests, the context in which the task is presented and certain characteristics of the task itself. The task should be meaningful, but not one the child has learned well already. It should have a series of steps, the number of which will be determined by the child's ability. The task should be easy to demonstrate to the child on a nonverbal level, and should include some tactile stimulation as well as eye-hand coordination. Some suggestions include: age three — placing blocks inside a pail, one at a time; age four — threading large beads or rings on a string one at a time; and age five — sewing cards may be used in the traditional manner.

While the child performs these tasks the therapist may observe the following:

I. Can he follow from one step to the next?
   Does he stop and ask for repeated instructions?
   Does he confuse the order of the steps?
   Does he make many false starts at a step and then change his mind?

II. Does he place things accurately?
    Does he often miss his target?
    Does he have difficulty making his hands work together?
    Does he become very frustrated in his attempts to perform the task?

If the therapist can answer I and II affirmatively the child probably does not have a severe motor planning problem — or the task is below his developmental level. If the subquestions are also answered "yes," however, the child may have a motor planning problem or he may be having a difficulty in another area, which makes him appear deficient in this area. Through further testing the therapist may validate or deny the existence of the other problems and by comparison and elimination, determine whether the child has a problem in the area of motor planning. Often a child who experiences difficulty in motor planning will say, "I know what I want to do, but I can't do it." Thus indicating that he is aware of his problem. If the therapist is unsure of the existence of a problem in this area it would be well for the child if the therapist gave him tasks which would improve his motor planning ability. This is a very basic and important skill and should not be ignored.

Suggestions for Enhancing Motor Planning Ability   When a child demonstrates difficulty in planning motor movements, one must start on a level at which he will have some success — that is, one must return to an activity with which the child is quite familiar and which is meaningful to him; the child must be aware of the goal. For example, if the goal is to have his jacket on, one first would ask him to imitate the therapist going through the movement, while she gives verbal reinforcement. Then, when it is obvious at which point he has difficulty, the therapist can assist him through these portions of the motor movement with simultaneous verbal and visual cues.

One might start with the use of a modified version of Simon Says. First, the child need only imitate the therapist's arm movements in the basic directional orientations. If the child has difficulty at this level, the therapist can move the child's arm for him so that he can feel the correct motor patterns. When he can imitate simple patterns, he can be asked to do these from verbal command. Then the therapist can increase the complexity of the patterns, using one hand or two, first in parallel and then in opposing movements and including crossing the midline. Another activity that might be useful is acting out routine activities such as brushing teeth, or combing hair, following the same sequence of imitation and then initiation on verbal command. Be sure to begin with activities that involve single units of movements or simple combinations of these. Then one can progress to more complicated sequences of motor patterning, such as dressing or pretending to iron clothes. Once the specific factors in motor planning (directional concepts, imitation and initiation) become established, accuracy of eye-hand coordination can be more easily attained through practice.

Motor Accuracy

Accuracy of eye-hand coordination can be viewed in several stages; each is based upon visual direction by the hand in motor activity.

Unilateral   One aspect involves the development of unilateral hand use — the child's ability to use either hand alone as is appropriate for a given task. Basic patterns of reach, grasp, release and control of individual finger movements should be established in each hand before one attempts to improve most intricate bilateral hand skills or to develop efficient use of one hand as the lead hand. The degree of accuracy expected by age five and one-half should be sufficient enough to allow the child to build ten-block towers of one-inch blocks, to pick up and adjust and place one-eighth-inch-long pegs in the pegboard (without using the other hand), to unscrew nuts from bolts in toy workbenches, or to toss a beanbag into a pail approximately ten feet away.

Bilateral   Once the child is able to control each hand sufficiently in order to accomplish such patterns, he is able to initiate bilateral hand skills — skills in which two hands are used together for a single activity, in either parallel or opposing or alternating movements. Activities involving parallel movements include throwing a ball with two hands, carrying an object with two hands from one place to another, using a rolling pin on clay and other similar activities. Activities involving opposing movements include unscrewing nesting kegs (where each hand must turn in the opposite direction) stringing beads (in which one hand holds the beads and the other directs the thread), or such activities as hammering a nail or cutting a piece of paper with scissors in which one hand must maintain the position of the material while the other hand acts upon it. Alternating movements are seen in beating a drum or a table surface with two hands alternately.

Hand Preference As individual hand skills become more refined and the bilateral use of hands develops, the child progresses toward finer, more precise movements. As more complex activities requiring greater dexterity and a higher degree of motor planning become necessary it is more efficient to learn these intricate patterns with one hand instead of both. This lead hand can then develop relatively greater skill for finer manipulation, while the other hand assumes an assistive role. Such a need for a lead hand is evident in such gross activities as feeding, and later in the development of coloring, drawing and writing or in the manipulation of tools (such as scissors).

There is still much controversy regarding what determines hand preference, when it is established, and its relationship to perceptual-motor function. It appears that even within the normal population some children seem to have an innate and strong drive to prefer either the left or right hand and that, barring physical impairment, they automatically and very early establish a preference, but who are easily influenced by the environment and thus adapt to the right-handed world. A third group, for some reason, do not establish an early hand preference spontaneously — nor are they easily influenced by their environment. Consequently, they continue to experiment with both hands without evolving a preferred hand in order to refine manual skills necessary for writing and other specialized pattern movements.

Evaluation of motor accuracy can be done on a clinical observation basis for the young child, using the Gesell Scale of eye-hand development as a guide. It is well for the therapist to learn this scale and devise games which enable the therapist to observe the child's skill and thus determine the developmental level of his ability in this area. Standardized tests include the *Southern California Motor Accuracy Test* by A.J. Ayres and the eye-motor coordination subtest of the *Marianne Frostig Developmental Test of Visual Perception*. Both are useful for children whose chronological ages fall between four and eight years. The therapist should not rely on these tests alone to provide an evaluation that will lead to a treatment program, but should give a functional evaluation as well to help understand the particular child's individual needs.

Suggestions for Developing Accuracy of Motor Skill
Developing efficiency of each hand separately should be considered first. One should begin with activities which require direct placement at close range, such as building block towers with increasingly smaller blocks until the child is able to build a tower with one-inch blocks, or placing pegs in a pegboard, gradually decreasing the size until success is achieved with one-eighth-inch diameter pegs. Then accuracy of placement can be increased by having the child touch a target suspended in space, such as tapping a balloon suspended from a string or poking bubbles blown from a wand. The next step would be to have the child toss a beanbag or a ball into a pail or at some other target that could be moved farther away as accuracy improves. Another aspect to be included in unilateral skills is the development of a strength and accuracy of fine finger movement. This accuracy can be accomplished through the use of finger painting, squeezing and pitching and pounding clay, pasting, and a variety of finger-play games.

In developing accuracy for bilateral activities, one must start with those which require parallel movements of both arms for direct placement at close range. Then activities which require one hand to hold material while the other does the manipulation, such as holding a board for pegs or holding the paper for coloring, should be attempted. A higher level of accuracy in bilateral activity can be attempted by using activities which require more refined manipulation of both hands, such as stringing beads or macaroni, unscrewing barrel kegs, tinker toys, and sewing cards. The highest level of bilateral manipulation requires that one hand develop an even finer degree of skill, while the other hand remains assistive. Such activities include hammering nails, using a screwdriver or coloring a complex picture.

It is often difficult to discriminate between the motor planning and accuracy aspects of an activity. The following example may help. The child who has not developed accuracy knows what he wants to do and executes his movements in the right direction and sequence but constantly overshoots the mark, being unable to place the peg directly into a hole or hit the nail directly on the head. The child who has difficulty with motor planning does not seem to know how to go about making motor movements in order to accomplish the activity; for example, the child who cannot wind a string on a spool because he either does not maintain enough tension in the string as he wraps it around the spool or does not see the relationship of movements required between the two hands.

A child who is having difficulty buttoning his jacket may be having difficulty with the motor accuracy involved in manipulating the button through the hole, or difficulty in planning his approach — including the motor sequence of grasping the button, placing it through the hole correctly aligned from the inside out, and retrieving it on the other side. By breaking down the activity, one can work on individual components before combining them into a final act. One may work on the fine pincer movements required to hold the button by having the child practice picking up pennies or poker chips or by pinching clay. The child can then develop the concept of aligning the button to go through the hole more easily by practicing putting the poker chips or buttons through a slot in the large container. The child must learn to align the edge of the chip to correspond with the slot in the container. When he has understood and can execute both the visual-motor match and the motor control necessary to carry out this activity, one can go back to the sequence of buttoning with more efficient learning of that specific task being possible.

Another skill which is helpful to break down into component parts is cutting with scissors — one must first learn the mechanical manipulation of scissors.

ADVANCED VISUAL-PERCEPTUAL-MOTOR FUNCTION

Advanced functioning denotes more integrated levels of visual-motor activity. Performance on such a level of integration is prerequisite to success in school. These functions will be described only briefly at this point, since they will be discussed in greater detail (including specific methods of remediation) in the next section.

Advanced Visual-Perceptual Task

The visual-perceptual skills outlined in this section require efficient integration of all the basic visual attention and discrimination skills discussed thus far, and in turn, will be utilized as a basis for the visual-perceptual motor skills to be discussed in the next section.

Organization of Forms in Space   This ability involves seeing the relationship between forms within a specific space. Forms may be arranged and varied in terms of area, quantity, direction, or position. The arrangement is affected both by the relationship of the parts to each other and by the relationship of the parts to the whole space. Examples of a child's ability to organize forms in space can be noted in his attempts to determine how many blocks might fit into a container, or how many two-dimensional forms might be placed on a page without overlapping each other or going off the page.

Visual Memory   This involves the ability to recall visual stimuli in terms of form, detail, position, and other significant features, on both short- and long-term bases. Development of visual memory is an ongoing process in that the length of time something can be retained and the amount retained must increase in order to make more detailed visual discriminations. Memory must eventually be efficient enough to enable the child to maintain an accurate visual image of a pattern in order to reproduce it or to associate its verbal label. While we are concerned with increasing both the length of time *and* the wealth of material that one might be able to remember, we must also be concerned with developing some organizational plan to allow for the material that is memorized to be retrieved efficiently and economically. This makes it possible for information with which one is dealing.

Sequencing   This process concerns the ordering of visual patterns in time and space. As one's use of spatial organization becomes more advanced and visual memory becomes more efficient, further elaborations can be achieved by sequential ordering. Temporal sequence involves concepts of first, second, third, and the concept that one event occurs before or after another. Spatial sequencing is a method of organizing according to a set pattern (top to bottom, side to side, left to right). One builds a block tower from bottom to top, but one might write a list of words from top to bottom on a piece of paper. At times it is important that a certain sequence be followed in order to achieve the finished product, in spelling words or dividing numbers, for instance. At other times it is not particularly important, but perhaps may be more motorically efficient to follow some predetermined sequence —as when drawing a single symbolic design.

The development of skills in organizing, remembering, and integrating information can be observed early in life as a child learns to identify and recall objects familiar to him or to empty and fill containers, build blocks, or assemble nesting cups. With nesting cups, he also becomes aware of the sequencing element. At first, this play is largely trial-and-error experimentation, but as the discrimination of form and memory increases and the methods of organizing material become more familiar, behavior becomes less and less trial-and-error and more and more purposeful. The child learns the sequence of visual cues and motor movements necessary to put the nesting cups one inside the other without any left over.

Advanced Visual-Perceptual-Motor Tasks

This area first demands planning and fine motor skill with a tool, such as a pencil or paint brush, but initially a crayon. In the use of a crayon, it is the form in space which directs the motor movements. Form will limit the extent of movement and dictate the direction of such movements. In coloring, the child up to three and one-half years will simply learn to confine his movements to the paper, rather than the wall or table. Soon he begins to recognize that the outlined form is the area in which he must operate and that his tool can reproduce marks that mirror his movements. The process of organizing or producing a visual-motor match begins when he attempts to localize the crayon marks within the form. As the space becomes more confined, movements must become more refined, and he soon becomes aware that it is more efficient to match the direction of his strokes to the type of form he wishes to color; for example, horizontal strokes for wide areas and vertical strokes for tall areas.

As skill becomes more refined, he may begin to attempt simple pencil mazes and then to trace on line drawings. At this point, it is necessary for the motor movements to follow the given visual form exactly. Next, the child can attempt to copy line designs. Finally, he develops the ability to recall the form and the motor movements required to produce a visual stimulus he has seen previously. First, he should be able to draw vertical lines, then horizontal, and on to the basic geometric forms: circle, cross, square, diagonal lines — and finally combinations of these to form more complex designs. One can observe the child's development in this area as he spontaneously begins to try to reproduce or copy the first forms he recognizes, such as straight lines and circles. We further see the efficiency and accuracy in this skill closely relates to the development of visual discrimination and memory of forms. Initially, the child makes only a scribble. As he begins to recognize letter forms and to develop the specific motor patterns necessary, his reproductions correlate more and more with the actual visual stimuli.

Once the child achieves a certain degree of accuracy in reproduction, he must learn to vary his reproductions in terms of size (making the same form, large or small), spatial aspects or placement (being able to draw the designs at the top, bottom, middle or sides of the paper) and sequence (being able to place forms in a specific order). If a child can control all these variables, he should be able to write letters (upper and lower case) in the correct sequence to form words (and finally sentences) in the proper place and direction on the paper. While activity at this stage remains mainly a copying activity, the child does begin to rely upon visual memory of form and the sequence of motor reproduction required to make these.

Finally, the child must learn not only to translate visual stimuli into motor patterns but also to add auditory stimuli into this sensory-motor process. He must learn to draw a circle or some specific letter form from verbal command. Then he must reproduce complex forms, including elements of size, position and sequence from dictation. At this point all the basic elements of visual-perceptual-motor skills required for writing activity have been established and integrated.

Summary   This section has provided an overall framework of looking at Visual-Perceptual-Motor functioning. The therapist must become acutely aware of the individual sensory awareness and the discrimination and eye-hand coordination components — as well as their combination into integrated visual-perceptual-motor function. Development within this framework occurs both simultaneously and progressively; by isolating the component parts, it is hoped that one will be able to observe a child's functioning at any stage of development, assess the various components of this development, and therefore obtain a point from which remediation or further stimulation can begin. It is hoped that this plan will give the therapist a rationale for working out and establishing a learning experience for a child, rather than simply having him repeat or practice a specific activity until he can achieve it. This task analysis approach should be more beneficial as well as more meaningful for both the child and the therapist.

EVALUATION AND TREATMENT OF VISUAL-PERCEPTUAL-MOTOR FUNCTION

This section is presented with two purposes in mind: the first is diagnostic, since the activities presented and functional skill levels discussed should be accomplished by a child before he begins first grade academic work. The therapist can determine whether or not the child possesses these skills by using the observational materials in this section. The second purpose is to help the therapist in the development of a program which will enhance learning skills. To do this he must have a clear picture of the basic processes and sequences involved in visual-perceptual-motor function in order to facilitate these aims and to provide the basis of an integrated treatment program, the format of this section is arranged differently from the previous one.

In this section the higher aspects of visual-perceptual-motor function (Part II: Eye-Hand Coordination, and Part III: Advanced Visual-Motor Function) are presented within a model to be used for treatment planning. This model describes the areas of visual-perceptual-motor function by first separating the visual-perceptual and eye-hand coordination elements (visual-motor) and presenting some of their individual developmental aspects, and the integrates of these two areas in combined visual-perceptual-motor tasks.

Within the three major areas, the model also breaks tasks down into three levels of complexity depending upon the amount of organization provided by the therapist (Table I). The highest level, Level I, includes activities which require the child to organize and integrate skill components to achieve a given goal in relatively unstructured situations. On the second level, Level II, a more specific goal is provided; the child again must develop the means of achieving a goal — but some structure is provided. On the third level a more highly structured approach is utilized to help the child develop the basic skills necessary to function on Levels I and II.

This model with the visual-perceptual and visual-motor (eye-hand coordination) areas separated first and then recombined in a visual-perceptual-motor section has been developed because it is necessary to focus upon both the component parts of the task and upon the process of integrating them into complex skills. All too often, current tests available for evaluating visual-perceptual-motor function give tasks which combine several skills at one time. Some do so without indicating the separate elements involved; others separate the elements but do not suggest how to refine the skills or integrate it with other areas.

Area I: Visual Perception

One assumes within this model that visual acuity and ability to match basic shape, size and color are intact. Part III of the first section of this chapter has already discussed the fact that this area is concerned with three elements in the visual-perceptual processing system which appear to be essential in the overall development of efficient visual-perceptual-motor skills: (1) organization of forms in space, (2) memory of visual form, and (3) sequence of visual material. Growth in skill in these elements occurs simultaneously, thus priority cannot be given to any single one. They have been isolated only in an effort to better focus attention on some of the dynamics involved in visual perception.

Area II: Eye-Hand Coordination

One assumes, once again, that there are no specific neuromotor problems present and that the basic hand patterns of reach, grasp, release, transfer, and prehension have been established. This area is concerned with two major aspects of motor control: (1) developing hand skill and establishing a preferred hand to increase refinement of manipulative ability, and (2) developing awareness and integration of the two sides of the body through experiences in parallel, opposing and alternating hand patterns. Again, development of these two aspects occurs simultaneously and undergoes continuous and ongoing refinement.

Area III: Combined Visual-Perceptual-Motor Tasks

There are three successive phases which seem basic to the integration of visual-perceptual and eye-hand (visual-motor) abilities in establishing prewriting skills. The first phase involves fine motor control as typified in coloring with a pencil or crayon. At this level, motor planning and accuracy are governed by the area enclosed by the form to be colored, and emphasis is placed upon the match of the motor pattern to the spatial area. The second phase involves the translation of visual image into a motor reproduction of the form; increased motor control and memory for motor patterns is essential. During the third phase, the child combines the elements of fine motor control, memory for patterns (shape and size) visual organization of form in space and visual sequencing.

To obtain an overall view of the child's performance in the visual-perceptual-motor area, the therapist should present activities on Level I from each subarea; he will then gain a profile of the child's skills, and will be able to plan his program so that it will emphasize the areas in which the child has difficulty. When a child has difficulty in any subarea, the therapist can move to activities on Levels II and III of that subarea to assess and develop the component parts of this specific skill. If the child is under five years or appears to be very impaired, the therapist may wish to begin his evaluation at Level II or III. Experience will guide the

TABLE 6-1

Model for Assessment and Training of Visual-Perceptual–Motor Skills

	Level I Unstructured	Level II Moderately Structured	Level III Highly Structured
Eye-Hand Coordination			
A. Increasing motor efficiency	Use of preferred hand for refined, repetitive movements; assistive use of other hand, i.e., hammering	Use of lead and assisting hands for less skilled activities, i.e., bead stringing	Fine finger dexterity prehand objects; Eye-hand coordination, direct placement
B. Awareness and integration of two sides of the body	Singing-action games	Modified Simon Says for crossing midline	Modified Simon Says no crossing, in parallel, opposing and alternating patterns
Combined Visual-Perceptual-Motor Tasks			
A. Fine Motor Planning with tool	Color in figure of child with adapted strokes and segmental awareness	Copy sample coloring to become aware of segments	Match direction of strokes to shape
B. Translation of Visual Form into Motor Pattern	Copy line designs	Imitate motor movements of designs	Trace or use stencils of designs
C. Elaboration of Design	Copy shapes of varied size in correct sequence and position on paper	Copy sequence	Copy size
A. Organization of Forms in space	Arrangement of precut shapes on paper as child desires	Arrangement of precut shapes on paper to match the sample	1. Match positional orientations of 3D objects 2. Copy placement of 3D object Indicate which one of three 3D objects has been removed
B. Visual Memory of Form	Remember details of storybook picture	Remember nine specific pictures (include 3 categories, 3 rows, 3 columns)	
C. Sequencing of Visual Material	Match sets of 3-4 sequential designs	Copy sequence of forms	Copy sequenced 3D objects

therapist's judgment regarding which level of evaluation would serve as a beginning level for a particular child.

Each specific activity presented should be considered as only one sample of the process. The essential principle of each activity is indicated 'in Table 6-1. The therapist can supply many additional activities of his own for each subarea based on the underlying principle.

Visual Perception

Organization of Forms in Space

The emphasis here is in helping the child realize the relationship of forms within a specific spatial area. The area may vary in plane (upright, as on a blackboard — or flat, as on a table), size, or shape. The problem is to determine how specific forms may be arranged in this spatial area, which requires an understanding of their size and number, their position, and their sequence. Arrangement is affected both by the relationship of the parts in and of themselves, to each other, and to the "whole space." The child must become aware of and then master such problems as: whether forms are too large to fit within a designated area and, if small enough, how many will fit within this space. He must also learn the primary sections (top, middle, sides) of an area. He must be aware of the positional orientation of forms that have a "right-side-up-ness," and, as well, the correct positional relationship of separate parts of a whole. Finally, he must learn to use the space provided in an efficient manner.

A child's ability to recognize spatial orientation of forms and to manipulate these is a gradual process which develops from awareness of his own body in space to appreciation of objects within three-dimensional space to then still finer discrimination of two-dimensional space. The child first learns to move himself around furniture, through narrow passages, and under or over obstacles without mishap. Next, he learns to manipulate objects in relationship to each other via building, nesting, take-apart and construction toys and objects; then he is ready to manipulate two-dimensional pieces on a flat surface, such as pasting pieces on paper or moving magnetic or flannel pieces on a board.

It is this latter aspect of two-dimensional organization which we are particularly interested in establishing before first grade. There are many activities that give the child experience in this area and provide the therapist with an opportunity to assess levels of competency. Suggestions are made for assessment in terms of the three levels of complexity outlined in Table 6-1.

Level I: Unstructured   At this level, spontaneous manipulation of the material within a broad framework is encouraged. This requires a degree of self-organization, since it is necessary for the child not only to establish his own specific goal but also to organize an efficient sequence to achieve it.

An evaluation activity may be to ask the child to arrange and paste a specific number of precut shapes on a piece of paper. The materials are: a piece of 8- by 10-inch paper, paste and a specific number of representational precut forms with definite positional orientations which can be related to each other. For example, a house made up of separate parts, a strip that could be a road, an animal, a tree, and so forth.

Have the child seated at a table with enough room to work unhindered. Say, "I am going to give you some pieces to paste on this piece of paper. You may paste them any way you wish, but be sure to use all the pieces." Observations are then made on the child's approach to the task during the activity and on his visual-perceptual skills. (These latter observations can be made later in the day from the finished product.) For ease of recording and reviewing it is felt that only problem areas should be recorded.

Approach

Does the child understand the task or do the directions have to be repeated several times?

Can the child organize himself to complete this task, or does he become distracted and/or forget what he is supposed to be doing?

Does he make an attempt at representational organization or does he make some effort to organize material by shape, size or color?

Visual-Perceptual Skills

Does the child use the total space provided effectively or does he use only one area or overlap pieces off the paper?

Are pieces appropriately organized on the paper?

Are pieces appropriately related to each other?

The objective of this activity is to observe a facet of the child's perception of space and the relation of objects in space, minimizing motor control. Thus, one can determine whether space has any meaning as a quality to be manipulated, whether the child is aware that some forms have a predetermined sided-ness or orientation, so that parts may be related in different ways to produce different effects.

If the child has difficulty in obtaining and maintaining an approach, the therapist should determine whether this is the case only when visual-perceptual tasks are involved — or whether such behavior is characteristic of his performance in general. In this way the therapist can determine whether the learning approach is the area in which he must concentrate, or if it is visual-perceptual skills he must develop.

In scoring the product, various possibilities of finished products are possible. The child should not be penalized if he does not make a representational product. However, if he does not, and the product is very abstract, activities (such as the one given in Level II) should be utilized in order to determine whether he can, in fact, cope with this type of spatial organizational problem when necessary.

Level II: Moderately Structured   Here the child is given a specific goal to accomplish, but still must organize the process himself. A sample which he must copy provides him with a moderate degree of structure.

For the evaluation the child is shown a picture which has been assembled by the therapist from the multiple precut colored construction paper shapes pasted on 8- by 10-inch drawing paper. He is given a duplicate set of pieces and told to paste these on his paper to match the sample. The therapist should observe whether the child attempts to copy the model and whether he is able to complete the task. Are the parts in correct relationship to each other? Is the whole arrangement in correct spatial orientation on the page?

Meaningful pictures rather than abstract designs are often easier to reproduce because familiarity with the object helps the child orient and organize the parts into a whole. If the child has difficulty at this level, one must first determine whether the problem involves the details of spatial organization or an inability to understand and follow directions and/or complete a task. When there is a basic problem in self-organization one must focus on these problems by using material or tasks already familiar enough so that they can be easily accomplished. The child can then concentrate solely on self-organization rather than on the visual-perceptual organization of the material as well.

When the problem appears to be essentially that of spatial disorganization, one must look further into the component parts of spatial organization, which is considered on Level III.

Level III: Highly Structured   Here specific skills required for organization in space can be assessed within a highly structured situation. Two important skills are (1) the ability to discriminate positional orientations and (2) the ability to locate spatial areas.

For evaluation, notice whether the child has difficulty with the positional aspects of form. He can be asked to match upside-down, left-right and diagonal orientations of objects, and then cut out pictures or felt pieces. First, he should be asked to point to the correct matches, later he can correct the item which is different from the others. If the child has difficulty in placing material in the correct spatial area he can be asked to copy placement of three-dimensional objects. Once the specific skills can be accomplished, they should be combined gradually, in order to enable the child to work on the integration of these skills (as in Levels II and I). This basic awareness and manipulation of space is fundamental to future efficiency in reading and writing.

Visual Memory of Form

The emphasis in this subarea is on helping the child develop retention and recall of visual material as he increases his discriminatory ability. Visual memory must evolve in terms of increasing both the amount and detail of material (eventually to forms in sequence; words, for example) retained, as well as the length of time which forms can be recalled. This short-term (and eventually long-term) memory process is essential to higher levels of visual perception.

A child must be able to remember increasing amounts of visual detail to allow him to compare and contrast complex designs. This is a prerequisite to future ability to compare words and thus achieve success in spelling and reading. When copying material from the blackboard, efficiency in transferring visual stimuli to motor patterns depends to a great extent upon the length of visual materials one is able to retain (short term). Otherwise, time and accuracy may be sacrificed in constant rechecking. The time factor is of further importance, since there is limited value in recalling items for only a brief period. Recall must eventually be long enough to allow one to retrieve a fund of material to use in any old or new combination. When writing spontaneously, one must be able to revisualize letters and word forms without any visual or auditory cues.

In order for the child to develop this short-term retention and long-term recall, he must evolve an organizational process which will enable him to cope with a large amount of material. This organizational process will utilize elements of perception and cognition. Perceptually, he must scan the stimulus to recognize positional and sequential aspects, and, as the amount of length of visual material increases, he must categorize this material in order to render it more manageable.

In order to assess the child's skill in this area the therapist can use a variety of activities within the classroom. Again these will be outlined on three levels of organizational structure provided by the therapist.

Level I: Unstructured   At this level the child has considerable freedom of selection, since there are a variety of items and he must organize himself to select and sort the stimuli into a framework so that he can remember them.

This activity is to evaluate the child's memory for details of a picture. The materials are a fairly complex picture from a storybook or magazine in which there is interaction between people and animals or objects.

Have the child sit in front of the therapist. Say, "I am going to show you a picture that has many things in it. I want you to look at it very carefully because when I hide it I want you to tell me what you can remember. Don't tell me now, look very carefully at everything in the picture." These instructions may be repeated wholly or in part until the child understands. Do not provide any description of the picture to help the child remember the items, if this is to be used for evaluative purposes. When the child has had a chance to view the picture carefully (about 15 or 20 seconds) hide it and ask him to tell you what was in the picture.

Observe both the child's approach and his visual-perceptual skills:

Approach

Does he understand the task?
Does he look carefully at the whole picture?
Can he wait until asked to tell what he remembers?

Visual-Perceptual Skills

How many items can he remember?
Are adjectives and adverbs of size, color and action used?
Does he simply list items or does he relate objects into a simple story? (By asking what he saw in the picture, both methods are made possible.) The criteria for this activity is visual number of stimuli recalled, not expressive language skills.

If performance is very poor, the therapist should ask the child to name the items in the pictures without memory involved. If there is no language problem present, then he must evaluate the visual memory process. This can be accomplished by first checking to see if the child utilizes any organized means of recalling visual stimuli (such as association of items into a category by use, color or other characteristic). It is important to note and encourage the child to use such methods, for memory is seldom enhanced by mere rote practice — we remember best that which we have made some association. The dynamics of organization can be observed on Level II.

Level II: Moderately Structured   The evaluative activity is to show the child a stimulus card with nine pictures arranged in three rows of three pictures each. These pictures should be taken from categories such as food, animals (familiar categories) with three objects in each category, one item from each category in all rows. The stimulus card is removed after fifteen to twenty seconds and the child is asked to name all the things he can remember.

The therapist should note whether the child looks carefully at the card as well as how many items he can remember. Most important, one should observe whether there is any apparent system of organization to the child's retention. If the child remembers fewer than four items, but there is evidence of organization in his attempt, he essentially needs more practice at this level to increase the number of items retained. If he is not able to succeed at this level after an attempt has been made to help him organize his memory process, the therapist should drop back to Level III.

Level III: Highly Structured   Here we check recognition of form, awareness of its absence, revisualization and the sequential aspects of a series of forms. First, the therapist should check to see whether the child understands the concept of something "missing" or "has been taken away" from a series of objects. It is advisable to begin with three-dimensional objects, since some children have difficulty in recognizing even familiar objects in the two-dimensional pictorial form.

Evaluative Activity   The child is given three familiar objects placed in a row on the table (have the child name all items to be used before you begin the memory task). Have the child hide his eyes or place a barricade between the child and the objects. Then ask the child to look and tell you which one is missing. (Be sure to vary position of missing items in subsequent trials. As the child is able to remember any single item removed, remove two items of the three possibilities and then all three. Continue to increase the number of items presented and removed. Positional clues and sequential order should be emphasized as a means of organizing the memory process. When a child has named missing item(s) correctly, ask him to point to where the item had been, and begin to establish labels such as "beginning," "middle" and "end" of row, etc. When retention of three-dimensional objects has been established, one may use two-dimensional representations of these objects, following the same progression.

One can also increase the complexity of the task by increasing the number of rows, as well as the number of items. As the number of items increases, one should introduce the importance or efficiency of categorizing the items presented as a further aid to remembering material. A higher degree of efficiency can be obtained when the child is able to utilize both the perceptual (position) and conceptual (categorization) aspects of organization, even when items are scattered within a specific area.

Sequencing of Visual Material

Another aspect important in visual-perceptual development is sequencing. Here the child must recognize a spatial-directional ordering of visual stimuli. The sequence may involve both three-dimensional and two-dimensional aspects. Material may be positioned in a vertical or horizontal sequence from left to right, in front, behind, beside, or top or bottom. In all cases, there are dimensions of "beginning" or "first," "middle," and "end" or "last," denoting sequential progression. Developing an awareness of sequence gives the child a systematic means of organizing, interpreting and transmitting information. Sequencing is, therefore, a higher level of manipulation of forms in space.

If the child has the concept of sequencing, he then knows where to begin and end, and what must occur between the two extremes. This, of course, is basic to reading and writing skills. The therapist must observe whether the child has basic awareness of the sequence and progression in visual materials. He must eventually be able to store or remember certain sequential patterns in order to use them in reading and writing.

Level I: Unstructured The following activity does not leave the child as much opportunity to organize himself as the prior, Level I, activities do. However, sequencing is a more exact skill requiring considerable built-in structure from the child.

The activity is to match sequencing of shapes. The materials are a pencil or a crayon and a ditto sheet on which one of three or four possible sequential sets of designs are to be matched with a sample. Four or five shapes or line designs should be included in the sequence. All sets should have exactly the same elements, the sequence of these being the only variable (see Appendix for sample).

Have the child seated at a table with enough room to work unhindered. Say, "Look at the first set of designs, up here at the top of the page (point to the first *sample*). There is one set of designs that is *exactly the same as* (just like) this one. There are two other sets which look *something like* the first one but are not exactly the same as this (point to all sets in the first row). Put a circle around the first set of designs and another circle around the one which is exactly the same as the first one. When you have finished, go to the next row, put a circle around the first set of designs and a circle around the one which is exactly the same."

Observations: Approach

Is the child able to listen to and follow directions for this type
   of activity?
Is he confused by so many rows and the fact that he must treat
   each separately?

Visual-Perceptual skills

Does he have the basic concept of matching sequence?
Does he miss part of the sequence (middle or end)?

If the child demonstrates a good basic concept of sequential processing and makes only incidental errors, he simply needs more practice at this level. If on the other hand, he shows poor understanding of this task, there are two major explanations. He may think all sets are the same because all *forms* are present, being oblivious to the order, or he might match sets only by the first and last elements, disregarding the middle elements. One could, therefore, use the second level to point out all the elements involved.

Level II: Moderately Structured   In this activity the therapist has a set of flash cards with forms drawn in different sequential patterns. The child is given a set of cards with individual forms drawn on each. He is to arrange his cards in the same sequential pattern as those of the therapist. The therapist can observe not only the finished product, but also the manner in which the child executes the sequence (proceeding from left to right or in random order).

If the child has difficulty at this level, the therapist may point out the first, middle and last positions — and that one generally starts at the left side and proceeds toward the right in order. If the child continues to have difficulty with this task, one might consider the possibility that the dual discrimination of form and sequence is too confusing. In such a case, one may have to resort to more concrete situations, such as the use of three-dimensional materials, where shape is constant and the sequential orientation is denoted by size or color (Level III). If, however, the child can manage this task successfully, the therapist might wish to vary the task by placing the child's cards in a random order and asking the child to correct these to match the model. This should prepare him for a return to Level I and the more rapid scanning and matching process of comparing one sample to three or four others, thereby building memory and speed as well as accuracy in sequential matching.

Level III: Highly Structured   The evaluation media is three-dimensional material (such as differently colored or sized blocks presented in vertical or horizontal arrangements). One should start with three items to establish the concept of first, middle and last. The child is to copy the arrangement, item by item, with the help of the therapist, who emphasizes the placing procedure as well as the placement of objects (the sequence of time as well as space). One should use the appropriate verbal directions to emphasize the process as he demonstrates. It would seem that the easiest pattern to copy would be an arrangement of three differently sized blocks into a tower. Next, the child can be asked to copy tower patterns by color using three blocks of identical size. Next he can be asked to copy horizontal patterns (trains), using colored blocks and progressing from left to right. When he is able to succeed at this level, copying item by item, then he should be asked to copy the pattern from the finished product.

These activities should help to establish the basic concept of sequential ordering. The process can be elaborated by increasing the number of items to be ordered and by varying the properties of the materials, using size and color simultaneously, or using beads to string or by placing familiar objects in a line.

Eye-Hand Coordination

This area concerns the basic motor aspects of perceptual-motor skills. These will be divided into two phases: the first phase deals with the increased motor efficiency of individual hands, and the second with the integration of two hands in more complex patterned movements.

Increasing Motor Efficiency

A certain amount of efficiency in each hand — whether it is to become the lead or the assisting hand — is necessary and must be achieved. Both hands must be able to grasp small objects and manipulate them (pick up, hold and place) in order to complete functional activities (playing with simple construction toys, feeding, and dressing). The degree of skill in each hand should be fairly equally developed until the activity becomes so complex that it requires either two hands (one to lead and one to hold), or such refined patterned movements that it is more efficient for one hand to learn and perfect that specific activity, and therefore become the preferred hand.

We are not concerned here with specific theories of hand dominance concerning which side or when dominance should be established. We *are* concerned, however, that a child establish a preferred hand before he enters first grade. It has been our experience that if a child has not established a hand preference by the time he is five, he also displays a delay in fine-motor coordination in general. Normally, as a child refines manipulative skills, he begins spontaneously to evolve a hand preference. It seems better, therefore, to help the child refine manipulative skills in both hands and allow a natural or spontaneous preference to evolve rather than preselecting a hand to be the lead or dominant one and prescribing practice with it. If, as occasionally happens, the child seems unable to determine a preference for himself through the above process, then a preference must be selected for him before he enters the first grade — for a continual switching of hands for pencil activities at this time (when he is learning many other new skills) will only confuse and inhibit his performance further. It would seem most logical that the right hand be selected in this case.

In order to assess the degree of skill established in either hand and the inclination toward a hand preference, activities will again be presented on three levels.

Level I: Unstructured   On the first level one should present an activity requiring refined and repetitive patterned movements of one hand and refined assistive manipulation of the other.

The evaluative activity is hammering with a Playskool nailboard. The materials are one-inch nails, hammer and a masonite board. The child may stand or sit as desired. Say, "Here is a board, hammer and nails, and some wooden pieces." Further instructions are up to the therapist, since variations in instructions will not affect the activity appreciably.

Observations: Approach

Can he stay with the task a reasonable length of time?
If he stops, is it due to behavioral or perceptual difficulties?

Motor

Does the child use one hand consistently for hammering?
If he still switches, is one hand noticeably more efficient than
the other?
Does the child hold the hammer toward the end and is the
hammering movement rhythmical?
Does the child have any difficulty picking up nails and
positioning them on the board?

If hand use is consistent, but accuracy or manipulative skill is
poor, then the therapist should provide the same type of activity,
but one which requires less accuracy (larger pegs and a pounding
peg bench). As skill improves, gradually reduce the size of the
pegs to be hit. A variation of this activity and probably one that
would be beneficial as an adjunct to hammering would be to
present a set of Playskool screwdriver and screws. This will
require a different type of motor manipulation and different
patterned movement, but would also be illustrative of the child's
control and choice of a lead hand. If hand preference is not
strongly established, drop back to Level II.

Level II: Moderately Structured   At this level two hands are
used in a similar pattern of lead and assist, but the skill required
allows for either hand to be the lead — with a lesser degree of
accuracy of both hands necessary. Activities include stringing
beads, popbeads, assembling tinker toys, nuts and bolts and the
like. These activities can be graded in difficulty by varying the size
and complexity of the materials used. The child can obtain much
manipulative practice and opportunity to experiment in
developing a lead hand. The therapist should note when there is a
tendency toward consistent use of lead and assistive hand
patterns, and also when accuracy of manipulation allows for the
handling of materials of small sizes.
    If the child can manipulate materials of this size easily with one
hand as lead, he is probably ready to proceed to Level I. If he
demonstrates poor coordination, drop back to Level III.

Level III: Highly Structured   At this level there are two
separate aspects which are important to achieve and then combine

in order to attain efficient eye-hand skills. One is fine finger dexterity, which involves fine prehension (either thumb to index and third, or thumb to index) and the control of individual fingers to allow an object to be repositioned or manipulated in the process of placing it. The other is eye-hand coordination, which involves the efficiency and accuracy with which the eye directs hand movement. Poor eye-hand coordination would be quickly apparent when over- or undershooting the target occurs. In both of these aspects, one should always work toward development of accuracy first and then toward increasing the speed at which the activity can be performed.

Observation and training can be carried out with the utilization of several activities, each emphasizing the use of one hand at a time to develop skill with both hands separately.

To observe individual finger control and manipulation (including prehension), one may present clay, finger-paints, pennies to be placed in a bank, picking up small pegs or marbles to be placed in specific spots, tiles, clothespins to pinch and place around the rim of some container, or tweezers with which to pick up small objects.

Observations   While engaged in these activities the child will use many different finger movements, thus strengthening and improving skill. Activities, of course, may be graded by size and degree of strength required to manipulate the object or tool. One should always begin with larger objects and/or those objects which do not require much prehensile strength — notice that some activities require only grasping and placing an object (blocks, transferring pegs from one board to another, marbles in a Chinese-checker board), while other activities require repositioning or additional manipulating of the particular object before final placement is achieved (tiles, pegs, pokerchips in variously slanted slots). Therefore, start with the more simple and work toward the more complex.

To observe the directness of eye-hand coordination, one may watch the accuracy of alignment of small blocks in a vertical tower, directness of placement of small pegs in a board and placement of round beads on top of these pegs, accuracy of hammering in pounding bench activity or tiles in tileboard.

Observations   Again, large objects should be used first. Distance from pickup to placement should be kept short at first and in one plane, horizontal to the body — lengthened and varied as skill improves.

Most activities require both elements of fine finger dexterity and direct eye-hand coordination. However, one should attempt to observe each aspect as sepatately as possible, in order to isolate the particular problem that a child may be having. If he has difficulty with both fine finger manipulation and placement, one should concentrate on only one aspect at a time. Have him practice picking up large pegs, simply dropping them into a container rather than placing them into individual holes; or have him practice placing material which he does not have to reposition first.

When each hand can perform these types of activities — smoothly and rapidly and with equal skill — one may move back to Level II, where both hands are required to carry out the activity, but neither needs to be more skilled than the other.

Awareness and Integration of Two Sides of the Body

At the same time as the child is refining individual hand use, he must also learn to control the two sides of his body in parallel and opposing and alternating movements, including crossing the midline of his body. This development generally occurs spontaneously, the child being unaware of specific patterns as he participates in the typical childhood games which range from active gross motor skills (hopping, skipping, jumping-jacks and jumping rope) to fine motor skills (handsies-clapsies (a sequential handball game), jacks and cats-cradle). What must evolve is the ability to isolate, choose and combine specific patterns, as they are appropriate, to carry out the smooth and controlled movements of skilled performance.

To assess these developmental aspects of arm movements, one can again look at this on three levels.

Level I: Unstructured

This level requires the highest degree of integration. The child should be able to control all types of movement in various sequential patterns, shifting to a different sequence as necessary. This control can most easily be observed, probably, through simple singing-action games (finger plays) which involve arm and finger movements, such as "This Old Man," "Peas-Porridge Hot," "Ten Little Indians," "I Am a Funny Little Dutch Boy," and so on.

The activity is any singing-action game. No materials are necessary. The child is seated near the therapist, who proceeds as one would when teaching songs or finger plays.

Observations: Approach

Can the child integrate motor movements with the words of the song?

Can he follow the motor sequence correctly?

Motor

Can the child perform motor patterns involving only parallel movements?

Does he have difficulty crossing the midline of his body?

Most children will have minimal difficulty with these activities. Some of them, however, will be able to perform specific movement patterns but will have difficulty in terms of speed — or in combining or shifting from one pattern to another. These children, essentially, need more practice at this level to build up speed or the ability to carry out the transition smoothly, or both. For those children who become disorganized and unable to carry out these patterns adequately, go back to Levels II and III in order to ascertain the nature of their problems.

Level II: Moderately Structured   On this level we are assessing the child's ability to cross the midline of his body when such movements are more efficient in carrying out motor activity. Difficulty may be evident when the child either (1) isolates the use of each arm to that corresponding side of the body (for example, when it becomes necessary to move an object across the midline, he transfers the object from one hand to the other in continuing the path), or (2) makes exclusive use of one hand (when it becomes necessary to cross the midline he uses his arm and whole body in parallel movements — instead of moving only his arm across his body.

Activity   Present such tasks as having the child draw a line on the blackboard between two targets placed approximately three feet apart. The first target should be placed to the left of the child and the second to his right. The child is to stand at a point in the center of these. The targets should be approximately at nose height. The child is requested to draw a line with one hand. He may choose which one he wishes to use; he should, however, be able to do this with either hand.

To determine whether the child can cross the midline with both hands simultaneously, the therapist can play a modified game of "Follow the Leader," using the arms. The therapist should perform patterned arm movements which require crossing the midline (both hands to opposite knee or shoulders, etc.) alternating with movements which do not require crossing from one side to the other.

Observation   The child may demonstrate difficulty in crossing with one or with both hands simultaneously. If the child has difficulty only in those activities that require crossing with both hands simultaneously, then it can be assumed that he is able to cross the midline but has difficulty in integrating the two sides, and that practice will be necessary, which can be accomplished on Level III. If he has difficulty in all patterns which require crossing, one still should refer to Level III in order to assess awareness and control of individual sides. If his skills are adequate at this level, the therapist will still have to spend time on development of crossing the midline. This can be done by utilizing activities which require the child to keep his hand on an object (such as a car) which is to be moved along a long road drawn on paper which crosses his body, or activities which keep one hand occupied. He can, for instance, hold a container in one hand while the other picks up small objects placed randomly on either side of his body.

Level III: Highly Structured   On Level III we are concerned with the child's ability to execute and control arm movements in simple patterns — which do not require crossing the midline, but which do require the control of both sides together, first in parallel and then in oppositional movements.

Activities   Observation and training can be carried out by using the same modified game of "Follow the Leader" mentioned on Level II, except that no patterns which cross the midline are used. The therapist should begin with simple symmetrical movements where both hands move in the same direction (both up, front, side etc.). When this is smoothly executed, he should progress to patterns in which one hand is moved to a position opposite the other. These should be carried out in sequences of continued movement to produce a pattern. The child should next be able to produce alternating movements, beating on a drum or on his knees. He should then be asked to follow patterns which are not exactly oppositional but differ in position — similar to patterns a flagman might use. Once this stage has been achieved the therapist can move back up to activities on Levels II and I.

COMBINED VISUAL-PERCEPTUAL-MOTOR TASKS

Three successive phases which seem essential in the integration of the perceptual and motor skills necessary for writing comprise this area. This discussion is an attempt to describe the progression involved in combining the component parts of any reproduction activity. Once a child has achieved a certain efficiency in both visual-perceptual discrimination and motor-control or planning, he is ready to explore the relationships between these two areas. While the therapist will provide a logical progression of activities to be used for the child who demonstrates difficulty in the area of visual-motor reproduction, this does not mean that he is to eliminate the child's spontaneous attempt at drawing. On the contrary, such activities should be encouraged, for his attempts at self expression are also important in developing perceptual-motor skills.

Fine Motor Planning with a Tool

In this first phase the emphasis is placed on the utilization of a well defined spatial area to provide a broad boundary within which motor movements are guided in terms of distance and direction. It is necessary that the child learn to perceive the relationship of movements to spatial area and begin to act upon this awareness. (This knowledge is functionally demonstrated when the child colors pictures with adapted strokes and clearly defines the separate parts of the picture. For example, when the spatial area is a vertical box, crayon strokes used to color in this area should be up and down. If the box is horizontal, strokes should adapt to this directional orientation.)

Level I: Unstructured   Coloring a simple picture is the evaluative activity. The materials are a simple picture, the form of which allows for vertical, horizontal, and diagonal stroke patterns and a box of crayons. Have the child seated at a table and say, "Color the picture as best you can." Pertinent observations are to perceive the child's ability to separate segments of the picture and to match motor patterns to the given spatial area or form.

Approach

Does the child attempt to color the picture?
Can he complete this activity?

Visual-Perceptual Skills

Does the child adapt the direction of the strokes to the forms provided, or does he continue the less efficient use of vertical strokes for all spaces, or does he rotate the paper as an alternative to adapting strokes?
Does he demonstrate awareness of separate sections of the picture by assigning different colors to these or by shifting strokes for different sections, or does he ignore the smaller area segments adapting strokes only to the larger ones?

If the child makes an attempt to adjust his strokes, but the lines extend beyond the area, his problem may reflect lack of motor control rather than the perceptual-motor match. This child would need practice primarily in confining motor movements to stay within specific boundaries. However, his problem may also be due to an inability to make a clear distinction between separate segments of this picture and thus, he adapts his strokes only to the larger areas. This child will need assistance in perceiving the separate segments (Level II).

Occasionally a child may indicate awareness of the separate segments and appropriately adapt his strokes, but utilizes several colors within one area, such as making the boy's shirt multicolored. This is felt to be part of an experimental and spontaneous stage during which the child's interest is primarily in the awareness and utilization of color rather than form. This child should be able to modify his performance when requested. There are, however, some children who do this work without apparent adaptation of strokes and who cannot modify performance when requested. These children may be focusing on color because of their difficulty in perceiving a perceptual-motor match. They will need help on Level III.

If the child simply scribbles over the whole area, it is evident he has no concept of confining and/or adapting strokes and thus, should be given practice in coloring at a lower level (Level III).

Level II: Moderately Structured   Activity   Ask the child to copy a model colored by the therapist. Different sections are designated by the use of different colors.

At this level, emphasis is placed upon helping the child who has begun to adapt strokes to major areas, but who has not yet been able to perceive the minor segments of a picture. The therapist should observe whether the child identifies segments by matching colors and whether he adapts strokes to form. If he does not copy colors exactly, one should check to see if he can match colors and simply did not achieve the correct set for this activity. If the child has difficulty identifying segments, a progression of pictures with an increasing number of segments should be presented. If he identifies the segments, but his strokes do not adapt to the forms, he will need practice on Level III.

Level III: Highly Structured   In order to test or train the child at this level, give to him a series or isolated geometric shapes to color — long and narrow vertical, horizontal, and/or diagonal boxes, for instance. If orientation of form is vertical in nature, then the movement of strokes covering this form should also be vertical, etc.

One would expect the child by kindergarten age to be able to adapt progressively to vertical, horizontal, and then diagonal spatial areas without rotation of the paper. If the child is able to color in the vertical orientation with evenly spaced strokes, but seems unable to spontaneously shift to the horizontal or diagonal, point it out to him and help him to initiate the correct movements by moving his hand in the proper directions. If he actively resists this progression to horizontal and then diagonal patterned movements, one must consider specific neuromotor difficulties which are preventing fine motor control.

Primary concern here is to help the child to achieve an exact match between the shape of the form and the direction of his strokes. When he has achieved these directional patterns he can be considered to have made the perceptual-motor match and can move to Level II where more intricate adaptation is required.

Translation of Visual Form Into Motor Patterns

In this second phase, emphasis is placed on the child's ability to visually perceive a line drawing and to translate this drawing into a motor reproduction. In this phase, the visual stimuli remains present during reproduction. Patterns must be predrawn so that children do not have the benefit of being able to imitate the teacher's motor movements. The focus is on accurate reproduction of each pattern in terms of form and position. Spatial organization of forms on the page or accurate reproduction of size are not of concern at this time.

Level I: Unstructured The activity used for evaluation is copying line patterns. The materials are a piece of 8- by 10-inch paper, a pencil and a set of nine 4- by 6-inch cards, each with a simple line pattern predrawn on it. The designs should include vertical, horizontal, diagonal and curved lines. Make sure the top of the card is visible to the therapist. (Numbering cards on the back may facilitate assessment later.)

Have the child seated at a table facing the therapist and close enough to see the stimulus cards, which can be held up or taped on a blackboard. Do not mount cards on a piece of colored paper, since some children will then draw a box around each of their reproductions.

Give the child his paper in a horizontal position and mark the top of the paper. Say, "Please leave your paper just as I give it to you and keep your hands in your lap until I say GO. I am going to show you some pictures one at a time. You are to draw each one on your paper. When you have finished put your pencil down." Hold up the first card and say, GO. "Take your time and do the best you can." When the child has finished proceed to the next card and continue the same procedure.

If a child does not have room to fit all the patterns on one side he may turn his paper over to complete the task. The therapist may wish to number the child's reproductions if they are beginning to be mixed together as the child draws. Do not draw patterns as the child watches, for it is important that the child make the patterns from a finished product without the help of watching the process of creating the pattern.

Observations: Approach

Can the child organize himself adequately to sit in a chair and carry out a pencil and paper activity which requires accurate perception of visual stimuli and motoric representation of this stimuli?
Does he understand the directions given?
Can he carry these through to completion?

Visual-Perceptual Skills

Apart from behavioral components, does the child have any specific perceptual-motor difficulties?
Can he make forms resemble the model closely enough for the therapist to recognize them?
Is the pattern in the correct position (right-side-up, not reversed or rotated)?
Can he achieve the diagonal orientation?

Perceptual observations can be made from the finished reproductions and recorded at the end of the day. Each child's paper should be assessed, item by item, in order to determine whether or not there is difficulty in one or more of the areas listed; these observations can be marked directly on the child's paper. To achieve a clear picture of the child's overall performance, one should note the frequency of a specific error — overall performance may then be charted on an accompanying check sheet.

As long as the essence of the form is achieved, the child is considered to be able to make the translation of visual pattern to motor pattern. However, if he has difficulty in achieving the essential form, one should drop back to the lower levels (II and III).

If the child makes numerous rotations or other positional errors (probably five or more is significant), the therapist should drop back to activities which give him practice in spatial orientation through manipulation of three-dimensional materials and discussion of their orientations. (Appropriate activities are outlined in detail on Level III of the section, *Organization of Forms in Space.*) When this level has been satisfactorily reached, the therapist may move on up to Level II of the present section.

The ability to recognize and achieve diagonal orientation seems to follow appreciation of vertical and horizontal lines. If this recognition has not been achieved by this time, possibly it would help to point out the differences between vertical, horizontal and diagonal orientations and use three-dimensional materials to demonstrate. One could draw lines on a piece of paper with a ruler, allowing the child to manipulate the ruler and, therefore, the lines.

If there is evidence of overlapping, size variation or irregular placement of forms, these characteristics should be noted as being a problem separate from misperception of the form, so long as the essence of form is achieved. In such cases, fine motor control or coordination and/or spatial organization should be assessed.

In all cases we are most interested in trends — or determination of the factors which may be causing the child to have difficulty succeeding. The therapist should be aware of all the components involved in these tasks so that he may determine just which aspects cause a child difficulty.

Precision of visual-motor reproductions is tested here and is directly related to the child's capacity to copy letters of the alphabet without rotations or reversals. If he cannot accomplish the above task easily, he certainly is not ready to learn to write letters.

Level II: Moderately Structured   The therapist draws simple designs, single vertical and horizontal lines, diagonals, and circles and combinations of these, one at a time, on a paper. The child should first imitate the movement of each line drawn for any design on a paper along with the therapist. When he is successful, he can attempt to draw each pattern on his paper as the therapist draws them on another piece. We are interested on this level in aiding the child who is unable to initiate independent copying of line patterns, which can be accomplished by giving him a clue of the motor pattern necessary, and by allowing him to imitate the therapist's movements. If the child still has difficulty, the therapist should provide activities on Level III.

Level III: Highly Structured   Allow the child to trace line drawings — with or without stencils. Within this level, and with this kinesthetic reinforcement, one could proceed from thick stencils to thin, to tracing line drawings, to completing broken line patterns to connecting dots. In this activity one assumes that the difficulty lies in motor planning, and that the child therefore needs a more constant structure to allow him to experience the visual image and the motor movements required in producing that image simultaneously.

Elaboration of Design

The third phase involves the combination of the elements of fine motor control, memory for patterns (shape and size), visual organization of form in space, and visual sequencing. The child will be expected not only to draw basic designs but to vary their size and organize them into specific sequential patterns as well as to cope with the placement of these on the paper.

Level I: Unstructured   *Activity*   Copying shapes of varying sizes in correct sequence and spatial orientation of the paper — is an activity very similar to the one described in copying line patterns. The same basic skills or self-organization and ability to deal with perceptual-motor material are required, but the task is complicated by the presence of more variables. The child must not only be able to draw basic shapes, but to make them the correct size, to place them in the correct order, and to place them in the proper place on the page. Additionally, he is shown a group of patterns and shapes on a whole page, not just one design at a time. All these variables must be considered before the child can reach any success in writing or copying letters and words. The ability to draw diagonal lines is not required in this activity. One may wish to use a triangle in place of the cross when diagonal orientation has been achieved, since this ability is necessary to writing many letters.

The materials to be used are an 8- by 10-inch sample card drawn off into three long horizontal spaces with three shapes (large and small) in each section, and a piece of 8- by 10-inch paper and pencil for each child (be sure to mark the top of each child's paper).

Have the child seated comfortably in a position where he can see the sample card easily. Give the child his paper in a horizontal position and a pencil. Say, "Please leave your paper just as I give it to you, and keep your hands in your lap until I say GO. I am going to show you another paper, like yours, with some shapes drawn on it. You are to make yours exactly the same as mine. When you are finished, put your pencil down and your hands back in your lap, so I know you are all finished." Show him the model and say "GO...Look very carefully. Take your time and make it exactly the same as this one."

Observations: Approach

Does the child appear to understand the task? The same observations concerning self-organization made in copying line patterns are to be assessed.

Visual-Perceptual Skills

These observations can again be made from the completed production and assessed in the same way as with line patterns; tendencies or types of difficulties should be noted. Does the child have specific difficulties with:

Drawing shapes accurately?
Achieving the correct size?
Achieving the correct sequence of shapes?
Positional orientation?

If the child has difficulty drawing shapes, drop back to Level III, in which he can trace shapes or use stencils. If he does not vary the size of drawn shapes, check his visual awareness of size (without the motor aspect). Checking for the visual awareness of sequence and position may also be necessary if either of these aspects is hindering his motor performance (refer to the Visual-Perception Section).

If the child can visually discriminate size, sequence and positional aspects of form, but has difficulty when motor reproduction is required, the therapist may utilize Levels II and III in which these aspects have been separated.

Level II: Moderately Structured   Have the child copy a model similar to one used on Level I, minus the size element. At this level, the size variable is eliminated, but we expect the child to be able to reproduce basic shapes. Here the emphasis will be placed upon the problems of sequencing: (1) position of forms within a row (first, second, third) and (2) position of rows on the paper (top, middle, bottom).

If the child still has difficulty with this task, the therapist may separate the elements further. One could start by presenting single strips of paper with two or three forms in sequence drawn on each. Give the child a strip of paper on which he can copy the model sequence. Gradually increase the number of forms on each single strip to five or more. (This activity may be presented not only with the paper placed in a horizontal position, but also in the vertical.)

A variation of this task which involves more emphasis on visual scanning and discrimination of forms in sequence — as well as a motor element — would be to have the child fill in the missing element of a sequence. The child will be given papers on which partial sequences have been drawn and the teacher holds up a completed model of these same sequences. In this task, it is important that missing elements do not fall in same position on each sequence.

Once the child resolves difficulty in this area, and if he has no difficulty with the size variable, return to Level I.

Level III: Highly Structured   The child is asked to copy large and small shapes. Emphasis is placed on effectively controlling the size of forms reproduced. If a clear distinction between the sizes is not evident, he will need practice refining control of motor movements. The therapist should exaggerate differences in size by having the child trace very large and very small forms. If needed, stencils could also be utilized — a "middle size" should be introduced to further refine control. When the child can manage this part of the activity, proceed to having him copy different size forms; then add another variable, and so on back to Level I.

Summary   The highest level of perceptual-motor reproduction ability has been reached when the child can integrate visual and motor components (as in copying); and can also produce motor patterns from memory and translate auditory stimuli into motor reproductions. In this latter, the child has to receive stimuli auditorily (with no visual stimuli present) and to recall visual stimuli. If a child is to succeed in academics, he will have to be able to integrate basic modalities in various combinations in this way. In order to learn letters and numbers, he must be able to match symbols visually, reproduce them from a visual or auditory stimulus (and eventually from memory), control spatial dimensions, and properly sequence the elements.

The activities mentioned for diagnostic purposes on Level I of each phase are not the only ones that could have been used. They were given in detail in order to demonstrate the method by which one may initially gain information concerning any subarea before teaching it. On Level I the therapist can observe each child's performance in activities during which the child has to organize himself to a great degree. It is of primary interest to note whether or not each child is aware of and can cope with the variables inherent in the task. To do this, the therapist is asked to minimize other elements (verbal, motor) and to observe the child's mastery of the elements being evaluated. One should not teach the activity first if he wants to use it diagnostically.

It has been found that performance is often quite variable in children with learning problems when their difficulties lie mainly in the area of self-organization. Performance can be quite different from day-to-day and depends to a great extent on what type of activity and whether success or failure has-preceded the evaluation. It may be profitable for the therapist to repeat the activity, varying the stimuli used, two or three times in one week to get a clearer picture of performance and to insure that the set is understood. It is still important to use the directions given, however, in order to avoid making the task too easy and therefore, not achieving the information desired.

Although the therapist is urged to follow the instructions given for initial diagnosis, we certainly do not mean to intimate that evaluation is not an ongoing process. Obviously after teaching or helping a child to achieve a certain skill, the therapist will want to retest the child's grasp of this skill. He should be careful, however, to see that the child does not learn to perform an activity only under certain circumstances and is, therefore, incapable of transferring the basic underlying skill to other situations.

Types of Dysfunction

Like other developmental processes, the impairments of the perceptual process are represented in varying degrees of severity. For the purpose of this discussion these deficiencies have been divided into four categories. These are not medical diagnostic categories, only roughly defined groups which one may use to organize his thoughts about the large number of varied handicaps in the perceptual-motor area. The categories identified are: (1) Serious Neurological Deficit; (2) Mild Neurological Dysfunction, (3) Isolated High Level Perceptual Handicap, and (4) Developmental Lag.

Serious Neurological Deficit   These children suffer a severe handicap because of lack of or damage to part of the central nervous system. The damage may have occurred pre- or post-natally as a result of faulty development or trauma. A large majority of children with a diagnosis of cerebral palsy, mental retardation and brain damage have very deficient perception and have great difficulty in perceptual-motor skills. Perceptual deficits in these children are often multiple, and begin at an early developmental level. They are only a part of a more global syndrome and are seldom- treated in themselves, but are treated as a part of the integrated therapeutic program which these types of children need. Evaluation does not involve standardized tests, but is usually a more global and functional form of evaluation.

Treatment, as defined by the evaluation, usually begins at an early developmental level; such as basic sensory awareness (Section One) and proceeds up the developmental scale at a rate determined by the child's own capacity and rate of development. Treatment of these children is usually a team effort and is guided by the philosophy of the clinic. A sound knowledge of normal development plus an understanding of the clinical condition of the child will be combined by each of the therapists to create the basis for a good treatment program.

Mild Neurological Dysfunction   These children constitute a less well defined group than the previous one. Much research and clinical practice is now being devoted to these children so that the problems may be further defined and better treated. Although they have a variety of minor problems for a variety of reasons there seems to be one factor which serves to define these children as a group: they all, in one manner or another, show deficiencies upon neurological evaluation. They typically show aberrance in the areas of balance, coordination and sensation. These indications are referred to by the neurologist as "soft signs," which means that there are minor indications that the nervous system is not sufficiently integrated or matured. Some indications of this problem are insufficient cutaneous innervation, tested by steriognostic tests and skin localization. Poor fine-motor coordination is discovered through tests of patterned prehension; poor kinesthetic and proprioceptive capacities are discovered by asking the child to balance on one foot with his eyes closed and a few similar tests. These tests are useful in that they indicate to the physician the presence of some neurological dysfunction. How this dysfunction relates to the child's performance can be only partially assessed at this time. Evaluation by other members of the medical team contributes information regarding the child's performance in several areas. These multidisciplinary teams often see the same patterns of dysfunction in different children — through this, observation theories are beginning to emerge which will contribute to the development of specific treatment techniques for the therapists to use with these children. Ultimately the new treatment techniques will be translated into teaching techniques for the use of the special teacher.

Isolated High Level Perceptual Handicap   Definition of this group is the least clear. There are many children who perform marginally well in the public school system, yet who score poorly on one or more of the subtests in *The Marianne Frostig Developmental Test of Visual Perception,* or on one of the A.J. Ayres tests. They may show normal to superior verbal intelligence, an excellent vocabulary and apparent speed in grasping abstract concepts. Typically they are discovered because they "can't read at the expected level." That is, that the teacher cannot understand the great discrepancy between the child's apparent cognitive skill and his difficulty in learning to read. These children have a handicap in one or more perceptual skills, and consequently are poor in the perceptual-cognitive skill of reading and in the perceptual-motor skill of writing. Educators refer to this syndrome as a learning disability, or *specific learning disability* or *dyslexia.* Some theorists hold that this is not a neurologically based problem; however, many of these children do show hints of neurological "soft signs." It is often noted that these children are "clumsy," a more appropriate term is probably "slight neuromotor insufficiency." In addition to these children, there are those whose severe emotional problems have prevented them from developing perceptual or perceptual-motor skills, thus presenting a double problem of both delayed development and emotional fragility. (There is also some evidence that seems to show that some children thought to be psychotic had severe perceptual problems, which made the child unable to interpret his visual world appropriately, and so developed an emotional problem.) Many of the mildly perceptually handicapped children develop secondary emotional problems and school phobias, since they are required to perform tasks which are intellectually beneath them but perceptually beyond them.

Evaluation   The evaluative procedures described in Section III are useful informal tests for evaluating these children. Standardized tests are available but tend to evaluate only limited areas of perceptual-motor function.

Treatment   The treatment procedures described in Section III should be used when appropriate. These tasks may also be used as models from which the therapist may begin to design his own treatment procedures.

Developmental Lag In contrast to the previous group of children, who are characterized by a rather uneven pattern of development, this group displays a very even one. The majority of each child's scores on developmental tests will fall at a certain age level, and vary not much more than a year from each another. The major difficulty here is that, although the child may be functioning adequately at a particular developmental level, he happens to be chronologically older than is typical for this level. These children may progress well in a less academically oriented society. However, American children are expected to be able to perform certain tasks by age six (reading, writing, etc.). If these children are discovered earlier than first grade, the best course to take is usually an extra year in kindergarten. If the child is in grade one, he should be given intensive developmental therapy in the areas in which he is experiencing difficulty, in the hope that by the time he reaches grade two he will be functioning at grade level.

Many of these children progress rapidly in therapy — and working with them is very rewarding. Some children appear to need help only for a short time, and then continue to develop on schedule. Most need a developmental program for about a year, while some continue in therapy for two or three years.

The therapist will find many children who do not fall into these classifications; it is hoped, however, that the conceptual framework brought forth here will give him some confidence in approaching such a diversified group of children.

Criteria for the Design and Construction of Perceptual-Motor Toys and Games

The therapist often finds himself making many of the materials for his young clients. This time-consuming activity may be frustrating or rewarding — at times it may even be fruitless. If the toy is improperly designed or poorly constructed, it may not serve the purpose for which it was intended. Whether he makes his own materials, adapts commercially produced ones, or buys special materials for the perceptually handicapped, there are some questions he should ask himself about the toy before he uses it. The therapist may need to use the toy with a few children first in order to determine the usefulness of the toy — but the following considerations should be of use in initially selecting the materials for the clinic.

What perceptual (or perceptual-motor) skill will the toy serve to develop? At what level? What other sensory skills does it employ to teach the desired skill? Are these skills commonly found in children lacking the target skill, or is this only compounding the difficulty?

Are the directions easy to follow? Is the process involved easy for the child to understand? Are the pictures clear and large? Are the pictures or pieces appealing to a broad range of ages and interests? Is it made of durable material? If it breaks, will the pieces be harmful? Is it attractive? (Does it *look* like fun?) Will it hold a child's attention? Specific considerations may also be added, but these suggestions should help the therapist to begin to evaluate the toy.

Bibliography

Ayres, A. Jean. "Occupational Therapy for Motor Disorders Resulting from Impairment of the Central Nervous System." *Rehabilitation Literature* (1960), pp. 302-310.

Ayres, A. Jean. *Perceptual-Motor Dysfunction in Children* (monograph from the Greater Cincinnati District Occupational Therapy Association Conference, Cincinnati, Ohio, 1964), p. 3.

Ayres, A. Jean. "The Role of Gross Motor Activities in the Training of Children with Visual-Motor Retardation." *Journal of the American Optometric Association*, 1961.

Ayres, A. Jean. *Southern California Perceptual-Motor Tests* (Los Angeles, California: Western Psychological Tests, 1969).

Baldwin, A. L. *Theories of Child Development* (New York: John Wiley and Sons, 1968).

Barsch, R. *Achieving Perceptual-Motor Efficiency, Volume I* (Seattle: Special Child Publications, 1967).

Barsch, R. "A Movigenic Curriculum." Bulletin Number 25 (Madison, Wisconsin: University of Wisconsin, 1965).

Cruikshank, W. et al. *A Teaching Method for Brain-Injured and Hyperactive Children* (Syracuse, New York: Syracuse University Press, 1961).

Denhoff, E. and Robinault, I. *Cerebral Palsy and Related Disorders* (New York: McGraw-Hill, 1961).

Frostig, M. *Developmental Test of Visual Perception* (Chicago: Follett, 1963).

Frostig, M. and Horne, D. *The Frostig Program for the Development of Visual Perception* (Chicago: Follett, 1964).

Frostig, M. "Visual Perceptual Development and School Adjustment and Progress." *American Journal of Orthopsychiatry* 33 (1963), pp. 367-368.

Gesell, A. *The First Five Years of Life* (New York: Harper and Row, 1940).

Kephart, N. C. *The Slow Learner in the Classroom* (New York: Charles E. Merrill, 1960).

Kohlberg, L. "The Cognitive-Developmental Approach to Early Education." In Elkind, D. and Flavell, J. (eds.) *Contributions of Jean Piaget* (New York: D. VanNostrand, 1967).

Muller, P. *The Tasks of Childhood* (New York: McGraw-Hill, 1969).

Piaget, J. and Inhelder, B. *The Psychology of the Child* (New York: Basic Books, 1969).

340

NOTES

Chapter Seven

The Development of Communication and Cognition

Barbara Sharpe Banus, M.A., O.T.R.

(November 1970)

Communication and cognition are two very important areas of behavior which were too often neglected by the occupational therapist of the past. Fortunately the importance of cognition is now being recognized, and cognitive development is being increasingly emphasized in occupational therapy as an independent entity — and as one which strongly influences the development of other behaviors. Speech and language continue to be a secondary focus of the occupational therapist. However, without knowledge of the development of speech and language, the therapist often meets with failure when trying to communicate with a child. In addition, without such knowledge he can neither observe nor communicate the speech and language needs of the child to the speech and language therapist, nor can he appropriately stimulate the speech of the child during therapy.

Speech and language and cognitive development will be discussed more briefly than neuromotor, psychosocial, and visual-perceptual-motor development because they usually fall in the domain of the speech and language therapist and educator, respectively. For the same reason, no recommendations for formal or standardized evaluations or highly specific treatment techniques will be presented. The responsibilities of all developmental therapists, however, include the stimulation of both speech and language and cognitive development. Consequently, a few tentative suggestions for developmental stimulation will be presented in order to encourage the therapist's use of this content.

THE DEVELOPMENT OF SPEECH AND LANGUAGE

The Relationship of Communication to the Other Developmental Processes

Development and function in all behavioral areas are crucial to communication and, therefore, can impede or facilitate its function. *Communication* as a concept encompasses speech and language, and is interwoven with all other developmental processes. Pronovost,[1] in his explanation of the communication process between two or more people, has described seven stages of communication. The *perceptual phase* of communication, is the perception of the other individual by the speaker through one or more stimuli (such as visual and auditory). Upon recognition of the individual, the speaker quickly transfers to the *psychological stage* and makes the decision whether to ignore or to approach the person and communicate verbally. The communication also may be nonverbal, as, for example, a gesture which expresses a speaker's feelings. If the communication is begun, the speaker's ability to express himself, his knowledge of the language and his emotional behavior will influence the content of the discussion. The *linguistic stage* is the meaningful sequencing of sounds to form words and then sentences. These are the structural elements of a language and are defined as the *phonemes, morphemes,* and *syntax.* Phonemes are the speech sounds which affect the meaning of a word. For example, as the phoneme "s" is changed to "t," the word "seas" changes to "seat" or "teas." Morphemes are combinations of phonemes which create the smallest unit of meaningful language in the form of a word. Syntax is the sequencing of words to form a sentence which is unique to a particular language. The process of converting the actual words into sounds which can be heard by the listener is the *neurophysiological phase.* The *acoustical phase,* which follows, is the point at which the vibrations created by the voice within the air move to the listener and form meaningful sounds for him. The *perceptual phase of the listener* occurs as he hears meaningful sounds and comprehends them via the auditory mechanism. He perceives the loudness, pitch and quality of the sounds and the location of the speaker through the use of both ears. The communication process shifts to the listener and begins again as he becomes first the listener and then the speaker. The *psychological phase of the listener* determines the degree to which he actually listens to the speaker, actively and concerned, or passively with disinterest. The effectiveness of the listening will determine the direction of the conversation and the effectiveness of continued communication beyond just the use of speech and language.

Definitions of Communication, Speech and Language

Communication is the exchange of ideas or feelings between people. These ideas and feelings may be exchanged via language on a verbal basis or through nonverbal gestures and expressions.

Speech is...
formalized oral communication; audible language, particularly that which is conventionalized into an arbitrary code, in contradistinction to emotional cries. There are four aspects of speech: (1) linguistic, including the thoughts underlying oral expression as well as grammatical form; (2) phonatory, including breath support for the tone as well as the laryngeal vibrations themselves; (3) articulatory, including control of the velum in regulating the nasal components of tone, as well as control of the jaw, tongue, and lips in shaping the breath stream, voiced and unvoiced, into vowels and consonants; (4) auditory, including control of articulation and pronation by means of sensory reports via the organ of hearing, as well as the understanding of the meanings of others through interpretation of the acoustic symbols that they produce.[2]

Language is a system which is the basis for oral communication within a speech community (a group of people who have developed a systematic way of responding to common verbal expressions). Language also can include the nonverbal expressions and mannerisms which accompany speech behavior.[3]

Language can be subdivided into three units: receptive, central, and expressive. These can be analyzed separately, but for the purpose of this text, the concepts of central language will be combined with those of receptive language. Central language can be described as the integrative element which perceives the meaning of the words prior to an appropriate response. This definition implies the comprehension or understanding element of language.

Receptive language includes the receiving of verbal or nonverbal stimuli which, in turn, includes the ability to comprehend or understand the meaning of its content. It requires the visual or tactile receptivity of the nonverbal stimuli and the auditory receptivity of the verbal stimuli. As the number of sensory receptors involved in the communication is increased, the likelihood of the message being understood and responded to increases. The extent of the development of a child's receptive language is evaluated through his verbal and nonverbal response to the stimuli.

Expressive and receptive language develop simultaneously, although receptive and central language precede expressive language initially and each develops at a different rate. For example, the child sees and recognizes his mommy before he can say "Mommy." The degree of speech and language development is assessed through the child's ability to respond appropriately to a given situation and in a way that can be understood by the child's speech community. If the communication requires words, they must be meaningful and sufficiently intelligible.

Expressive language demonstrates a person's comprehension and thought process through his motor response. This response can be verbal, as illustrated in speech or nonverbal as in body language. In standardized testing, expressive language is usually evaluated by the child's response to verbal questions — the identification of words common to his speech community and within the range of his developmental age. Because receptive and expressive language are strongly influenced by the environment in which the child lives and functions, a problem arises when the language of the home in which he lives differs from the environment in which he functions, such as the neighborhood or school.

The degree to which the child develops speech and language is influenced by numerous factors. He may demonstrate temporary immature speech patterns because he focuses on other developmental behaviors at some time during the preschool years. He may show limited development in speech because of mental retardation, in which case his developmental and chronological age in speech may never become parallel. Underdeveloped or dysfunctioning speech and language can have a pathological basis because of emotional problems, brain damage, hearing loss, aphasia and so forth, or an environmental basis, such as poor teaching methods in school, poor speech standards, or a poor or unfavorable environment.

Language is an important unit of the child's development; it is one of the most effective and acceptable means of expressing one's needs. The child who says, "Tummy hurts" receives quicker treatment in the area of the pain than the child who cries extensively or who withdraws and gives only general nonverbal cues. All therapists assess language function in order to determine the child's ability to communicate both receptively and expressively. Language in the early years is in a rapid state of change and is easily influenced by the child's immediate emotional and social situation. When a young child is under stress, he frequently regresses in language behavior. He may stop talking and instead communicate through body language and crying or other sounds — depending upon his development and the degree of stress. In evaluation and early treatment sessions, the child may refuse to communicate verbally, and it may be very difficult, therefore, to evaluate his language skills during the initial observation. The greater the amount of pressure applied to him to speak, the less likely he is to respond. In some testing (the Gesell Developmental Appraisal, described in Chapter Eight for instance) the unit in which the language is to be evaluated is placed in the middle of the examination, after the child becomes comfortable with the examiner and before he needs gross motor activity.

The therapist also has the responsibility to help a child develop adequate speech patterns and language during his treatment of the child. This can be accomplished readily by knowing the receptive and expressive language developmental sequences with which to stimulate the child's speech and language. The developmental ages which are identified in the following developmental scheme highlight the beginnings of some of the language behaviors.

A Sequence of Speech and Language Development
The First Six Weeks of Life
Receptive language: The child may show a total body response or startle (moro reflex) to loud or sudden auditory or visual stimuli. His vision is nonspecific in its direction and shows the absence of his awareness of his surroundings.
Expressive language: The newborn makes sounds reflexively, with no intention of expressing his needs and combines them with

other behaviors, such as crying, which are often paired with total body activity. He smiles reflexively to tactile and kinesthetic sensation. By the end of two or three weeks, a person who knows the child well can distinguish among the cries of the infant — the cry for food, for pain and so forth. The sounds that the child makes are internally motivated and produced rather than externally stimulated. Although most of the sounds in the first month are crying sounds, an occasional vowel can be heard in addition to the small grunts, gurgles, and sighs.

Recommendations for stimulating sound production: A child should be encouraged to vocalize (cry and make sounds). This permits him to develop the vocal and respiratory coordination for breath control which is prerequisite to speech. However, too much crying inhibits the child from making useful sounds. There seems to be an association between nonpurposeful sounds and later speech. Perhaps this is related to a critical period, since it has been found that orphanage babies talk later than those brought up in a home.

Six to Eight Weeks of Age

Receptive: The child begins to focus visually and appears alert to his surroundings. He attends to a person's voice and shows an awareness of his own sounds.

Expressive: Babbling usually begins about this time and is a continuous experimentation with speech sounds. This includes nasal front sounds rather than real speech sounds. The child makes sounds that are common to a variety of cultures and uses them randomly. (It is at a later time that he begins to associate the specific sounds with his parents or the community around him.) It is thought that until this time the deaf child and the hearing child perform the same behavior in making sounds, since the deaf child does not need to hear to vocalize because the behavior is reflexive.

Recommendations: At this time the child is self-stimulating and attempts to make the sounds in his vocal play. If interrupted by an adult, he may cease to vocalize. Permit the child time to play alone and experiment with sounds in addition to talking to him when interacting with him.

Sixteen to Twenty Weeks of Age

Receptive: The child can turn toward a noise and visually fixate on an object. He watches people and objects held in his own hand; he cannot yet differentiate sounds or behaviors more explicitly.

Expressive: Cries are specific to the infant's own physical needs and he begins to use his vocalization as a means of communication. Babbling continues.

Recommendations: Beginning vocal-social association should be encouraged through smiling and increased varied verbalization by the adult.

Six Months of Age

Receptive-expressive: The child begins to make spontaneous sounds and gestures in relation to objects around him and to repeat the sounds he hears over and over for the pleasure derived from his own self-stimulated performance (this repetition is known as *lalling*). This process indicates that the child is making associations between his receptive (what he hears) and expressive language (the sounds he can make). In addition to the social response he receives from others, this repetition encourages him to continue the behavior. Most of the mimicking is a repetition of the same syllable, such as *ma-ma* or *da-da*. Toward the end of the first year, the child combines two different syllables—such as *ma-da*. Receptively the infant reacts distinctively to angry and happy talk of others and listens to himself.

Recommendations: Teaching the child language and words begins at the vocal play stage as the adult imitates the sounds made by the infant, and he in turn imitates the adult's sounds. For example, the child who says *ma* or *mama* is immediately imitated by the mother who says *mama* so the child begins to associate her with the sound. Although the child does not know that *mama* symbolizes the person who cares for him, he does receive pleasure from making the sound and the social response from mother after he has made it.

Seven Months of Age

Receptive-expressive: About this time there is increased facial expression and specific movements of the body parts. The infant auditorially attends to the speech of family members and visually attends to the environment. He expresses emotions of pleasure and displeasure vocally and imitates sequences of sounds. In other words, the child's expressive body language is becoming more refined.

Eight Months of Age

Receptive-expressive: The child begins to make inflections in his speech which gives it an adult-like quality from the way in which the sounds are combined. Perhaps this can be associated with his increased attentiveness to his surroundings. There is an increase in the back vowels and the front consonants in syllables such as *ba, da,* and *ka*. The child is making more sounds and crying less. He also continues to make sound which is not culturally recognizable.

Recommendations: Encourage the child to respond socially. He may not use the same sounds as the adult, which is irrelevant at this time. The objective is for the child to associate speech with other people and to begin developing a communication link.

Nine to Ten Months of Age

Receptive-expressive: Speech has an additive function — as new speech patterns begin, the others which preceded them continue to develop and become refined. Although there are both qualitative and quantitative changes, the quantitative changes are most apparent. The child responds to an increased number of meaningful words and gestures from the adult. He attempts to name familiar objects and he may imitate others motorically: *bye-bye, pat-a-cake,* and *so-big.* This is a step beyond the lalling which he did previously for his own pleasure. The stimuli are now external human or nonhuman objects, and the motivation occurs from the reactions of others. This results in *echolalia,* the child's ability to hear others, to hear their sounds correctly, and to echo them automatically.

Recommendations: The adult or parent imitates the child in order to stimulate his sound production. In addition, simple musical songs or lullabies which require multi-inflections and rhythms are better stimuli than the flat, concrete, spoken word produced in a monotone. The nonverbal language games, such as those described previously, stimulate social response and attention to the adult and help develop the child's nonverbal receptive language.

Van Riper suggests that these developmental needs have implications for the treatment of children with defective speech.[4] These children need to hear expressive speech in terms of inflection in order to make their speech training interesting and exciting. The therapist motivates the child through his own dynamic speech and avoids monotonous drill whenever possible.

Ten to Eighteen Months of Age

Receptive-expressive: At some time during this period, the normal child learns to say his first real words and begins to talk: he forms words or sounds that are recognized, though not clearly enunciated, and have meaning within his home and environment (this might include a day-care center or nursery). By the age of eighteen months he may have five or six words. He understands many action words so that the behavior which he demonstrates in response to the stimuli is congruent with his language. An example of real understanding or receptive language might be the child's response to the mother's use of the word "up" (without a gesture), to which the child immediately lifts up his arms to be picked up. It must be remembered that the child integrates the meaning before he is ready to say "up," and that he should be encouraged to imitate verbally but should not be forced to verbalize.

Recommendations: One objective for the adult is to teach the child to use words for specific communication about a specific thing which performs a specific function. The objective is accomplished through the imitation, exploration and repetition of both verbal and action behaviors. Van Riper describes the teaching-learning procedure between adult and child which achieves this goal: as the child first begins a vocalization, the adult cuts him off, repeats the same sounds and waits for the child to imitate him. If the child says *mamamama*.....the adult cuts off the echolalia after the first *ma*, he says *ma* again, and waits for the child to imitate him—as though the vocalization was new to the child and being learned initially.

This teaching process has several purposes. The child has a very short memory and he may forget what he has vocalized. Through the adult's repeated stimulation of the behavior (this is also true for nonverbal behavior) the child learns the sounds and eventually integrates them into his own thinking. The adult is responding to the child's level of ability and, consequently, the child is able to respond.

Another purpose is to develop an association between the child and the adult from whom he is learning which will serve as a stimulus for the child to continue the behavior through the social-emotional interaction. Otherwise, the behavior would diminish rapidly (seen in children who have limited interaction with adults).

This pattern is continued until the child responds to the adult's interruption by consistent imitation of the adult's sounds. After that, the adult interrupts the child's silent periods and makes sounds for the child to imitate directly without his first initiating them. In continuing the reinforcement of this behavior, the adult gradually extends the child's sounds to include simple words in conjunction with appropriate gestures.

It is important that gestures remain secondary to words in order to prevent the child's learning the response to the nonverbal gesture while ignoring the words and thus not learning words. For example, the mother may lift the child from the crib, the couch, the floor or the playpen and unconsciously say, *mama*. Through such repetition, the child may learn to associate the action of being lifted up with the word *mama* rather than with the person who is performing the lifting action.

The child learns to speak via multiple stimuli. He interprets speech through *gestures* in combination with the *intonation* of the sounds and the number of *syllables* which he has recognized through his previous use. To learn the meaning of *bye-bye*, for example, a series of nonverbal actions may occur: the adult may put the child in his bed, wave his hand, and go to the bedroom door. At the same time, the adult may say *bye-bye* with the identical intonation that he uses each time the situation occurs, always combining the same two syllables in the same unit. As the adult generalizes this behavior to many situations, the child begins to associate the word with a variety of actions such as putting on his coat, getting into the car, daddy's putting on his coat. Initially the child uses the one word to represent a *total* unit of ideas or a whole sentence.

In stimulating the child to speak, therefore, it is a developmental prerequisite that the therapist use single words and short phrases, such as a sibling's name or saying, "time for supper"; and that he make no demands on the child to use words that are not within his level of understanding. To complicate a verbalization and at the same time nonverbally imply that a response is required confuses the child. He understands the context of the situation and may respond to the single words, the gesture and the sound in combination with the immediate situation. Not only does the child use one word to express an idea, but he probably understands a sentence only through recognizing the one word and the context in which it is used. Thus, in introducing a new word to the child, the sentence must be short and clear with the emphasis on the word and the gesture which defines the object. "This is a *BOAT*, David," is said in conjunction with pointing to a real boat or picking up the toy boat.

Eighteen to Twenty-four Months of Age

Receptive: The child's level of comprehension is seen in his ability to follow directions. He recognizes names of familiar objects such as *dog* and *baby*. Through the words and content of the situation, he may understand their meaning. Also, he begins to associate pictures, through visual receptive language, with the real objects in his environment as they are identified by the adult. The child may or may not have the words for these objects, but he will imply recognition as he points to a picture or as the adult says the name which he auditorially understands.

Expressive: The vocabulary usually consists of ten to twenty real words which indicate primary needs and wants, such as *cookie*. This word, cookie, may mean any breadlike sweet substance because the child extends the meaning of one word to multiple and sometimes unassociated situations. The words are interspersed in jargon which is a transition between sounds and fluent speech. Jargon is unintelligible continuous speech which has the fluctuations and intonations of real speech. It is important at this time in the child's learning to connect words fluently and to put sounds together into different intonations and lengths of sentences which will be appropriate to later speech with real words. Echolalia continues and reinforces the learning, which is now developing at a fair rate.

The process of generalization occurs at the same time, since the child uses one word to describe multiple events, objects or situations. Generalization may result from the phonetic similarity of words or the similarity of objects, such as the categorizing of both *cats* and *dogs* as *bow-wows* because they both have four legs, a tail, and move rapidly along the ground. The child learns the new and appropriate words when he arrives at a point of desiring to know the word. This process is assisted by the adult who interjects the correct words. If the child understands the word, relates it to his immediate situation, and produces the word (in other words, if the word is useful to him) he is more likely to maintain it in his new vocabulary than to return to the old vocabulary which was not useful to him. For example, if mommy says, "No, John, that isn't a dog. It is a cat, which says *meow*," the child will remember the explanation if he has discriminated between the sounds of the dog and cat and wants to express the difference.

The child's learning to discriminate words verbally is based on factors beyond a single experience. Perhaps in John's case, there is a dog in his home and a cat at the house next door; by learning the two words, therefore, he is able to explain a situation more clearly to his parents.

The adult's consistent and clear verbal intervention at the appropriate point stimulates the child's own natural responsiveness or his desire to use a word. Usually the new words are accompanied by a gesture and are repeated over and over in play for solidification in his memory. This can be seen in the child who is learning the location of and words for *eyes, ears, nose,* and so forth. He will point to his own eyes, his mommy's and his doll's as he learns to identify them.

Recommendations: From this age through the preschool years books and pictures are often used by adults and therapists unknown to the child for the development of rapport with the child. The natural inclination of the adult is to pick the child up, hold him on the lap, and say, "What's this?" while pointing to a picture, or reading a story word for word to the child. More often than not, this action creates problems. Although the child will talk freely with family and people who are familiar, he is shy and fearful of strangers and should not be forced to talk with them. In addition, he may not understand all the words of the story and rapidly loses interest in it. For this approach to have any effectiveness, the therapist must first respect the child's fear and recognize his level of understanding; he then can talk to the child and make demands on him *only* when the child indicates his readiness through verbal or nonverbal cues.

The therapist's lack of knowledge of the child's jargon may also inhibit communication when the therapist does not properly reinforce the child's verbalizations. For example, when Sarah sees a picture of a frog, she says, "ribbit," a word her Daddy taught her meaning the sound a frog makes: "ribbit, ribbit." Most adults probably would assume she was trying to say *rabbit* and would respond with, "No, Sarah, that's a frog." Because of her limited understanding, this correction would confuse Sarah, and could possibly lead to her silence if incorrect interpretation of the communication persisted.

The child's limited and poorly enunciated expressive language may create frustration as he tries to explain something. As one of the characteristics of this age is to pull the adult to show him something, the adult can most easily incorporate this action into the interaction by saying, "Show me."

Two to Three Years of Age

Receptive-expressive: At two years of age the child uses egocentric speech for the first six months, such as "Me cookies" and simple questions, such as "Where doggie?" More explicitly, jargon is discarded except when the child reverts to it in stressful situations. At about two and one-half years of age, the child begins to understand sentence structure and relays "telescoped" messages to another person. He uses three-word sentences, the pronouns *I, you,* and *me* and identifies objects, people and actions with nouns and verbs. Confusion occasionally persists as the child refers to himself by name or in the third person. Verbs and their tenses also remain confused.

Recommendations: The child is beginning to understand the meaning of the words and the reasons for the language and, therefore, enjoys using them meaningfully and in hearing stories which are in relation to himself. Emotional expression is extreme in noise and activity. He is becoming explicit in his use of words, such as *no,* which have gained meaning for him beyond the imitative process. With this increased meaning, he transfers very specific words and situations to other situations that may not be present. He is to be encouraged, therefore, to describe what he needs and to put together simple sentences which are meaningful, rather than imitative or repetitious in sound. The content of the sentences obviously must be within the realm of the child's experience in order to prevent eliciting extreme frustration when the child does not understand or cannot communicate clearly.

Three to Five Years of Age

Receptive-expressive: The third and fourth years are very important in speech development for two reasons. The child's voice begins to develop the characteristics which will be common throughout the rest of his life; indeed, many speech disorders may begin at this time. The three-year-old begins to use speech to express himself as a transition from the nonverbal expression of feelings and, therefore, needs to develop a vocabulary and the ability to use it fluently. At this time the child is beginning to acquire the adjectives, adverbs and so forth, which will permit his putting words together in a comprehensive context. He uses plurals and knows a couple of prepositions—as will be seen when demands are made which require him to respond to prepositions: put the ball *on* the floor, *under* the table, *in* the closet. He is slowly beginning to develop ideas and relationships. His vocabulary, which may have increased to about one thousand words, includes sounds which are within the incipient stage of learning and others which are well established and frequently used.

The nonverbal behavior and imitative play through which he develops his vocabulary continues and includes total concepts, rather than fragments—the child, for example, who imitates mother's total routine for the day when he plays house. This is a means of practicing and incorporating behavior into his thought process and integrating it with the language process. As Gesell [5] said, "he learns to listen and he listens to learn." The child really begins to make use of what he hears, listens closely and will change his behavior readily in response to the comments or actions of another person.

Questioning is a constant and typical behavior of the four-year-old child. Through constant talking, he becomes fluent in his speech, which may be a combination of social communication and attracting attention. The child is not always interested in answers to his questions. According to Gesell:

Much of his questioning is virtually a soliloquy by means of which he projects one verbal construction after another, concurrently rearranging his images and reformulating relationships. He is not building coherent logical structures, but combining facts, fancies, and phrases to strengthen his command of words and clauses. He makes declarations and running comments as profusely as he frames questions, using with aptness (and sometimes with marked ineptitude) such expressions as, I don't *even* know that. You *almost* hit him. *Now* I will make *something* else.... [6]

Recommendations: In order to develop good speech, the child needs good adult models which he can imitate. If the adult model uses *baby talk* (a falsetto or unnatural tone of voice and inflection), the child develops speech patterns with similar sounds and does not develop good articulation, vocabulary or intonation. On the other hand, the adult who speaks to a child in complex sentences and long paragraphs inhibits the child, because he cannot hear, interpret and respond as rapidly as the adult. The child needs to hear short sentences and phrases so that he can respond to them directly and verbally or indirectly through the appropriate action.

Adults must also avoid finishing sentences for children. This habit decreases the child's speech practice and inhibits learning of speech. If a child's speech is constantly corrected, he may begin to develop emotional reactions, stuttering or hesitant speech instead of fluent speech, for example. The development of fluency in language can be compared with the development of fluency in other behaviors such as learning to walk: the child begins slowly and progresses at his own rate in spite of his being prodded. Gradually, through practice, the child becomes fluent and coordinated. Therefore, the adult must speak with the preschool child in short, concise sentences; he must use words known and understood by the child or else explain their meaning; and he must use simple syntax. The child can then develop speech without excessive frustration and avoid speech problems.

When teaching vocabulary, it is useful to provide multiple stimuli for the child, combining a word with a visual image, an action or tactile sensation. As the child learns the word *walk,* he performs the movement, watches himself and others walk, and feels it. To learn the noun *table,* he touches a table, puts objects on it and sits at it. Each time the child performs the appropriate behavior and is praised, or each time he is requested to perform, the adult says "walk" or "table." Again, descriptions are within the child's developmental framework and are kept simple.

Five Years of Age

Receptive-expressive: The infantile articulation is diminished; the child can ask direct questions and can give answers. He asks reasonable questions for the purpose of learning, and not just for gaining attention and social interaction. He uses less imagination in his speech, and because of increased knowledge and experience is more practical in relation to the everyday world than the four-year-old.

Language is now essentially complete in structure and form. Five has assimilated the syntactical conventions and expresses himself in correct, finished sentences. He uses all types of sentences, including complex sentences with hypothetical and conditional clauses. He uses conjunctions somewhat more freely than Four, but in general the relative frequency of parts of speech is similar to that of Four. Vocabulary is greater by several hundred words...; usage more accurate and much more elaborate. Five follow linguistic custom rather than the naive movement of thought which determines word order in Two.[7]

Communicative Disorders

Speech Disorders

Three general areas of speech disorders can be categorized into defects of articulation, rhythm and voice production. *Articulation* refers to the production of speech sounds. Disorders in this area evolve from the substitution, omission, distortion or addition of sounds. The cause of the defects may be psychological or the result of a learning disorder (baby talk), or an anatomical problem based on a structural defect in the child's oral structure (lisping, for instance, in which the child has a slow-moving tongue tip). The articulatory defects may be multiple, as in the case of the child who lisps *and* baby talks. Examples of articulatory defects include baby talk, lalling, lisping and jargon when it is inappropriate to the chronological age of the child. If poor articulation persists it is considered a defect; if extreme, poor articulation can create frustration for a child as he tries to express himself, but is unable to make his message known.

A second disorder is found in the timing or *rhythm* of speech. When an individual is not able to execute a smooth, continuous rhythm in his own characteristic manner, a defect is apparent. (This is not to say that a person speaks in the same rhythm all the time, but that he speaks fluently using an organized pattern of words, phrases and sentences.)

Among the disorders in timing are the stutterers and clutterers. The stutterer is an extreme case of the average individual who sometimes speaks slowly, repeats himself, and hesitates. His speech rhythm is quantitatively and qualitatively different from the usual person. It is often related more closely to emotional problems than speech problems, or it may be the result of developmental problems in language. The clutterer speaks too rapidly so that words are expressed unclearly and are poorly sequenced; his speech is chaotic and he may not be able to speak slowly. In addition, some of his sounds may be slurred or omitted, so that the listener does not hear meaningful information.

Voice disorders are those which are related to the tone of the voice, meaning the loudness, quality and pitch. There is a broad range of individual differences in voices which is acceptable until it interferes with the person's social, emotional or work performance. At this point, the person is diagnosed as having a defective tone or voice disorder.

Pitch refers to the variation in sound from the very low sounds usually found in the adult male to the high sounds of a female or young child. Acceptable variations in pitch include the woman with a low voice or the man with a high voice or the adolescent boy whose voice is not controllable and breaks as a change in pitch is developing. The range of loudness or intensity varies according to the individual. An individual may speak very loudly as the result of an emotional problem or speak very softly because of deafness—or may not speak at all, (aphonia) as in laryngitis. Any of these characteristics can be a problem to the person who is trying to communicate.

Quality of the voice refers to the actual sound of the voice and to some extent depends upon the anatomical structure of the individual's head, the size and shape of the resonating cavities, the patterning of the overtones and the variable intensities. Voice qualities may be pleasant, but when distorted may be irritating to the listener. Husky, breathy or nasal qualities in a voice are not often appealing.

Language Disorders

Language disorders are related to the process of symbolization, or symbol formation and expression. The disorders are known as *aphasias* and may occur in children, although they occur more often in adults and in people who have had cerebral vascular accidents. There are three kinds of aphasias: the person with (1) receptive aphasia can hear sounds but cannot interpret their meanings; the (2) expressive aphasic hears and understands the sounds adequately, but is not able to form words or respond to sounds; and (3) central aphasia is disturbance in the inner symbolic function, so that neither receptive nor expressive function develops.

Multiply Handicapping Conditions

People who have a combination of any of the above described pathological conditions are multiply handicapped in speech and language. The deaf or hard-of-hearing child may have a combination of pitch, rhythm and articulation errors which depend somewhat upon the degree of deafness. The child with cleft palate may have articulation problems, such as nasality in his use of consonants, and the rhythm of his speech may be affected by breathing problems. The individuals with cerebral palsy, in which a problem with muscular coordination occurs, may have problems in pitch, quality or articulation. Finally, multiple developmental speech defects and delay may be evident in the child who is slow or retarded in other areas of development. The child will develop speech only to the degree of his capability—as is true in each of the other developmental areas.

A Language Development Inventory

The following inventory questions are the descriptive statements of language development framed in the form of questions. They may be used by the therapist in talking with parents or health care staff to determine the child's approximate language performance. In addition, the therapist may use them reflexively for himself as he observes the child.

Boston University Speech and Hearing Center
A Language Development Inventory
(Original Source Unknown)

Four Weeks
Expressive
1. Does he cry?
2. Does he cry a great deal?
3. Is his cry loud and strong?
4. Does his cry change with environmental conditions?
5. Does he make throaty noises?
6. Does he make front vowels?

Receptive
1. Does he react to your presence?
2. Does he startle when a loud noise is introduced?
3. Does he blink his eyes at a loud noise?
4. Does he follow you with eyes as you walk around the room?
5. Does he smile when you talk to him?

Sixteen Weeks
Expressive
1. Does he coo?
2. Does he smile at your approach?
3. Can you get him to talk back to you?

4. Does he talk to himself in the morning?
5. Does he seem to play with his voice?
6. Does he chuckle?
7. Does he squeal when he gets excited?
8. Does he anticipate the sight of food by vocalization?
9. Does he anticipate with excited movement?

Receptive
1. Does he laugh out loud?
2. Does he respond to his image in the mirror?
3. Does he seem to play peek-a-boo?
4. Does he listen to your voice?
5. Does he listen to a rattle?
6. Does your talking or singing to him quiet him?
7. Does he turn his head in the direction of your voice?

Twenty-eight Weeks
Expressive
1. Does he talk to his toys?
2. Does he grunt or growl?
3. Does he make sounds consisting of several vowels?
4. Does he make syllables?
5. Does he make consonants?
6. Does he vocalize "m-m-m" when crying?

Receptive
1. Does he turn his head to a bell?
2. Does he know you?
3. Does he discriminate strangers?

Forty Weeks
Expressive
1. Does he say "dada?"
2. Does he mean you when he says "mama?"
3. Does he imitate sounds?
4. Will he imitate a cough or clicking of the tongue?
5. Will he wave bye-bye?
6. Does he play pat-a-cake?
7. Does he play nursery games ("So Big," etc.)?
8. Has he any words?
9. Does he use any sounds to mean something even though it doesn't sound like the real word?
10. Does he shake his head "yes" and "no?"
11. Does he vocalize with the above response?

Receptive
1. Does he seem to understand when you talk to him?
2. Does he respond to his name?
3. Does he respond to "no-no?"
4. Does he understand if you say, "Where's Daddy?"

Twelve Months

Expressive

1. Does he say any words besides "mama" and "dada?"
2. Does he know some of his toys by name?
3. Does he jabber?
4. Would he look if you said, "Where is the bell?"

Receptive

1. Does he respond to music?
2. Does he understand if you tell him to: Look up? Look down? Look at me?
3. If you ask for something in his hand, will he give it to you?
4. Would he look if you said, "Where is the bell?"
5. Does he seem to know some of his toys?

Eighteen Months

Expressive

1. Does he exhibit a jargon type of speech?
2. Does he use four or five words?
3. Does he indicate his wants by pointing?
4. Does he vocalize with pointing?
5. Does he name or point to one picture in a book?
6. Does he use gestures?
7. Has he any words for his toys (ball, car, etc.)?
8. Has he any words for his food?
9. Does he have ten words?
10. Does he have any words for his clothes (shoes, socks, etc.)?
11. Does he pull you or indicate that he wants to show you something?

Receptive

1. Does he throw a ball on request?
   Put it on the table?
   Give it to "me?"
   Give it to mother?

Twenty-seven Months

Expressive

1. Does he name three pictures when a book is shown?
2. Does he have 25 words?
3. Is he beginning to join two words together: two words that join two ideas like "daddy go" or "bye car?"
4. Does he refer to himself by name?
5. Does he refer to himself as "I" or "me?"
6. Does he ask for food?
7. Does he verbalize toilet needs?
8. Does his play include domestic mimicry?
9. Is the jargon discarded?

10. Does he have sentences of three words?
11. Does he have 50 words in his vocabulary?

Receptive

1. Does he throw a ball on request?
    Give it to "me?"
    Give it to "mother?"
    Put it on the table?
    Put it on the floor?
2. Does he point to the picture if you say, "Show me the_____?"

Thirty-six Months

Expressive

1. Is he beginning to use sentences?
2. Does he give his name if you ask him?
3. Does he give his last name?
4. Does he give his sex if you ask him?
5. Can he name five pictures in a book?
6. Can he give the use of objects?
7. Can anyone understand him?
8. Does he know nursery rhymes?
9. Does he cooperate in play with other children?
10. Does he talk when he plays alone?

Receptive

1. Does he seem to remember directions?
2. Can you give him two directions at once?
3. Upon command will he put the ball:
    On the chair?
    Under the chair?
    In front of the chair?
    In back of the chair?
    Beside the chair?
4. Does he listen to stories?

Four to Five Years

Expressive

1. Can he count to three?
2. Does he tell tales or stories?
3. Does his vocabulary reach 1,000 words or more?
4. Does he use words such as "and" or "but?"
5. Does he question a great deal?
6. Are his responses often silly and his language silly?
7. Does he show interest in new words?

Receptive

1. Does he listen to stories or readings with sustained interest?
2. Does he enjoy being read to? [8]

COGNITIVE DEVELOPMENT

Jean Piaget, a Swiss psychologist, has developed a theory of intellectual development which many American educators, psychologists and occupational therapists regard as the most plausible theory in existence today. Piaget has interests in both biology (the study of life) and epistomology (the study of knowledge). As a result, many of his principles are applicable to the biological behavior of man as well as to his psychological behavior. This chapter will focus on the psychological-intellectual behavior and the constructs which Piaget has developed to explain the behaviors.

The theory is very complex because of the problems of translation, vocabulary, the changing character of the theory and the intricacies of the cognitive process. The purpose of this chapter unit is to familiarize students with the basic concepts of Piaget's theory, the sequence of cognitive development, and the vocabulary, which are all vital to an understanding of a child's cognitive behavior. Before reading this chapter unit, it is suggested that the student review Chapter One, and particularly the discussion of learning theories. It is expected that the student will need to pursue Piaget's work further — and it is hoped that the familiarity with his theory will make that task easier.

Intrinsic motivation, as described in Chapter One, is the child's desire to experience a situation for the sake of the experience itself, not for the external reward. This is the basis of Piaget's concept of development. According to him, learning occurs through the child's active pursuit of knowledge. Children desire to expand the capacities of their bodies and minds — and accomplish this goal through the exploration of their environments. Therefore, in order for learning to occur, the environmental stimuli must be appropriate to the developmental age of the child.

Piaget has divided the sequence of cognitive development into four stages: *sensorimotor intelligence* is the first stage and includes about the first two years of life; the second stage is *preoperational thought*, which ranges from about two years of age to about seven years of age; the third stage is *concrete operational thought*, which occurs between seven or eight years and about eleven years of age; and the last stage is the period of *formal operational thought* which begins about eleven years of age and continues throughout life.

The sequence of these developmental stages is invariant (constant or unchanging). The child progresses in turn through all the stages in sequence and does not omit any stage (although the length of time a child spends on mastering each developmental stage may vary). Development is gradual and continuous; one behavior pattern is not necessarily completely mastered before the child begins the next stage. This process results in the child's developing multiple behaviors at the same time and in his retaining and using previously learned behaviors.

Definition of Cognition or Intelligence

Piaget has described three characteristics of intelligence in order to avoid the creation of a limited and binding definition. *The characteristics which comprise the sum of intelligence are content, structure and function.* Ginsburg and Opper have summarized the qualities of each of Piaget's characteristics of intelligence.[9] The *content* of thought is the material about which an individual is thinking. Content differs at each age and may be changed rapidly, or may be sustained. The two-year-old identifies objects in his immediate environment through the use of his visual, auditory and other senses. For example, for the two-year-old a truck contains only the properties which the child can see and hear and touch. A truck is a truck that moves on wheels and perhaps can be filled with sand and then emptied. Between the early years and adolescence a transition occurs, which results in the content of thought becoming abstract and critical. The adolescent can think about trucks in their absence. His thoughts of trucks may focus on the driver's license which he will obtain in six months, and on the evaluation of the pros and cons for his becoming a truck driver.

In looking at the characteristics of *structure* and *function,* one must first consider the biological structures and functions which are invariant. The phrase *hereditary physical structures* refers to these structures which the human inherits both as a member of a species and as an individual. These inherited structures, such as the automatic behavioral reactions and reflexes described in Chapter Four, broadly influence all developmental functions. Different structures are dominant in different stages of a person's life — reflexes, for example, dominate at birth but later diminish in importance.

The *basic tendencies or invariant functions of organization and adaptation* are also ascribed to inheritance by Piaget. These functions are invariant because they pertain to the organism throughout the life cycle. They are constant in the way in which they are expressed at different stages of the life cycle.

Piaget states that *organization* is the inherited tendency for all members of a species to organize all their structures into a coordinated whole. This characteristic is always present and the same for all the members of a species at an identifiable point of development. The reflexes of a newborn function independently, but are coordinated with each other for the infant's survival; the newborn does not willfully coordinate all its structures or functions. As children develop, organization continues but advances toward cognitive sophistication. This level of development begins as the infant becomes aware of the way in which his eyes serve as a guide for his hands and his hands become capable of bringing food to his mouth. Ginsburg and Opper state that organization is the "tendency for all species to systematize or organize their processes into coherent systems which may be either physical or psychological."[10]

Adaptation as a construct is described as an invariant function because all organisms tend to adjust to their environments by learning. In adapting to the environment, the organism performs two kinds of processes: assimilation and accommodation. The individual *accommodates* itself to environmental demands by changing itself either physiologically or psychologically. *Assimilation* is the complementary process of incorporating useful material from the environment into the child's present structure. These two processes can be understood in terms of changing the self to meet the demands of the environment (accommodation) and consciously or unconsciously using the environment to meet the needs of the self (assimilation).

Although Piaget uses these terms to describe both physical and psychological development, discussion here will be limited to the development of intelligence. In the process of intellectual adaptation, for example, a child who is given a new toy accommodates his behavior to meet the requirements of its characteristics and the environment in which it is found. A child can only use a unilateral, refined grasp pattern to pick up a safety pin; a child cannot build a tower with balls or roll blocks; and a child must use a bilateral grasp pattern to pick up a beach ball with a 24-inch diameter. The child is accommodating to the properties of the particular object and probably to the environment in which the object is found (on the table, on the floor, in a spacious playroom, or on the beach).

Assimilation requires the child to apply his past knowledge and experience to the new situation. The child will manipulate the toy according to the intellectual framework, which he has developed prior to the time that he is confronted with the new toy. He will assimilate information about the toy from the properties he recognizes from past experience with it — or with similar objects and from his present exploration of it. The child who sees the beachball with a 24-inch diameter for the first time tries to throw or kick the ball because of the characteristic roundness which he has experienced before in the form of a ball.

The processes of assimilation and accommodation complement each other in the process of adaptation and are present in many actions of the individual. There must be a combination of accommodation and assimilation in order for the child to be able to adapt to his environment. It is useless for the child to assimilate information continually if he is unable to accommodate the assimilated structures in response to the demands of the environment. For example, it is useless for the child to learn the numbers from one to ten by rote if he is unable to use those numbers appropriately in his daily experience. The interacting processes can be seen in most behavior. In the physical process of digestion, the body accommodates to the foreign matter, food, and then assimilates it through the digestive process. In the social process the child accommodates to the manners required by the culture (learning to eat with a spoon, for example) and then assimilates this response into his own behavior.

The processes of organization and adaptation result in the development of *psychological structures,* which are the basis of Piaget's theoretical framework. The psychological structures are variant — they differ with each age — and they are constantly interacting with the physical structures. These psychological structures are the bases of Piaget's sequence of intellectual development. They explain the behaviors of the individual which cannot be explained on the basis of inherited characteristics — such as reflexes, or automatic movements. The reflex behavior of sucking is innate. However, the behavior of bringing the thumb to the mouth — which is repeated frequently by the infant — is not a reflex. Therefore, it must be explained in terms of a child's learning, and is placed in the framework of psychological structures. Piaget describes organized patterns of behavior (logical and orderly behavior) as *schemes* and enumerates their characteristics. A scheme describes a child's action, whether it is easily observable or not; it may be the act of watching, listening, smelling, playing or thinking.

The scheme describes the basic components of a behavior, not the subtle variations which occur at each execution. For example, the scheme of drawing for a fifteen-month-old child might include the grasping of a writing object and the making of scribbling marks. These are the basic components of the behavior. The variables illustrate the child's knowledge of the concept and his ability to apply it to many situations (from scribbling on the wall next to his bed to scribbling on daddy's newspaper to scribbling on drawing paper). The scheme of drawing for a four-year-old would incorporate a regular or consistent way of holding the writing object and the making of recognizable forms, such as circles or vertical lines. The schemes of the fifteen-month-old and four-year-old child differ because each developmental age has its own common behavioral characteristics.

Schemes develop progressively from the overt, physical acts of the newborn to the covert, intellectual behavior of the adolescent. The child may use all his previously learned schemes in addition to those he is learning at his particular stage of development. The infant uses sensorimotor schemes exclusively; the adolescent can use sensorimotor, preoperational and concrete operational schemes — in addition to the formal operational schemes which he is presently developing.

All of these constructs which Piaget developed to describe intelligence are relevant to all four stages of cognitive development and are referred to in the following description of the developmental sequence.

Sensorimotor Intelligence

Sensorimotor intelligence is dominant in the development of cognitive functions from birth to about two years of age. The child responds to or acts upon those stimuli which he can touch, see, hear, or experience kinesthetically. The development of these responses has been subdivided by Piaget into six stages.

Stage One

The first stage is called the *reflex stage.* The physical structures of innate and acquired reflexes, organization, and adaptation facilitate the function of the newborn until psychological structures become available to him through maturation. Reflexes, therefore, are the infant's means to survival. In addition — and more importantly — they are maintained and developed through use, and they serve as the foundations for the development of schemes of assimilation. Assimilation at the level of the newborn is known as *functional or reproductive assimilation.* This means that when an infant has a structure present or available, such as the sucking reflex, there is a basic tendency for him to use it. Those schemes, such as sucking, are developed through exercise, because of the tendency of schemes to function.

Generalizing and recognitive assimilation occur as a result of functional assimilation. According to Piaget, the child is intrinsically motivated to exercise his scheme and, as a result, discovers new stimuli, such as the thumb which he then uses for sucking. This is *generalizing assimilation.* With the accumulation of varied experiences, the infant begins to discriminate crudely between meaningful objects and nonmeaningful objects in the first month of his life. This discrimination is *recognitive assimilation* and differs in character from the sophisticated discrimination of the adult. The infant, for example, learns to distinguish between the nipple which provides him with milk and the thumb which does not. Recognitive assimilation also is applicable to the groups of sensations which an infant receives from a variety of stimuli at one time. The infant posturally and kinesthetically recognizes the feelings of being held by mother while tasting the milk from her breast and seeing her face. This sensory experience differs considerably for the infant from the kinesthetic feelings of a hard crib mattress, the taste of his own finger and the absence of the mother's body.

Stage Two

The *first habit stage,* which generally falls between the age of one and four months, is a raw description of sensorimotor behavior which is acquired and repeated. The infant is not able to distinguish between the end result of his behaviors and the means through which he learned the behavior. The *primary circular reactions,* such as thumb sucking, are the psychological structures which describe the infant's random behavior and its reinforcement. Once a behavior is reinforced, the child attempts to duplicate the response through trial-and-error experiences. If the child is successful in repeating the necessary response, he learns the process and finally develops an organized scheme or habit. The circular reactions are called primary because the focal point of the action is the infant's body, his primary environment.

Stage Three

The period between five and seven months of age has been described by Piaget as *secondary circular reactions* or the third stage which "introduces the next transitions after the beginning of coordination between vision and prehension." [11] In this stage the infant attempts to grasp and manipulate everything that is within his immediate environment. Each time he produces a result, he again attempts the task. In other words, the result motivates repetition of the act (which refers to the circular reactions), and they become secondary because they are related to objects apart from the infant. The nonreinforced responses will be extinguished.

As described by Piaget, *the child is on the threshold of intelligence at this time* (the combination of content, structure and function) because he uses the same means to achieve different ends. The child consistently accommodates his hand movements and visual pursuits at the same time to produce the desirable results. Once the child has learned to pull a toy on a crib-gym, for example, and has assimilated the action through receiving a desirable result, he will again pull any object which is in the same position over the crib — whether or not it is the identical object and whether or not the end result is the same. It is the scheme which the infant uses (reaching, grasping and pulling), and the response to his use of the scheme (bell ring), which are most important to the child's intellectual development, not his awareness of the object for its own sake (block, ball, rattle).

The child is encouraged to explore a variety of materials which are separate from his body and which actively stimulate his senses. Preferred materials are toys and objects which he will experience in his own home. The child is encouraged to decide how he wants to explore and use his environment and the people in it; whenever possible he is permitted to choose whether he wants to be cuddled or whether he wants to crawl or sit.

Stage Four

The period from approximately seven to eleven or twelve months of age may be described as the period of *coordination of secondary schemes*. At this point a child perceives the object he is responding to as his known goal, whereas in stage three the child accidentally discovered the goal through his explorations and manipulations. He now uses his known schemes in attempting to assimilate the goal; he also uses generalizing assimilation to develop ways of overcoming obstacles which would prevent his achieving that goal. For example, the adult may place an obstacle, such as his hand, between the desired toy and the child. The child first reaches for the toy, but upon the discovery of the obstacle he stops. By coordinating two secondary schemes, the child may be successful in overcoming the obstacle and reaching his goal. The first scheme for the child might be to hit the adult's hand and thus knock it out of the way; the second scheme would be to grab the desired toy. Prior to this stage, hitting and reaching would have been two independent goals or secondary schemes — now one scheme has become the means and the other has become the goal. Neither scheme is new to the child's repertoire of behavior. *The originality and consequent first use of intentional behavior occurs in the combining of the two schemes. According to Piaget this behavior defines the beginnings of intelligence.*

Stage Five

Stage five, between eleven or twelve months and about eighteen months of age, is often called the period of *tertiary circular reactions.* At this time the child searches for new ways to achieve the desired goal by choosing from already assimilated schemes or by randomly finding a scheme and achieving his goal. For example, Piaget describes the child's use of a rug as an extension of his arm which helps him reach the desired goal: the child unsuccessfully attempts to grasp an object which is placed on a rug out of his reach; by chance or intent, the child grabs the rug and pulls it slightly toward himself. As the child perceives that the rug and the object are getting closer, he intentionally pulls the rug toward himself and succeeds in taking the object from it.

The stage of tertiary circular reactions has also been described by Piaget as a time when the child is very curious about objects and their qualities and searches for novel uses of them. In this stage the child's interest shifts from the self (such as grasping) to the object (such as the block) and the phenomenon which can be created by it (such as falling). (Prior to the tertiary circular reactions, the child was intent upon the process of releasing the object or other actions which were directly concerned with himself.) Because of his curiosity about the objects and falling, the child drops many of them from many positions and heights. Thus, tertiary becomes referent to the object itself and its characteristics which the child explores apart from his effect on them.

Stage Six

In the sixth stage, approximately the period between eighteen months and two years of age, the child passes from the exclusive development of sensorimotor behavior to the *beginnings of thought.* The transition is from a stage of the singular use of sensorimotor behavior to a stage in which the additional use of symbols and signs in language in order to define absent objects occurs. The child begins to use more than the physical or sensorimotor trial-and-error approach to learn about his environment: he begins to think before he responds verbally or motorically. In other words, the child mentally performs a behavior before performing the physical behavior. Piaget has called this *insight;* he describes the way in which the child of this age initially uses a trial-and-error approach to problem solving. If he is unsuccessful in performing the task, the child stops his actions, apparently to think about what he is doing. He looks at the object and may, physically but silently, go through the desired motions as though imitating the behavior. For example, he may open and close his mouth before attempting to open a box. Then he proceeds to perform the task without any overt trial-and-error experience. Although the child may not appear to be in thought, he should not be hurried or interrupted until the adult is reasonably sure that he will not interfere with the child's covert thought. Otherwise, the child who is mentally exploring new territory may be sidetracked in his problem solving, and unable to refocus on it.

In addition to the child's ability to think about and act upon an object which is within his immediate visual-motor field, he is able to think about objects which are not present. Furth describes this process clearly as he distinguishes between *acting*, which is sensorimotor behavior, and *knowing*, which is operational behavior. The child begins to acquire an awareness of *object formation*, which results in a scheme of *object permanence* (see Chapter Five). In other words, the child knows that an object exists outside of his immediate temporal and spacial environment. This is a distinct development at the end of the sensorimotor period — and a prerequisite to cognition. The simple example of hiding a desirable toy shows the child's cognitive awareness or knowing of an object's permanence (for the child of less than about eighteen months the toy that is hidden from his sight no longer exists; the child of more than eighteen months will search diligently for the desired object). In understanding the meaning of object permanence for the toddler, the adult can appreciate the hospitalized child's fear of separation from his parents and his diligent search for them when they desert him without his knowing about it.

The display of insight and knowledge about an object's permanence graphically demonstrates the transition from the sensorimotor schemes to preoperational thought. The child begins to learn by thinking about the object rather than by acting upon it.

The stimuli which are presented to the child in the sensorimotor period should be used repetitively to permit the infant's and child's thorough exploration of their properties. Early in the development of object awareness the child will be interested in exploring objects one at a time; later in the development of the coordination of secondary schemes and tertiary circular reactions he will combine objects in his play. Initially the child is interested only in the object itself; he later becomes interested in what he can do with the object. Obstacles which present a challenge to the successful completion of a task are incorporated into the child's play at the later time also. These obstacles include the hiding of favorite toys initially in one place — under a single box — and then alternately in, under or behind several places.

Sensorimotor intelligence and initial thought (the use of symbols and signs) evolve into preoperational thought, concrete operational thought, and, finally, formal operational thought. *Operations* are actions which the child performs mentally. Preoperations indicate the early manifestations of mental thought; concrete operations are thoughts occurring in conjunction with concrete events or objects; and formal operations advance to abstract thought. Each of these stages incorporates a multitude of behaviors, some of which are more significant at one stage than at another.

Preoperational Thought

The most important occurrence during the stage of preoperational thought (two or three to six or seven years of age) is the development of *representational thought.* In this stage the stimulus gathers a meaning which the child can represent through other objects or situations. For example, a child uses the doll to represent a baby. The behaviors in the first two or three years of this stage resemble sensorimotor behavior, whereas the child's behavior in the last three years shows an early resemblance to concrete operational thought.

Semiotic function is prerequisite to representational thought because it "enables us to represent objects or events that are not at the moment perceptible by evoking them through the agency of symbols or differentiated signs. Symbolic play is an example of this process, as are differed imitation, mental images, drawing, etc., and, above all, language itself." [12] A *symbol* is a differentiated signifier which is motivated by the child. It has some resemblance to the object which is being signified but, because it is perceived by the child or person to meet his own needs, it has its own variations. A child's teddy bear, for example, may symbolize different people and objects — such as a playmate one day and the child himself as a baby (which he would like to be) the next day. These symbols are differentiated from the object which they represent and, as such, serve as a bridge between sensorimotor knowledge and representational knowledge. On the other hand, a *sign* represents the conventional expression of the signified. The child learns signs, or incorporates them into his own behavior, through imitation. Words such as *mama, baby,* and *cookie* are all signs which are learned early and which have the same meaning throughout a culture.

The period of preoperational thought is identified as the transition between sensorimotor functions and mental or intellectual functions. This transitional period itself is imbued with some problems for the child because of the adult's unrealistic expectations of the child's cognitive abilities. First of all, the child has what is frequently called a *motor memory*. He is not able to mentally represent that which he has absorbed on the level of action. The child may be able to perform an action motorically in response to a verbal request, but probably will not be able to describe the answer verbally. For example, the child may be able to find his way around a hospital ward but would not be able to duplicate his path or the layout of the ward graphically or with blocks. He could not give someone directions to find a specific place although he probably could take the person's hand and guide him to the place. Therefore, the therapist incorporates the child's use of his motor memory in communication and says "show me" when exploring the child's needs, rather than requiring a verbal description.

Another problem in the transitional stage of preoperational thought is the child's egocentric view of the world in which his point of reference is himself. The child must *decenter* his learning, from his own body to an objective form of thinking; to do this the child must completely dissociate himself from the materials about which he is learning. In other words, he must learn to understand the meaning of objects in his environment independently from his relationship to them.

"Preoperational *egocentrism* is a very general characteristic with numerous sequelae. First and foremost, the child repeatedly demonstrates a relative inability to take the role of the other person, that is, to see his own viewpoint as one of many possible and to try to coordinate it with these others.

There are two other difficulties which derive directly from the child's egocentrism...First, the child — lacking other role orientation — feels neither the compunction to justify his reasonings to others nor to look for possible contradictions in his logic. And causally related to this, he finds it exceedingly difficult to treat his own thought processes as an object of thought. He is, for example, unable to reconstruct a chain of reasonings which he has just passed through; he thinks but he cannot think about his own thinking.

One of the most pronounced characteristics of preoperational thought is its tendency to *center* (centration), as Piaget says, attention on a single, striking feature of the object of its reasoning to the neglect of other important aspects, and by so doing, to distort the reasoning. The child is unable to *decenter*, i.e., to take into account features which could balance and compensate for the distorting, biasing effects of the single centration." [13]

Perhaps the most vivid expression of the egocentrism of a two-year-old child is his frequent use of *"Mine!"* All toys belong to him whenever another child is around, and it is this behavior which must be resolved into "This is mine and this is yours." Social decentration is encouraged by stating the limits for the child through telling him facts in a simple way: "This is not your toy, it's Gregory's," "You have to go with us; you can't stay alone," or, "You must stop playing and eat." Decentering is necessary for the child's increased utilization of objects, as well as for the child's communication with people. For example, the child first understands the words *right* and *left* in relation to his own body. He cannot objectively dissociate the meaning of the terms from himself to the objects — he cannot talk about the relationship of objects in terms of right and left, unless in terms of his spacial relationship to them.

Within the second year a series of behaviors occur which indicate the beginning of mental representation of objects and events which are absent. These representations are seen in the appearance of the signifiers (symbols and signs). Piaget has described the elements of semiotic function or the use of signifiers as appearing almost simultaneously, but in the following order of increasing complexity.[14]

Elements of Semiotic Function

Deferred imitation is the imitation of gestures, and which is initiated after the disappearance of the model. This is an advance over sensorimotor imitation, in which the imitation began in the model's presence and continued after the model disappeared. Deferred imitation (accommodation to reality) implies the beginning of thought and the beginning of representation because only thought can connect a real situation with that imitated at a later time. The imitative aspects demonstrate the beginning of differentiated signifiers. The child paddles the puppy after watching mommy paddle the dog because he made a puddle on the floor; or the child hears a shout or laugh and at a later time repeats the action. In other words, the child is becoming very aware of adults and other children in his environment. These adults (in real life, movies and television) are the models of behaviors which the child develops.

Symbolic play is pretending. The child may pretend that he is eating or sleeping or that his toy rabbit is eating. This play "...transforms reality by assimilation to the needs of the self, whereas imitation...is accommodation to external models."[15] Rather than accommodating to the demands of the environment, symbolic play is an assimilation process in which the child manipulates his environment to match his needs. This symbolic play helps the child relive an event or enact it symbolically for clarification of his understanding. Because his language (which signifies thought) is limited, the child creates the symbols to express those ideas or situations which he cannot put into words. In other words, this is nonverbal, symbolic imagery. Symbolic play is particularly important for the young child who is sick or disabled. For example, it helps him assimilate new and painful situations at a time when his language is too meager to express his ideas and feelings.

The child may imitate behavior without realizing it. Symbolism which surrounds the child and his life is based not only on the conscious material and experience, but also on the unconscious material described in the psychoanalytic theories in Chapter Five.

Drawing, which is described by Piaget as the intermediate stage between play and the mental image, occurs at about two or two-and-one-half years of age. It combines the functions of both symbolic play and mental image. Drawing resembles symbolic play in the pleasure which the child derives from it in the process of assimilation and through the stimulation of autonomous behavior. On the other hand, drawing is similar to mental imagery because it suggests the imitation of the real events rather than the imaginative situations.

The *mental image* may be described as internalized imitation. It fluctuates, and may include auditory, visual and motor movement images. There is some discussion in learning theory about the derivation of the image and the actual type of mental image that is formed. Piaget notes that people can have mental images of objects, situations or sensations; however, people do not have a mental image of concepts or judgments which determine the reality of the image itself. In other words, one can have mental thought without the formation of an image.

There are two kinds of mental images. *Reproductive images,* which include the mental reproductions of past experiences (known objects or situation), are the first images to develop. "Reproductive images may include static configurations, movements (changes of position), and transformation (changes of form), for these three kinds of realities occur constantly in the perceptual experience of the subject." [16] At the preoperational level of thought, the child is primarily limited to the static images. In concrete operational thought, the child can reproduce the movements and transformations and can anticipate imagery transformations and movements. *Anticipatory images* envisage movements or transformations as well as their results, although the subject has not previously observed them (as one can envisage how a geometric figure would look if it were transformed)." [17]

Memory as a part of mental imagery is categorized in two ways: the memory of *recognition* and of *evocation*. Recognition is a less advanced form of memory and is even found in the infant. Through the recognition memory the child who has encountered an object before he recognizes it upon a second encounter and responds to it appropriately. The higher order memory of evocation is that in which the child can recall or evoke the object in the absence of any stimulus through image memory.

The elements of memory affect the child's reasoning. Although the child may be unable to progress logically from step to step in his thinking (similar to the problems of motor memory), his memory of evocation will provide him with some information. The hospitalized child will remember that mommy comes to visit every afternoon after naptime, but he will not logically understand why she comes only at that time or how she comes. He must accept the facts on their face value because of his preoperational function.

The preoperational child cannot yet anticipate the future outcome of an immediate situation. He does not know the value of performing a task today for a reward tomorrow. Conversely, he does not understand that he feels okay today, but that his body will hurt tomorrow after surgery. He may hear the words of the adult who describes the future, but he understands them only in the context of his own past experience.

Language also becomes an important part of semiotic function early in the second year. The use of conventional language by the therapist helps the child identify signs and learn the significant language of his speech community.

Flavell has further described some of the psychological structures which are present at the time of preoperational thought. These structures clearly demonstrate the absence of mental operations in the child between two or three and six or seven years of age and clearly indicate the limits of possible semiotic functions.

States and Transformations — Characteristics very closely related to the phenomenism or configuration-boundedness just described concern the child's reactions to states versus transformations of states...The child is much more inclined to focus attention upon the successive states or configurations of a display than upon the transformations by which one state is changed into another (the experiment with the liquids involves this kind of display: an initial configuration A', a terminal configuration B, and the process of transformation of A′ to B). Preoperational thought, then, is static and immobile. It is a kind of thought which can focus impressionistically and sporadically on this or that momentary, static condition but cannot adequately link a whole set of successive conditions into an integrated totality by taking account of the transformations which unify them and render them logically coherent.

Equilibrium — A principal characteristic of preoperational thought is a relative absence of stable equilibrium between assimilation and accommodation...The assimilatory network — the child's cognitive organization — tends to rupture and dislocate itself in the process of accommodating to new situations. The child is unable to accommodate to the new by assimilating it to the old in a coherent, rational way, a way which manages to preserve intact the fundamental aspects of the previous assimilatory organization... It is a useful and only slightly misleading generalization about the preoperational child that he has no stable, enduring, and internally consistent cognitive organization, no system-in-equilibrium, with which to order, relate, and make coherent the world around him. His cognitive life, like his affective life, tends to be an unstable, discontinuous, moment-to-moment one.

Action — ...Preoperational thought tends to operate with concrete and static images of reality rather than with abstract, highly schematic signs. Thus, although the child does represent reality rather than simply act in it, his representations are much closer to overt actions, in both form and operation, than is the case for older children and adults. Piaget believes that much of the young child's cognition takes the form of what he calls *mental experiment*...: that is, an isomorphic, step-by-step mental replica of concrete actions and events. Rather than schematize, reorder, and generally refashion events as does the older child, the young child simply runs off reality sequences in his head just as he might do in overt action. Thus, preoperational thought is extremely concrete.[18]

Because the child cannot reason, he cannot be expected to give logical reasons for the behaviors of people or environmental occurrences. One must accept the child's reasoning and explain reality step by step at the child's level. Reasons or explanations are given according to the vividness of the child's recall of past or present experiences: "You can't play with Chris because he is *isolated*" (abstract, nonmeaningful term). "You can't play with Chris because he is *sick* and *coughs*" (experienced by the child). Familiar action words are appropriate to the child's preconcepts. If the child has not experienced the situation, a short, concrete statement is given. In telling the child about therapy, for example, the therapist might say, "You and I are going to play with toys."

The child's concrete interpretation of words can create frustration for him and amusement for the adult. In his response to the adult's slang expression of annoyance, "Oh, nuts!" the four-year-old girl looked around the room with a frown on her face and said "Where are the nuts?"

Irreversibility — Perhaps the most important single characteristic of preoperational thought for Piaget is its irreversibility...For present purposes, suffice it to say that a cognitive organization is reversible, as opposed to irreversible, if it is able to travel along a cognitive route (pursue a series of reasonings, follow a series of transformations in a display, etc.) and then reverse direction, in thought, to find again an unchanged point of departure (the beginning premise, the original state of the display, etc.). Again, it is reversible if it can compose into a single organized system the various compensating changes which result from a transformation and, by seeing how each change is annulled by its inverse (the one which compensates for it), insure an underlying constancy or invariance for the whole system. In a general way, a thought form which is reversible is one which is flexible and mobile, in stable equilibrium, able to correct for distorting superficials by means of successive, quick-moving decenterings. But the turgid, slow-paced, and extremely concrete *mental experiment* of preoperational thought is not reversible, parroting as it does irreversible events in reality.

Concepts and Reasoning — Piaget refers to the first, primitive concepts used by a young child as *preconcepts*...In keeping with the general character of preoperational thought, these preconcepts tend to be action-ridden, imagistic, and concrete, rather than schematic and abstract. But they have one specific peculiarity as well: they refer neither to *individuals* who possess stable identity over time and in different contexts nor to genuine *classes* or collectivities of similar individuals...the preoperational child has difficulty in recognizing stable identity in the midst of contextual changes.

Piaget uses the term *transducive* for the types of reasoning by which the preoperational child links various preconcepts...Neither true induction nor true deduction, this kind of reasoning proceeds from particular to particular. Centering on one salient element of an event, the child proceeds irreversibly to draw as conclusion from it some other, perceptually compelling happening. Piaget makes the important point that the factual correctness of the child's conclusion (and of course the child is sometimes correct) is by itself no guarantee that the mechanism for arriving at it was logical rather than transducive...Just as an incorrect conclusion can sometimes reflect a deductive or inductive logical orientation, a correct conclusion can follow from a basically transducive one." [19]

Concrete Operational Thought

Ginsburg and Opper have defined the individual words in the term *concrete operations* (the period between seven or eight years of age and about eleven years of age). Operations are the "actions which the child performs mentally and which have the added property of being reversible." These mental actions are *concrete* since the child can apply them only to objects which are immediately present." [20]

To facilitate operational thought, the structure of *groupings* evolves. This structure permits progressive and logical sequencing involving various combinations of operations. The importance of the concept of groupings cannot be overemphasized. Sanford and Wrightsman have clearly defined the value of groupings in the process of conceptualization.[21] Because of the continuous and variable nature of the world, it is impossible for an individual to respond separately and distinctly to each event, object, or person. The quantities of details which would be required of the human mind if there were no grouping would be so overwhelming that a person would have little time to devote to anything beyond the sorting of minutiae. For example, the therapist would not describe a four-year-old's behavior as being *normal* or *average*; instead, all the details of the four-year-old's behavior would have to be described each time the therapist had to describe the four-year-old children he was treating. In addition, one could not use abstract values on a continuum to describe behaviors, such as the *A, B, C, D, E, F* used in grading classwork; a description of the specific performance of each student would have to be given by the teacher each time he graded the students. To alleviate this impossible situation, the child develops the ability to group objects or to categorize them in different ways and, therefore, to perform varied operations with them.

Because the child is in the period of transition between motor learning and abstract thinking, learning tasks relevant to grouping and other structures must be sequenced accordingly. The child is encouraged to act upon his environment motorically in the early phase of concrete operations in order to learn about its properties. Gradually, thought is emphasized and action de-emphasized as the concrete operational abilities develop.

An example of the development of a structure in the period of concrete operations — which is based on groupings — is *conservation*. This concept is based on the understanding of all conservations — continuous quantity, volume, substance, weight and length. The child must recognize that in the transfer of an object or substance to another shape or size (with no additions to or subtractions from the original material), there is no change in the original qualities of the material; the original amount is conserved. For example, the quantity of water in a tall thin glass remains the same when it is transferred into a short, fat glass. Or, the substance of Plasticene in two balls remains the same when the shape of one is changed by squeezing.

In the early stage of the development of conservation, which occurs about the fourth or fifth year of age, the child does not conserve. This stage of development is probably the result of his being able to concentrate on only one of the dimensions of a property at a time. For example, the child may say that the weight of the Plasticene which is squeezed into the form of a hotdog is heavier than that which remains in the form of a ball because the former is longer.

The five- or six-year-old child still does not conserve the original weight, but vacillates between the two possible responses. Sometimes, for example, he believes that the ball is heavier, at other times he is sure that the hotdog is heavier. By six or seven years of age, the child finally does conserve the weight and recognizes that the weights of both are equal, regardless of the shape.

The psychological structures which have developed during the period of concrete operations account for the conservation. The child has become *decentrized*. He can understand the dynamics of a task which is not directly related to himself. He can follow directions for a step-by-step procedure which involves two or three problems. He can now focus on and work with several areas of a problem at the same time. However, the child still cannot resolve an unexpected problem if it should arise. Although he can perform the operations mentally, he may need a demonstration of a task in order to help him organize his thinking by providing the concrete stimulus for that thinking.

The increase in the child's logical reasoning and anticipatory images permit concrete explanations about familiar situations and projections into the future. "If you do this exercise it may hurt your arm today, but your arm should feel better tomorrow." No theoretical description of the reasons for therapy can be given, however.

Dynamic transformations are evidenced as the child focuses on the change as it occurs in the content of a material, such as the change from the ball shape of Plasticene to the hotdog shape. He is aware of the dynamics of the transformation and is reasonably accurate in his interpretation of them.

The characteristic of *reversibility* also is available to the concrete operational child. "Cognitive organization is reversible...if it is able to travel along a cognitive route (pursue a series of reasonings, follow a series of transformations in a display, etc.) and then reverse direction, in thought, to find again an unchanged point of departure (the beginning premise, the original state of the display, etc.)" [22] For example, the concrete operational child realizes that pouring from glass C to B reverses or negates the action of pouring from glass B to C. He is aware that it is the same action performed in another direction. By carrying out the action mentally, that is, by reversing the pouring in his mind, he is able to ascertain that the quantity of water in C (the lower, wider glass) is the same as in B. He can perform a mental operation which leads him to a certain conclusion, and then reverse this operation, which enables him to return to his original starting point.

"The concrete operational child can also perform another type of reversibility when operating on relations. This is reciprocity. For instance, in the example of liquid quantity, when the child says that one glass is longer and thinner, whereas the other is shorter and wider, he is canceling out the differences between the two glasses by an action of reciprocity. One difference balances out the other, with the result that they have a reciprocal relationship." [23]

Horizontal decalage is the phenomenon in which a child does not achieve success at the same time in all problems which require similar mental operations. Although one does not anticipate consistency in developmental performance in diverse areas of behavior, such as in motor and social behavior, it might seem logical to expect continuity within a narrow range of behavior.

This continuity, however, does not always occur, as illustrated by the results of Piaget's research on the appearance of the different conservations. The conservation of substance appears at about seven or eight years of age; the conservation of weight at nine or ten years of age; and the conservation of volume at about eleven or twelve years of age. Therefore the child's understanding of a resolution to one concrete problem does not necessarily transfer to a similar problem, and may require either an additional explanation and demonstration by the adult or additional maturation of the child.

Formal Operational Thought

Formal operational thought begins during the eleventh or twelfth year. It is

... "characterized in general by the conquest of a new mode of reasoning, one that is no longer limited exclusively to dealing with objects or directly representable realities, but also employs 'hypotheses,' in other words, propositions from which it is possible to draw logical conclusions without it being necessary to make decisions about their truth or falsity before examining the result of their implications." [24]

The reasoning to which Piaget refers is called *hypothetico-deductive reasoning*. The adolescent is no longer constrained by the apparent realities of an object or situation. Instead, the raising of many possible questions about and solutions to a problem dominates his thought. The adolescent makes many hypotheses from his observations and through the canceling out of the poor hypotheses, makes deductions about the problem. The adolescent is encouraged to work toward completion of a task and competence in his work. He can correct errors and follow a problem to its solution, but may be inclined to explore multiple new areas, mentally resolve a problem and not complete the immediate project.

In creating a hypothesis, the adolescent institutes the *combinatorial system*. Instead of being limited to looking at only a single property of a given situation, as was true of the child in the stage of concrete operations, the adolescent looks at each property both singly and in combination with many other properties. This permits the combining of physical objects or ideas from which the hypothetico-deductive reasoning is initiated.

"...It is remarkable that at the level at which he becomes capable of combining elements (objects) by an exhaustive and systematic method he is also capable of combining ideas or hypotheses in affirmative or negative statements, and thus of utilizing propositional operations hitherto unknown to him: implication (if-then), disjunction (either-or, or both), exclusion (either-or) or incompatibility (either-or, or neither-neither), reciprocal implication, etc." [25]

The adolescent can combine and work with multiple factors when problem solving; he can make logical decisions when given multiple choices or options; he has begun to see cause-and-effect relationships. The adolescent, therefore, should be included in the decision-making processes which affect his own welfare. When situations occur in which he cannot make the decisions, such as the choice of surgical procedures, he still needs to be informed of the procedures and to be encouraged to raise questions about them and their potential results.

In addition to the characteristics of hypothetico-deductive reasoning and combinatorial thought, the adolescent is working toward the equilibrium of thought. By about sixteen years of age, the adolescent can adapt to many problems. He can now easily assimilate new material and has to accommodate less extensively to new problems. "Piaget does maintain...that, by the end of adolescence, the individual's ways of thinking, that is, his cognitive structures, are almost fully formed. While these structures may be applied to new problems with the result that significant knowledge is achieved, the structures themselves undergo little modification after adolescence. They have reached a high degree of equilibrium." [26]

Other characteristics ascribed to the adolescent as a result of formal operations are flexibility of thought, absence of confusion upon reaching unexpected conclusions due to the anticipated possibilities and a single system for the reversibility of thought. The last characteristic means "that his thought can proceed in one direction, and then use several different methods for retracing its steps in order to return to the starting point." [27]

Piaget has noted the influence of the adolescent's development of cognitive powers on other areas of his development. The youth is no longer constrained by concrete operations and therefore thinks beyond his family and their beliefs. In the attempt to exercise his new abilities, the adolescent raises questions about religion, politics and moral judgments. He searches for more satisfactory answers to the problems of society. He begins to think and hypothesize about the future, and, through this process, he is able to explore many previously unrealized possibilities. As described by Piaget and Inhelder:

"This is the age of great ideals and of the beginning of theories, as well as the time of simple present adaptation to reality. This affective and social impulse of adolescence has often been described. But it has not always been understood that this impulse is dependent upon a transformation of thought that permits the handling of hypotheses and reasoning with regard to propositions removed from concrete and present observation." [26]

Problems in Cognitive Learning

It is generally assumed that operational thinking is more difficult than sensorimotor thinking. However, the dimensions of abstractness or concreteness (referring to action learning, not concrete operational learning) usually are not the primary factors which determine the ease or difficulty in learning. Instead, as indicated in the research compiled by Sanford and Wrightsman in 1970, the crucial element in learning is the stimulus and the number of possible conflicting responses which it elicits. This conflict can appear at any developmental age. Perhaps difficulty in learning becomes more obvious in the period of concrete operational and formal operational behavior because society now expects more of the child cognitively than it expected of him in the sensorimotor and preoperational stages.

Because concepts such as numbers, colors, shapes or sizes can be applied to multiple objects or situations which may not be related, learning the associations between them and multiple other stimuli is difficult. For example, the stimulus word *red* elicits multiple possible responses: animate and inanimate objects, situations and feelings. A child may not clearly see the relationship between objects in a group which are varied shades of red from orange to pink or between objects in a group that all possess the common element of red (as in pictures of a house with a *red* roof, a person with *red* hair and a *red* apple). The child must learn to abstract the commonality for the operational process of grouping.

These concepts of learning do not conflict with Piaget's sequence of cognitive development, but they do require a teaching approach which emphasizes clarity in the presentation of learning tasks more than the sequential presentation of cognitive tasks. Instead of emphasizing the sensorimotor aspects of a task or the preconceptual elements of learning, the therapist focuses on alleviating the child's confusion when learning. [29]

There are factors other than conflicting responses which impede a child's conceptualization. Levi (1969) has described these as "error factors." [30] The child may be distracted by interesting but irrelevant stimuli. He may attempt to narrow the stimulus field and consequently ignore some of the stimuli necessary to the completion of the task. He may revert to a previously successful verbal or nonverbal response. The child may use an unknown concept which he magically thinks may be the answer to all the questions which he cannot answer. He may be unable to shift to a new problem because of perseveration. He may avoid repeating a previous response. He may show temporary physical fatigue when he is unsuccessful — or he may show daily changes in his physical state which may reduce his ability to function at his best.

Briefly, there are some ways to reduce the child's confusion in cognitive learning. Levi has suggested a logical procedure for the teaching of the concept of grouping. First, the child must develop the idea of category — the class in which a group of objects belong. Next he acquires a limited number of categories. He then learns to scan these categories and to choose the one which best answers his problem. A simple example might be the child's learning to identify the category *red* and thus the group of objects which are red (not pink or purple). Next he learns one or two other categories of color, such as green and yellow (two colors which can be distinguished easily from each other and from the original stimulus). Then the child may learn to match objects which initially are identical to red, yellow or green and then are graded into shades of red, yellow or green, such as pink and greenish-blue.

Sanford and Wrightsman have described other ways to reduce the child's confusion in learning which supplement Levi's concepts. Children learn concepts of color and form most easily if the similar parts of the stimuli are related to knowns. One would use the example of robin *red* breast or *green* grass rather than a *red* lobster or a *yellowtail* fish. A plate or glass which has a round rim is a preferable comparison to a smokestack or silo, which are both round, but which are unfamiliar to many children.

In teaching concepts, other variables initially are kept constant in order to reduce the possibility of raising conflicting responses, as may be seen in the examples of the house with the red roof, the person with the red hair, and the red apple. Instead, through the picture of a solid red ball, a single red door and a solid red apple, the concept *red* would be more easily learned.

Another important element in the teaching of mental operations of abstracts or nonpresent objects is to be positive in the description of what the concept *is*, rather than negative in defining what the concept *is not* — even though people do learn from negative experiences. It is more effective to say to the child "It looks like..." or "It tastes like..." than to say "It is not at all like..." For example, "An apartment is like lots of houses put together without roofs. They are on top of each other and next to each other." The statement, "An apartment is not like your house and it is not like the stores downtown," gives the child information to eliminate while trying to conceptualize an apartment, but gives him nothing on which to build the concept, *apartment.* There are still too many possible responses.

In summary, it has been found that communication and cognition are closely linked; the use of one readily affects the development of the other. Only for ease of learning have these two developmental processes been separated from each other. Suggestions for the stimulation of cognition and communication are brief, but general enough for the therapist to be able to make both broad application from this material and to make further study into the subjects.

References

1. Pronovost, W. and Mulholland, A. *Communicative Disorders— Development, Assessment, Therapy, Education* (Boston: Allyn and Bacon, in press).
.2. West, R. W. and Ansberry, M. *The Rehabilitation of Speech,* Fourth Edition (New York: Harper and Row, 1968), p. 501.
3. Carroll, J. B. *Language and Thought* (Englewood Cliffs, N. J. : Prentice-Hall, 1964).
4. Van Riper, C. *Speech Correction Principles and Methods,* Fourth Edition (Englewood Cliffs, N. J.: Prentice-Hall, 1963).
5. Gesell, A. L. *The First Five Years of Life* (New York: Harper and Row, 1940), p. 44.
6. Gesell, A. L., *The First Five Years of Life,* p. 49.
7. Gesell, A. L., *The First Five Years of Life,* p. 55.
8. Blatt, Burton. *The Intellectually Disenfranchised Impoverished Learners and Their Teachers* (Boston: Commonwealth of Massachusetts Department of Mental Health, Community Mental Health Monograph Series, 1966), pp. 184-186.
9. Ginsburg, H. and Opper, S. *Piaget's Theory of Intellectual Development: An Introduction* (Englewood Cliffs, N.J.: Prentice-Hall, 1969), pp. 15-18.
10. Ginsburg, H. and Opper S., p. 17.
11. Piaget, J. and Inhelder, B. *The Psychology of the Child* (New York: Basic Books, 1969), p. 9.
12. Piaget, J. *Science of Education and the Psychology of the Child* (New York: Orion Press, 1970), p. 31.
13. Flavel, J. H. *The Developmental Psychology of Jean Piaget* (Princeton, N. J.: D. VanNostrand, 1963), pp. 156-157.
14. Piaget, J. and Inhelder, B.

386

15. Piaget, J. and Inhelder, B., p. 58.
16. Piaget, J. and Inhelder, B., p. 71.
17. Piaget, J. and Inhelder, B., p. 71.
18. Flavell, J. H., pp. 157-158.
19. Flavell, J. H., pp. 159-160.
20. Ginsburg, H. and Opper, S., p. 150.
21. Sanford, F. H. and Wrightsman, L. S. *Psychology: A Scientific Study of Man,* Third Edition (Belmont, California: Brooks and Cole, 1970).
22. Flavell, J. H., p. 159.
23. Ginsburg, H. and Opper, S., p. 168.
24. Piaget, J., p. 33.
25. Piaget, J. and Inhelder, B., pp. 135-136.
26. Ginsburg, H. and Opper, S., p. 204.
27. Ginsburg, H. and Opper, S., p. 204.
28. Piaget, J. and Inhelder, B., pp. 130-131.
29. Sanford, F. H. and Wrightsman, L. S. *Psychology: A Scientific Study of Man*; Gibson, E. J. *Principles of Perceptual Learning and Development* (New York: Appleton-Century-Crofts, Meredith Corp., 1969).
30. Levi, A. "An Approach to the Remediation of Cognitive Deficit." In *Professional School Psychology, Volume III* (New York: Grune and Stratton, 1969).

Bibliography

Athey, I. J. and Rubadeau, D. O. (eds.) *Educational Implications of Piaget's Theory: A Book of Readings* (Waltham, Mass.: Blaisdell, 1970).

Beard, R. M. *An Outline of Piaget's Developmental Psychology for Students and Teachers* (New York: Basic Books, 1969).

Bearley, M. and Hitchfield, E. *A Guide to Reading Piaget* (New York: Schocken Books, 1966).

Berry, M. F. and Eisenson, J. *Speech Disorders: Principles and Practices of Therapy* (New York: Appleton-Century Crofts, 1956).

Furth, H. G. *Piaget for Teachers* (Englewood Cliffs, N. J.: Prentice-Hall, 1970).

Gesell, A. L. and Amatruda, C. S. *Developmental Diagnosis,* Second edition (New York: Paul B. Hoeber, 1947).

Human Communication and Its Disorders: An Overview (Bethesda, Maryland: U. S. Department of Health, Education and Welfare, 1969).

Sharp, E. *Thinking is Child's Play* (New York: E. P. Dutton, 1969).

Smith, E. B.; Goodman, K. S.; and Meredith, R. *Language and Thinking in the Elementary School* (New York: Holt, Rinehart and Winston, 1970).

NOTES

NOTES

Chapter Eight

The Integration
of Development

Barbara Sharpe Banus, M.A., O.T.R.

(November 1970)

INTRODUCTION

It should be evident by this time that the boundaries between developmental areas as I have outlined them in this text are superficial, and have been used only to assist the therapist in becoming aware of and alert to the different segments of a child's behavior. This approach might be described as a divergent thought process, through which the therapist analyzes the segments of child behavior.

The thought process of the therapist now converges all the child's behaviors into an integrated, functional whole. The degree of interdependence and interaction among all behaviors varies at different times throughout the process of continuous maturation and development toward the refinement of skills. This is an important concept. My purpose has been to stress behavior of the child within the first five years of life, since most of the basic developmental processes have been stabilized during this time. The refining of behaviors is continuous, of course, as may be seen in the adolescent who learns how to type rapidly and accurately (neuromotor refinement); or the adult who learns a foreign language (language development); or the student who proceeds into advanced study (cognitive expansion).

The multiply handicapped child shows more developmental problems than a normal child because of reciprocal relationships. I believe that handicapped children, particularly, need more developmental guidance so that maturation and learning will occur, for these children may not be able to cope physically or emotionally with their environment, and may, therefore, withdraw from it. They may not know which stimuli to choose for the enhancement of their development. For example, the child with paraplegia may not be able to crawl and because of his disability may not explore his environment; someone must bring the environment to him. The emotionally disturbed child might choose stimuli which reinforce his regressive social behavior rather than those which will gradually lead him into group behavior. Thus, the therapist must assist in the analysis of the child's total developmental process, in order to provide stimuli which are meaningful and developmentally appropriate.

These children also need guidance because they may avoid treatment which is difficult, possibly due to physical fatigue or emotional intolerance for a situation. The child may gain a broad developmental experience from the task he chooses, but he may not be therapeutically benefited in the specific direction of his problem.

THE INFORMAL DEVELOPMENTAL EVALUATION

The informal developmental evaluation can be a brief assessment of the child's overall developmental function, in order to expedite the choosing of the most appropriate formal or standardized evaluation for that particular child. A danger of the brief or single observation in the assessment of total development is the inaccurate judgment of the child's overall behavior. The child's total gross motor function and development cannot be determined from a single observation of his walking; his cognitive development cannot be judged from the completion of one task. A child's performance may vary over a wide range within a day or an hour depending upon his comfort in a situation. On the other hand, the child may focus only on a single task (splinter skill) which is not indicative of his overall behavior.

The informal developmental evaluation, which surveys all aspects of the child's performance, can be lengthy (Figure 8-1). This evaluation can be a tool used to scan several areas of development or to focus on a few specific behaviors within the total performance.

This evaluation is used most effectively by the therapist who knows the highlights of the developmental sequence for quick identification of the critical stages, such as the time for sitting, standing independently, walking or rolling over. This knowledge provides him with the cues which determine the direction in which he will guide the evaluation, and the tools which he will use to elicit the desired behaviors.

Figure 8-1 illustrates a general framework of behaviors to be observed in the informal evaluation. Its purpose is only to identify general developmental areas so that no critical observations will

Reflex patterns
   spinal
   brain stem
   midbrain
   cortical

Lower extremity development
   crawling
   walking
   sitting
   posture
   balance
   running, jumping, hopping

Upper extremity development
   arm function
   pronation, supination
   rotation
   reach
   grasp
   release transfer

Speech and language development
   receptive
   expressive

Cognitive development
   sensorimotor behavior
   preoperational thought
   concrete operational thought
   formal operational thought

Visual perceptual-motor development
   visual area
   sensory awareness
   eye-hand coordination
   visual discrimination
   basic motor planning
   advanced visual perceptual
   advanced visual motor

Social development
   solitary play
   looking-on play
   parallel play
   cooperative play group
   monosexual gang
   heterosexual adolescent group

Integration of above behaviors in development of self-care behaviors
   feeding
   dressing
   toileting
   grooming

FIG. 8-1. Possible behaviors to be observed in informal developmental evaluations.

be ignored. No test materials are required or suggested. These are chosen by the evaluator according to the purpose of the evaluation and his knowledge of the child. The behaviors are listed at random, with no consideration for their place in the order of the evaluation. All the areas of development on the form can, but need not, be evaluated — this, too, is determined by the evaluator. Once the therapist develops a mental image of the content of the evaluation, a written format may not be necessary. Seldom does the skilled clinician use a written form in the informal evaluation.

A Format for Recording the Results
of a Comprehensive Informal Developmental Evaluation

The comprehensive report presented here is a compilation of all observed behavior, the developmental level at which the behavior occurs, the immediate sequential behavior for each, and the media used to elicit the behavior. The objective is to contain all the evaluation data in an organized unit which can be expanded over a period of time (Figure 8-2).

The *description of observed behavior* is a detailed report of the observed behavior. It emphasizes the child's qualitative response in each behavioral area. A "yes" or "no" comment is unacceptable, since it does not give sufficient information about the performance. To say the child has "grasp" means nothing; to say that "the child demonstrates opposition of the index finger to the thumb" explicitly describes the observed behavior. Only from the latter description can the therapist make intelligent decisions about the successive developmental steps for treatment planning.

The therapist makes qualitative judgments about the temporary or permanent aspects of the behavior based on the frequency of its appearance in the child's repertoire and the maturity of its function. The positive responses (in other words, the behaviors which the child demonstrated adequately), are noted. Those which were not attempted, or which were attempted, but not successfully completed, are not described unless this process in itself demonstrates a developmental level. It is of no value to know that Sam, aged two years, cannot walk, run, or ride a tricycle. It is essential that the therapist recognizes that he uses a four-point crawl, pulls himself up into a standing position by using furniture, and stands only when holding onto objects. The extraneous information about the child's inabilities may mask his actual function. Performance is identified only to obtain a developmental profile. The report would lose its discriminative function if all nonperformed but attempted behaviors were included as well.

Description of observed behavior	Test media	Development level	Sequential development	Date accomplished	Sequential development	Date accomplished

Name of child: _____ Date of Evaluation: _____

Age: _____ Evaluator: _____

Diagnosis: _____

Number of days hospitalized: _____

Precautions and restrictions: _____

Reflex patterns

   spinal
   brain stem
   midbrain
   cortical

Lower extremity development

   crawling
   walking
   sitting
   posture
   balance

Upper extremity development

   arm function
   pronation, supination
   rotation
   reach
   grasp
   release
   transfer

Speech and language development

   receptive
   expressive

Cognitive development

   sensorimotor behavior
   preoperational thought
   concrete operational thought
   formal operational thought

FIG. 8-2. Comprehensive informal developmental evaluation format.

Name of child: _____ Date of Evaluation: _____

Age: _____ Evaluator: _____

Diagnosis: _____

Number of days hospitalized: _____

Precautions and restrictions: _____

Description of observed behavior	Test media	Development level	Sequential development	Date accomplished	Sequential development	Date accomplished
Visual perceptual-motor development						
visual area						
sensory awareness						
eye-hand coordination						
visual discrimination						
basic motor planning						
advanced visual perceptual						
advanced visual motor						
Social development						
solitary play						
looking-on play						
parallel play						
cooperative play group						
monosexual gang						
heterosexual adolescent group						
Development of self-care behaviors						
feeding						
dressing						
toileting						
grooming						

(Pertinent information gathered from clinic records, staff or family or both to be included within the appropriate section above.)

Summary

Recommendations for treatment in occupational therapy and further evaluations or treatment in areas such as speech and physical therapy.

FIG. 8-2. (continued)

The *test media* are the stimuli (chosen by the evaluator or the child) which elicit the developmental behaviors described in the second column of Figure 8-2. If the informal evaluation is extensive and communicates information to other involved personnel, the description of the test media is requisite. By identifying the media with which the child performed, a specific answer can be given to the individual who asks, "What, specifically, was used to elicit the response?" With the specific information available, a vague reply, such as, "I think it was the ball" or "It might have been a couple of things..." is eliminated In addition to verifying the type of stimuli, the description provides a specific visual image of the evaluation media, and leads to an accurate analysis of the child's performance in relation to the media: a red ball with a two-inch diameter. The identified test media suggests stimuli which might be employed or which should be avoided by other staff in their own evaluation or treatment of the child. Finally, it indicates those materials which presently are being used for initial and ongoing evaluations and, consequently, those which are not appropriate for treatment.

The *developmental level* denotes the level of the child's performance in each behavior or area of behavior. From this information a developmental profile can be constructed to assist in the diagnosis of a dysfunction or a developmental problem. For example, a child who is chronologically five years old but developmentally only two years old according to his developmental profile, probably has problems in socialization typical of his developmental age of two years. He may play only on a parallel basis with his peers and not interact with them. However, a child whose developmental profile is within the acceptable range of five-year behavior in all areas except social behavior may have a functional problem in socialization. Through further diagnosis it may be found that it is a temporary problem because of the child's lack of exposure to other children. Only minimum support by an adult may be necessary to assist the child in developing social skills. This would not be true, however, in the case of the child whose overall function is within the two-year range. By identifying the extent of the developmental delay both longitudinally and cross-sectionally in combination with the diagnostic reports, an educated guess may be hazarded about the degree to which the child may progress through treatment. The identification of a developmental level also guides the therapist in planning treatment. It excludes vague information which leads to vague treatment planning. The therapist is objective and accurate in choosing the sequential goals and the media for reaching them.

It is difficult to find normative data on the materials or media frequently used by children. Because of the lack of information, it is well for the therapist to use some materials in informal evaluations which have developmental levels assigned to them through prior standardization — in addition to using nonstandardized materials. Information on developmental levels can be extracted from standardized data, such as that obtained from research at the Gesell Institute, from the therapist's own experience, and from his informal research over a period of time.

Sequential development describes the behaviors which immediately succeed the described observed behavior. These behaviors are the immediate goals for the child's performance toward which the therapist directs treatment, and from which he assesses the child's progress. The sequential patterns are essential to the planning of specific treatment sessions (as opposed to the vague planning of treatment sessions based on vague goals). Also, they show the milestones of progress in an ongoing evaluation by identifying the date and point at which the child performs the desired behavior. With the collection of this data over a period of time, the degree of the child's accomplishments and the rate of his progress are evidenced.

This method of data collection is detailed, and, therefore, a time-consuming process. It is one approach to record keeping for the long-term collection of research information on development and for an ongoing evaluation of the child's progress.

The *summary* succinctly organizes the behavioral observations into a composite picture of the child. It may be used by the individuals who want to survey the child's total performance, or by those who are evaluating the possibility of a problem in a particular area. In addition, it assists the therapist in summarizing his own thoughts about the child.

Recommendations provide information pertinent to the planning of the child's treatment, and may or may not be a part of the informal developmental evaluation. Because the primary objective of an evaluation is to plan treatment, the recommendation from the informal developmental evaluation gives the therapist guidelines for both further testing and for total developmental planning, both remedial and prophylactic.

An example of a comprehensive informal developmental evaluation which is almost identical to the one stated in the format is illustrated in Figure 8-3. It was performed and recorded by an undergraduate occupational therapy student. This is one way to learn about informal developmental evaluation and to solidify one's own knowledge of developmental concepts, sequences, levels, and so forth. It would be unrealistic to expect that every

Name: Ann Franklin
Birth date: 10/28/63   Age at testing: 3½ years   Evaluator: Beverly Gladstein, O.T.S.
Diagnosis: mental retardation associated with disease and conditions due to unknown prenatal influences (genetic): Mongolism—Down's Syndrome.
Admission to hospital: 5/2/65

Observed Behavior	Test Media	Development Level	Sequential Development
Reflex patterns Observation of Ann's reflex patterns place her at the midbrain level with some deviations to the brain stem level.			
POSITIVE SUPPORTING REACTION— Ann held her feet in constant extension while being bounced.		Brain stem level	Midbrain level: while being bounced, the child will have leg flexion when in the air, and extension when her legs touch ground.
LABRYINTHINE RIGHTING ACTING ON HEAD (SUPINE)— While being held by the therapist in a vertical position, Ann leaned back and would have fallen if not held; she did not right her head forward while falling back, hence, she showed a negative reaction. (PRONE) When placed on her stomach, Ann lifted her head and thorax by resting on her elbows. Later, when held in a prone position under the thorax and leaning forward, she lifted her head to right.		Midbrain level	Cortical level: this reflex later helps in enabling the child to assume an upright posture and free gait.

FIG. 8-3. Comprehensive informal developmental evaluation.

400

FIG. 8-3 (continued)

Observed Behavior	Test Media	Development Level	Sequential Development
PROTECTIVE EXTENSOR THRUST—While in the above position, Ann extended her arms forward to protect her head.		Midbrain level	
AMPHIBIAN REFLEX—When pressure was applied to the hip, there was no visual flexion in the elbow and knee of that side, hence, a response was not observed or recorded.		Midbrain level	This reflex is a prerequisite for crawling.
BODY RIGHTING—When the pelvis was turned to one side, the thorax and head followed.		Midbrain level	
LANDAU REFLEX—When held in a prone position under the thorax, Ann lifted her head while her spine and legs extended.		Midbrain level	
Lower extremity development Although she leaned forward in an exaggerated thoracic curve, Ann was able to assume a steady and controlled sitting position.		9 mo.	Is able to sit and pivot.
Ann is able to stand erect and steadily if holding on to something and, it is stated in her chart, she is able to stand without support for a few seconds. It is not known		9½ mo.	Once she is able to pull herself up and lower herself down, Ann will lift and replace her foot until she is able to walk around holding bilaterally onto a rail.

if she is able to assume this position by herself since she was not really given the opportunity.

It was stated by the aide that Ann is learning to walk.

Upper extremity development

Although there was no evidence of deliberate pronation-supination (when presented with filling and emptying activities, she threw the cup away), Ann showed some wrist rotation while bringing her hands up in front of her face or reaching for an object.

cup filled with crayons		
Ann's reach is direct with a unilateral approach which involves the entire trunk. She is also able to cross the midline.	7 mo.	Well-coordinated reach for near objects, showing better balance; the whole trunk not involved in reach.
The child exhibits a pronated palmar grasp except when holding a block; the grasp then is one-quarter supinated with the 5th finger up in the air. Most objects held are mouthed. Ann also is able to slowly transfer objects; a doll is held unilaterally (left hand), then bilaterally, then unilaterally (right hand). — blocks	6 mo.	Inferior scissor grasp: thumb to one side of curled index finger. Transfers are made more easily.
Release is total involving extension of all fingers. — Teddy bear		Deliberate and controlled release.

FIG 8-3 (continued)

Observed Behavior	Test Media	Development Level	Sequential Development
Speech and language development Ann listens when being spoken to and appears to understand simple words such as "sit." When hand gestures are used along with statements, the child is better able to understand. For example, if hands are extended out to Ann while saying, "Do you want to get out of the crib?" she will respond by lifting her shoulders and extending her arms. Ann cries if frustrated and smiles at facial expressions or in response to physical activities such as being bounced or, twirled, but makes no laughing, babbling, or cooing sounds.		7 mo. 2 mo.	Has a better understanding of words and statements. Makes laughing noises and babbling sounds.
Perceptual-motor development VISUAL AREA—Ann shows visual acuity and, except when her eyes are fixated on an object, she shows short periods of localized visual attention. She also is able to track an object using maximum head movement.		Stage II: Uncoordinated level of development (Komich)	Longer visual attention and ability to track moving objects using minimal head movement.

| | 7 mo. | Kinesthetic perception—the child becomes aware of body position in space and direction and can realize he is in an upright position and does not lose his balance.

Once unilateral skills are obtained (supination-pronation, reach, grasp, release), bilateral hand use (parallel and opposite movements) is learned.
The child begins to develop body image and becomes aware of parts of the body.

Once prehension patterns are established, the child attempts to hold a cup, spilling most of its contents. |

SENSORY AWARENESS—Ann showed slight evidence of kinesthetic perception. When held by the therapist, the child made no attempt to balance herself and did not seem to realize she would have fallen if not held. However, she is able to sit in an upright position without falling backwards.

No tactile discrimination was observed since all objects held elicited the same response.

EYE-HAND COORDINATION—Ann is at a unilateral level where her eyes guide her hand movements until the object is reached. Then, visual attention is lost.

BASIC MOTOR PLANNING—Ann is beginning to explore her environment in relation to herself: objects held by her are brought up in front of her face and examined; she spends a lot of time looking at her own hands and moving them in front of her face.

Development of self-care skills

It was reported by an aide that Ann is unable to dress or feed herself at this time. It also was reported by the aide that Ann is beginning to become toilet trained; she is placed regularly on the "potty."

FIG. 8-3 (continued)

Observed Behavior	Test Media	Development Level	Sequential Development

Social development
 	
    Ann is at an egocentric level: she was somewhat receptive to the silly noises and faces made by the therapist, but she does not initiate communications such as laughing, babbling, or cooing. When placed next to another child, there was no evidence of recognition of that other child. Ann's chart records her social behavior at a 7-month level. The discrepancy between that report and the level reported here could be the result of Ann's unfamiliarity with the therapist.
 	
Emotional behavior
 	
    Ann was cuddly and maintained a pleasant temperament throughout the session. She became frustrated at one point when not allowed to leave the crib and responded by crying for a short time.
		2 mo.	The child initiates communication when approached by familiar people or situations.
			
			The child learns to laugh and shows anger; crying and smiling are not the only forms of communication.

Summary

In reviewing the preceding evaluation, Ann's performance averages between a 6- and 9-month level of development, with some deviations of 2 months in the areas of speech, social, and emotional development. The child is at a quadrilateral midbrain level of reflexes and exhibited responses to the labyrinthine righting acting on the head (prone), protective extensor thrust, body righting, and Landau reflexes. There was one deviation (positive supporting reaction) to the brain stem level. None of the above reactions elicited any gross response.

Ann's gross and fine motor skills show development of large muscles with the hand muscles still weak. She is able to assume a steady and controlled sitting position and can stand with support (9 mo.), however, she is unable to walk. Her manual development is recorded at a 6- to 7-month level: reach is direct and unilateral and can cross the midline, a pronated palmar grasp is shown, and release involves total finger extension.

Perceptual-motor development ranges between the stages of the uncoordinated level of development and the poorly coordinated level (Komich). Ann's best development is in the visual area: she is able to localize her vision and to track an object using head movement. She also is able to reach for an object with some visual attention.

Speech, social and emotional development are immature (at 2-month level). Although she is receptive to conversation and facial expressions, she is not able to express herself and does not initiate communication, such as babbling or laughing. Ann maintained a pleasant and quiet temperament throughout the session.

A.D.L. is minimal: she is unable to dress or feed herself; however, she is now becoming toilet trained and is placed on the toilet regularly. Her self-feeding is recorded at 7 months and is congruent with her upper extremity development.

Recommendations for treatment

Goals of treatment for this child are to (1) advance her skills from a 6- to 9-month level to a 10- to 12-month level of development, and (2) to provide numerous experiences for manual, perceptual-motor, speech, and social advances.

Opportunity for large muscle development is needed to facilitate walking. An area having space for exploration and objects for pulling herself up should be provided. (It is wondered how much incentive is given to the child to stand up when a net is placed tightly over her crib.)

Bright and colorful rattles and toys that squeak should be made available. Here, the child would receive tactile and visual (color and form) stimulation and motivation for reach, grasp, and release development. Different filling and emptying activities, such as buckets of sand, marbles, or blocks, could be presented to afford experiences of pronation-supination, exploration, manipulation, and tactile stimulation. Bright and colorful mobiles, which also provide visual stimulus, give the child practice in visual tracking, scanning and spatial perception.

Time should be spent with Ann in conversation and play to encourage expressive communication and social development. Objects should be slowly named and sounds made to give opportunities for imitation by the child. Once babbling begins, adult verbal responses are needed to help her language development. The approach used should include consistency and patience to encourage further development and autonomy. As much physical contact as possible, such as cuddling, rocking, and holding, should be given.

evaluator will remember specific dates and developmental levels for every child and disability. Also, most evaluations which are extensive in content are formal or standardized if they are to be reported in writing. Most important, this sample is an example of the content to be included and process through which the evaluator proceeds in an informal developmental evaluation.

THE FORMAL DEVELOPMENTAL EVALUATION

The formal developmental evaluation is devised for the assessment of specific developmental functions within the context of the institution's specific functions. This evaluation would include parts of the developmental areas described in Figure 8-1, but probably not all of them. For example, the therapist working in child psychiatry might devise a formal evaluation to assess each child's social-emotional, language, and cognitive development; the therapist in a cerebral palsy clinic, however, generally evaluates a child's motor control and might devise a neuromotor evaluation for reflexes, upper and lower extremity function and posture. The therapist always assesses the other areas of development informally, but may not formally include them in the report of the evaluation. If the child's other behaviors would conflict with recommended treatment, this is explained in the informal or standardized evaluation. The results of the developmental evaluation in child psychiatry may indicate a need for aggressive outlets. However, gross motor activities would be contraindicated if the child had a neuromotor dysfunction which would inhibit gross motor behavior.

Frequently the subtests from a variety of standardized tests are combined to form a new and institution-specific developmental evaluation. Sections on speech and language from the Gesell Developmental Appraisal, the WISC and the Stanford Binet test, for example, might be compiled to explore children's language function in depth. This approach is applicable for the therapist who is treating a defined population for which no test has been standardized.

From the analysis of the formal developmental evaluation, the therapist plans the specific treatment for the defined developmental problems. The method of treatment planning is similar to planning any developmental treatment. One difference found in the planning for the child's overall development (as compared with the planning for the treatment of a specific developmental problem) is the scope of treatment. A five-year-old child may be receiving his education in a public school, his social experience in recreational activities, his motor activity through outdoor play, but he may need special visual-perceptual-motor training prior to his learning to read and write. In this case, evaluation and treatment are specific, and focus on the development and visual-perceptual-motor skills as described in Chapter Six and not on the other behavioral areas.

THE STANDARDIZED DEVELOPMENTAL EVALUATION

The Gesell Developmental Appraisal

The primary *purpose* of the Gesell Developmental Appraisal is to assess change in direction and rate of the child's development over a period of time through intermittent evaluations. The appraisal was constructed to determine the degree of a child's development in each of four behavioral areas at the time of the testing: motor, adaptive, language, and personal-social. It is not primarily a prognostic tool which, from one test, can be used to make projections about the child's performance in later years; it can be used to determine treatment over a period of many years only through repeated testing.

Ames [1] feels that the determination of rate and sequence of development are the primary objectives of the Developmental Appraisal, not merely the definition of a developmental level at a specific chronological age. The continuous study of the relationship between the chronological age and behavior maturity demonstrates the pattern of the child's development and behavior. The ongoing evaluations determine whether developmental behavior continues progressively and remains parallel with chronological age, or whether there is a lag in behavioral maturation which increases over a period of time so that the developmental age becomes increasingly discrepant with the chronological age.

The formal *structure* of the Gesell Developmental Evaluation divides behavior into four major areas: motor, adaptive, language, and personal-social. Motor behavior which denotes gross bodily control and the finer motor coordinations includes postural reactions, prehension, locomotion, general coordination, and specific motor skills. Adaptive behavior is a convenient category for perceptual, orientational, manual, and verbal adaptations which reflect the child's ability to initiate new experiences and to profit by past experiences. The adaptivity also includes alertness, intelligence, and various forms of constructiveness and exploitation. Language behavior encompasses all visible and audible forms of communication, whether by facial expression, by gesture, or by postural movements; and it includes mimicry and comprehension of communication by others. Personal-social behavior includes not only the child's reactions to other persons and to his cultural environment but also his adjustments to domestic life, to property, to social groups, and to community conventions.

Dr. Gesell has stated that this categorical classification was established for convenience and to facilitate observation and diagnostic analysis (1940, p. 14). Although a distinction is made between the four major areas, an overlap in behavior occurs and is recognized even though the tasks used to evaluate the behavior may appear only in one category. For example, the copying of the model of a bridge in block building has both adaptive and motor significance. The child's ability to perceive the model and copy it indicates his adaptive level, and his ability to construct the bridge shows his motor level. In addition, as the child builds the bridge, the examiner may make general observations regarding his language skills and his social interactions. Developmentally, the emphasis is on the adaptive skill, consequently, the child receives credit for his performance only in that area.[2]

From the results of this developmental appraisal, a *developmental quotient* (to be referred to as a *DQ*) can be determined. This is a composite average of all the behaviors. Ames stresses that a DQ is a rather gross assessment of the child's behavior because it is a composite number which masks the discrete behaviors of the child in each area of development.[3] "It (the Gesell Developmental Appraisal) does not attempt to quantify an all-inclusive function in a single formula."[4] Therapists, ideally therefore, should evaluate each area of development separately and the performance of the skills within each area individually so that the child is not labeled inappropriately. The purpose of the evaluation by the therapist usually is to plan appropriate treatment, he consequently is more concerned with the child's current developmental status than with his specific chronological or overall developmental age.

Although two of the three children in Figure 8-4 have the same average developmental age and theoretically can be compared, the results of such a comparison may be misleading. They have varied profiles which coincidentally result in the same developmental age and composite DQ. The other child has a developmental profile which shows parallel developmental behavior in all areas and approximately the same DQ as those of Chris and Tor. To understand the child and plan treatment, the individual assessment of each item in relation to the others within each of the developmental areas must be considered. This includes an analysis of each of the four broad areas of behavior and of the performed items within each area, such as all the motor behaviors (see Figure 8-6 of Lisa's Gesell Developmental Appraisal). By analyzing the relationship between the items, problems can be defined which become masked when the DQ is the single expression of the performance.

There is much variation in normal individual maturation: when the performance of a 28-week infant is evaluated, any behavior within the range of 24 to 32 weeks is within the normal range; at 18 months, the normal range is from 15 to 21 months; at 36 months the normal range is from 30 to 42 months. The overall DQs and performances in each of the four areas of Tor and Chris are within the normal range for their chronological ages, but it is important to note the slight lag in Tor's speech and Chris's motor performance. These behaviors are observed routinely over a period of time to determine any increased discrepancy between the chronological and developmental ages. In most cases a lag of this dimension is minor and probably would not be re-evaluated unless there were further indications of language or motor problems. It is possible that Tor is motor-minded and temporarily not interested in speaking and that Chris is verbally and socially attuned to his environment with less interest and development in motor activity.

Intellectual development as defined by the intelligence quotient (to be referred to as *IQ*) is not comparable with behavioral development: an *IQ is not equivalent to a DQ*. Ames discusses this at length; she believes that behavioral tests and intelligence tests

	Tor — 18 months	Chris—18 months	Beth—18 months
Motor	21 months	15 months	18 months
Adaptive	21	18	18
Language	15	21	18
Personal-social	18	21	18
Average Developmental Age (D. A.)	18.75 months	18.75 months	18 months
$\dfrac{\text{D. A.}}{\text{C. A.}}$ =D. Q.	104	104	100

FIG. 8-4. A comparison of results from the Gesell Developmental Appraisals of three children.

represent two distinct evaluations, and that an IQ cannot necessarily be predicted from a behavioral test such as the Gesell Developmental Appraisal. "What is being measured by such tests as the Gesell Behavior Tests is behavior maturity, not intelligence." [5] Intelligence can be described as a part of the child's total behavior, and might be partially assessed in the Gesell Developmental Appraisal, through the language and adaptive behavior units. But total behavior is not a unit of intelligence. Neuromotor behavior is not dependent upon intelligence for its basic function, nor is social behavior entirely dependent upon intelligence. It is recognized that increased interdependence in all behavior occurs as each develops and becomes refined. Ames states that:

> The relationship between age and intelligence is hard to define. It is meaningful to the experienced clinician, but most difficult to explain to the layman or to the beginning student. Roughly we may say that the two measures need not be related. Behavior tests measure maturity — how far in age behavior has developed. Intelligence tests measure intellectual level.
>
> An infant or child can be, for example, superior in intelligence and mature in behavior, superior and immature, below average in intelligence yet mature in general behavior, or below average in intelligence and immature in general performance. Thus, although it may be assumed that the child who is mature in infancy will also be mature for his age later on, there is no guarantee that the child whose *behavior* is at or above age in infancy will also be at or above average in *intelligence* later on. [6]

Although the assumptions for these factors are related to Ames' work with infants which has been described in "Predictive Value of Infant Behavior Examination," it seems logical to assume that behavior is a broader concept throughout the child's life than is intelligence. Usually the therapist, except the educational therapist, is concerned with aspects of the behavior other than intelligence, and works with the educator on the development of skills which will affect the child's use of his intelligence. The therapist does not specifically work toward the development of intelligence.

The Gesell Developmental Appraisal (the *GDA*) was developed to assess a child's developmental progress and to broadly identify neurological, intellectual, emotional, comprehension, and perceptual problems. It was not developed for the *differential diagnosis* of the discrete handicaps of a child, such as brain damage, cerebral palsy and childhood psychosis. The Gesell Institute suggests only a few adaptations of the test for use in the testing of dysfunctioning children in *Developmental Diagnosis*. Ames clearly states that other tests are of greater value in determining specific diagnoses (such as the Koppitz version of the Bender Gestalt test, which has norms for immaturity, brain injury, and emotional disturbance; and the WISC and Bender Gestalt, which are valuable in differentiating immature children who are bright between five and seven years of age).[7]

The *materials* which accompany the developmental appraisal, or materials which are equivalent, must be used to obtain valid results in the testing of the child with a dysfunction. For example, if one-inch red blocks can be manipulated by a child with spastic hemiplegia to determine his neuromotor ability, his performance can be compared developmentally with the norms based on the performance of nonhandicapped children. However, if he is not able to grasp the one-inch block and a two-inch block is substituted, the child's performance is no longer comparable to the norms.

Through experimentation at the Gesell Institute, it was found that the variations in the *testing conditions* or situation did not substantially change the child's performance.[8] However, it must be remembered that the children on whom the tests were standardized were within the normal range of behavior and, consequently, may not have been as easily distracted by unusual situations as some handicapped children are.

The *appropriateness of the original normative data*, obtained in the 1930s and 1940s at New Haven, to the present population has been questioned in recent years. It is felt by some therapists that many children are developing faster in 1970 than in 1940, and that the norms should be revised accordingly. Others feel that, because of the discrepancies in development between the culturally deprived child and the nondeprived child, that norms should be developed for specific rather than cross-sectional populations.

Ames has stated in a personal communication that the norms and tests are as valid for environmentally deprived children as they are for advantaged children because the limits on a child's behavior are more biological than environmental. Gesell has said that development is not generated by environmental factors — it is only modified and supported by them. The human organism has an impulse to grow and change.[9]

Knobloch and Pasamanick tested a cross-sectional population of forty-week-old infants with the Gesell Developmental Appraisal and, as a result, suggested some new norms for that chronological age. Their analysis found that the infants performed tasks about four weeks earlier than stated on the original norms in gross motor, personal-social, and language behaviors. It is suggested that earlier development may be the result of several factors which reduce the possibility of neurological damage: better prenatal care, delivery and postnatal care than in the 1930s, and better nutrition. The researchers speculated on the lack of change in fine motor function and suggested that this area may not be as susceptible to changes resulting from improved nutrition or external factors, and that fine motor function may have developed to its maximum in the human organism at this age.

Knobloch's and Pasamanick's work implies the need for restandardization of the Gesell Developmental Appraisal norms, at least at the forty-week level. However, until this is done, the evaluation continues to be a good tool for the assessment of sequential development, and for the planning of sequential treatment. The age of performance may change over a period of years, but the sequence of behavior — and therefore, treatment — remains the same. The present norms do not affect the evaluations of multiply handicapped children, since the discrepancy between the normal and handicapped child is already great. The small discrepancies between the old and new norms are still within the range of normalcy for the age group tested. In addition, the new norms would show advanced behavior which usually would not be important to the patient population of most occupational therapists; the therapist is not trying to identify the developmentally advanced child.

The recommendations or suggestions of the Institute for individuals using the Gesell tests are the same as those for any professional examiners: that the person has basic knowledge in tests and measurements; understands and applies the normative data and statistical information correctly; practices it and becomes thoroughly familiar with it before presenting it; and follows the specifications for the presentation of and analysis of the test.

Ames feels that the Developmental Appraisal can provide a broad perspective of the child's development; however, she has stated that much is dependent upon the expertise of the examiner, his experience and knowledge of children, and his ability to analyze the child's behavior. The primary variable in determining the amount of information gathered about the child is the way in which the examiner uses the test, not the test itself.

A professionally competent person can use the total test or sections of it, as is appropriate to his particular situation. Dr. Ames feels that any one test material may be quite useful in determining the child's maturation (the observation of the child's use of a few blocks, for instance), although each additional test item in an evaluation provides more complete information. One section or test unit can be used independently or can be combined with items in that test or other tests.

The first step in *preparing to give the Developmental Appraisal* is to determine the child's general developmental performance, as it has been described in the informal evaluation. Then the outline for the appropriate sequence for presentation of evaluation items is chosen.[10] This is based on the developmental range of the child's behavior as illustrated in Figure 8-5 for Lisa, age 24 weeks.

This particular sequence was chosen for Lisa because of her good postural adjustment and ability to sit without becoming fatigued within the period of time required for testing. In the test sequence for the previous ages, emphasis was placed on the supine position and the appropriate tasks for it.

Following the choice of test sequence, the evaluator studies the method of presentation for each item. A sample test procedure for the presentation of the rattle in the supine position according to Gesell follows. Although the evaluator need not follow this format rigidly, he does review it to determine the kinds of behaviors to be explored with this tool, and for the logical sequence for involving the child. Even the simple direction, "the examiner holds the rattle in his left hand..." has a rationale. When standing at the child's left, the evaluator will not obscure his view of the child and will reduce the magnitude of visual stimuli (the arm of the examiner which may or may not contain distracting jewelry, such as a watch) for the child by holding the object in his left hand and bringing it forward to the child's hands from his feet.

24–28–32 weeks		
Cube 1, 2, 3	Supine	Pull-to-sit
Massed cubes	Dangling ring	Sit–supported
Pellet	Rattle	Mirror
Bell	Bell ring	Stand–supported
Ring and string	Social stimulation	Prone

FIG 8-5. Developmental appraisal sequence for presentation of evaluation items within the 28-week zone.

At four to twenty-eight weeks of maturity, the examiner uses the following format:

The rattle is held in the examiner's left hand and presented within reaching distance over the upper chest of the supine infant. His perceptual response is observed, and the rattle may be moved into the line of vision if the infant's head is averted, or it may be gently shaken to elicit attention. The infant is allowed to grasp the rattle if he can, or it is brought near his hand, or finally placed in his hand. The hand most favorable for rattle regard is selected and the fingers may have to be opened. His exploitation of the rattle is observed and also his response to loss of the rattle. If he retains it, it is gently removed and placed at his side to determine his ability to pursue the lost rattle.[11]

Once the preparation is done and the test given, the results of the GDA can be recorded, as illustrated in Figure 8-6, or as suggested by the Gesell Institute. Although the results were not recorded according to the format used at the Institute, the report is useful and appropriate because it provides a functional profile of Lisa's performance.

The specific developmental ages were derived from the Gesell Developmental Schedules (see Figures 8-7 and 8-8). In the columns to the left of the behavior, the evaluator identified the child's actual performance with minus or plus signs. The double plus indicates a well-integrated performance; the plus indicates a beginning or early behavior; and a minus indicates the absence of the behavior (this is omitted in Figures 8-7 and 8-8 to illustrate clearly the actual performance. The minus signs may be used to remind the evaluator that the behavior was tested.)

The asterisk and age in parentheses on the Gesell Developmental Schedules indicates the termination of a transitional period. From the time at which the behavior appears on the schedule until the time appearing in the parentheses, it is appropriate for the behavior to occur (perhaps this has implications for the critical period hypothesis).

Developmental treatment at the Gesell Institute encourages children to experience a broad spectrum of behavior rather than a limited and highly specific or structured program. A wide range of materials stimulates a broad range of development in all areas of behavior, and avoids the development of splinter skills. The Institute stresses that children grow at their own rates through maturation. They generally follow the same sequence, though each will vary somewhat from the specific set of norms — both in types of behavior and quality of performance.

Lisa: age 24 weeks	
Motor	
Prone: arms extended	20 weeks
Prone or testing table (TT): scratches TT or platform	20 weeks (28 weeks)
Pull to sitting: lifts head, assists	24 weeks (40 weeks)
Sit chair: trunk erect	24 weeks (36 weeks)
Standing: maintains briefly, hand held	32 weeks (36 weeks)
Adaptive	
Bell-ring: facial response	8 weeks (24 weeks)
Dangling ring, rattle: regards immediately	16 weeks
Dangling ring, rattle: arms activate	16 weeks (24 weeks)
Dangling ring, rattle: regards in hand	16 weeks
Rattle: visual pursuit lost rattle	20 weeks
Dangling ring, rattle: grasps near hand only	20 weeks (24 weeks)
Language	
Vocalizes: grunts, growls	24 weeks (36 weeks)
Vocalizes: spontaneous, vocal-social (includes toys)	24 weeks

Personal-Social	
Play: hand play, mutual fingering	16 weeks
Social: discriminates strangers	24 weeks

Summary of Lisa's performance: Lisa shows good postural and lower extremity development. However, she is just beginning to be aware of and use her arms in a functional manner, as seen in her contacting the blocks proximal to her hands. Frequently, she reverts to the more immature pattern of attempting to mouth objects directly. Response to the bell also is immature, although it is appropriate and indicates an awareness of sound. Her ability to perceive the direction of sound is questioned (this development should be noted in future evaluations).

Language and personal-social development, not involving hand function, are appropriate to the 24 week infant.

Lisa's behavior generally ranged from 16 to 24 weeks, with the more immature patterns in the area of hand function. It is suggested that she be placed in the functional sitting position frequently, for the development of eye-hand coordination. To encourage development in this area, she should be stimulated repeatedly with play materials, such as a crib-gym and rattles, in both supine and sitting positions.

It is recommended that Lisa be re-evaluated within three months primarily to determine further development of hand function.

(Film which demonstrates this Developmental Appraisal is available through the Boston University, Sargent College of Allied Health Professions, Division of Occupational Therapy.)

FIG. 8-6. The recording of a Gesell Developmental Appraisal.

KEY AGE: 16 Weeks

Motor

12 Weeks		16 Weeks		20 Weeks
Su: head predom, half side (t-n-r) (*16w)		Su: midposition head predominates		P.Sit: no head lag
Su: midpos, head & symm. pos. seen		Su: symm. postures predominate		Sit: head erect, steady
Sit: head set forward, bobs (*16w)		Su: hands engage (*24w)	X	Pr: arms extended
St: small fraction weight briefly		Sit: head steady, set forward (*20w)	X	Pr or TT: scratches TT or platform (*28)
St: lifts foot (*24w)		Pr: head Zone III, sustained		Cube: precarious grasp (*24w)
Pr: head Zone II sustained		Pr: legs extended or semi-extended (*40w)		
Pr: on forearms (*20w)		Pr: verge of rolling (*20w)		
Pr: hips low (legs flexed) (*40w)		D. Ring: retains		
Su: hands open or loosely closed		Su: fingers, scratches, clutches (*24w)		
Ra: holds actively				
Cup: contacts				

Adaptive

12 Weeks		16 Weeks		20 Weeks
D. Ring: prompt midline regard	X	D. Ring, Ra: regards immediately		Ra, Bell: 2 hand approach (*28w)
D. Ring: follows 180°	X	D. Ring, Ra, Cube, Cup: arms activate (*24w)	X	Ra, D. Ring: grasps near hand only
Ra: glances at, in hand	X	D. Ring, Ra: regards in hand	X	Ra: visual pursuit lost Ra (*24w)
Cube, Cup: regards, more than momentarily		D. Ring: to mouth		Cube: holds 1st regards 2nd
		D. Ring: free hand to midline (*28w)		M. Cubes: grasps 1 on contact (*24w)
		TT: looks down at TT or hands		
		Cube, Cup: looks from hand to object (*20w)		
		Pellet: regards		

Language

Vo: coos (*36w)
Vo: chuckles
So: vocal-social response
Su: predom, regards Ex.
Play: hand regard (*24w)
Play: pulls at dress (*24w)

Express: excites, breathes heavily, strains (*32w)
Vo: laughs aloud

Vo: squeals (*36w)

Personal-Social

So: spontaneous social smile
So: vocalizes or smiles, pulled to sit (*24w)
Feeding: anticipates on sight food
Play: sits propped 10-15 min. (*40w)
Play: hand play, mutual fingering (*24)
Play: pulls dress over face (*24w)

X X

So: smiles mirror image
Feeding: pats bottle (*36w)

FIG. 8-7. The Gesell Developmental Schedule for behavior ranging between 12 and 20 weeks.

24 Weeks			KEY AGE: 28 Weeks		32 Weeks
			Motor		
Su: lifts legs high in ext.			Su: lifts head (*40w)	X	Sit: 1min., erect, unsteady (*36w)
Su: rolls to prone			Sit: briefly, leans fwd. (on hands) (*32w)		St: maintains briefly, hands held (*36w)
P. Sit: lifts head, assists (*40w)	X X		Sit: erect momentarily		Pr: pivots (*40w)
Sit chair: trunk erect (*36w)	X X		St: large fraction of weight (*36w)		Pellet: radial raking (*36w)
Cube: grasps, palmarwise (*36w)			St: bounces actively (*32w)		Pellet: unsuccessful inferior scissors grasp (*36w)
Ra: retains			Cube: radial palmar grasp (*36w)		
			Pellet: rakes (whole hand), contacts (*32w)		
			Adaptive		
D. Ring, Ra, Cube, Bell: approaches & grasps			Ra, Bell: 1 hand approach & grasp		Cube: grasps 2nd cube
Ra: prehen, pursuit dropt Ra			M. Cubes: holds 1, grasps another		Cube: retains 2 as 3rd presented
Cube: regards 3rd cube immediately			Cube: holds 2 more than momentarily		Cube: holds 2 prolongedly
Cube, Bell: to mouth (*18m)			Bell: bangs (*40w)		Cup-cu: holds cube, regards cup
Cube: rescues dropt cube			Ra: shakes definitely		Ring-str: secures ring
M. Cubes: holds 1, approaches another			D. Ring, Cube: transfers		
			Bell: transfers adeptly		
			Bell: retains		

Language				
X	X	Bell-r: turns head to bell	Vo: m-m-m (crying) (*40w)	Vo: single syllable as da, ba, ka
X	X	Vo: grunts, growls (*36w)	Vo: polysyllabic vowel sounds (*36w)	
		Vo: spontan, vocal, social (incl. toys)		
Personal-Social				
X		So: discriminates strangers	Feeding: takes solids well	Play: bites, chews toys (*18m)
		Play: grasps foot (supine) (*36w)	Play: with feet to mouth (supine) (*36w)	Play: reaches persistently for toys out of reach (*40w)
		Play: sits propped 30 min. (*40w)	Mirror: reaches, pats image	Ring-str: persistent
		Mirror: smiles and vocalizes	Ring-str: fusses or abandons effort (*32w)	

FIG. 8-8. The Gesell Developmental Schedule for behavior ranging between 24 and 32 weeks.

The Denver Developmental Screening Test

The Denver Developmental Screening Test (the *DDST*) was developed to quickly detect gross dysfunction or developmental delay in the first six years of life in order to promote early therapy and thus improve the child's present performance and future prognosis.

As the name of the test implies it is a screening test which is intended as a quick tool for assessing the asymptomatic population to determine which subjects have the high probability of being significantly delayed in development. The test, therefore, differs from the Gesell Developmental Examination and many other tests, because the latter type of tests are intended as *diagnostic* tools to determine the exact developmental level of a particular child.[12]

Briefly, the original DDST evolved from a survey of twelve developmental tests and preschool intelligence tests from which 240 items were selected. These items met the criteria for the final test, which required minimum and relatively easy equipment for both the evaluator's administration and interpretation of the child's behavior. Through the process of administering the items, analyzing the results, and deleting those items which were not discriminatory or did not meet the criteria for testing, 105 test items were chosen and administered to a new sample of children — 1036 Denver children — and were standardized for the ages between two weeks and 6.4 years. The DDST might be described as *a formal or standardized means of organizing the informal observations of the therapist in the screening of gross delays or developmental dysfunction.*

The format of the Denver Developmental Test was devised to present all the normative data for the total sample...in a graphic manner so that the user can quickly compare an individual child's performance with that of the children on whom the items were standardized. Each item is represented by a horizontal bar placed along an age continuum. Various points on the bar represent the specific ages at which 25 percent, 50 percent, 75 percent, and 90 percent of the sample of children pass an item.[13]

The 1969 revised screening test form has each item arranged along the developmental continuum in one of four categories: personal-social, fine motor-adaptive, language and gross motor Figure 8-9).

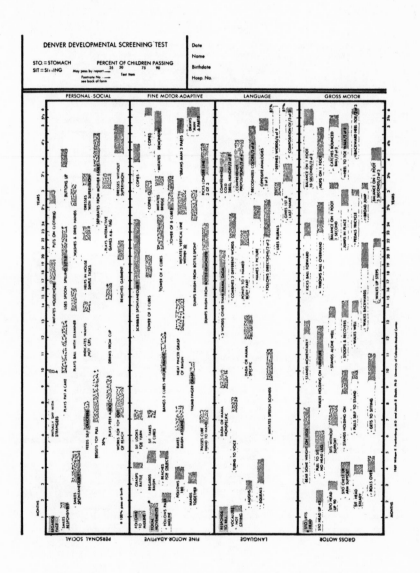

FIG. 8-9. Denver Developmental Screening Test.

1. Try to get child to smile by smiling, talking or waving to him. Do not touch him.
2. When child is playing with toy, pull it away from him. Pass if he resists.
3. Child does not have to be able to tie shoes or button in the back.
4. Move yarn slowly in an arc from one side to the other, about 6" above child's face. Pass if eyes follow 90° to midline. (Past midline; 180°)
5. Pass if child grasps rattle when it is touched to the backs or tips of fingers.
6. Pass if child continues to look where yarn disappeared or tries to see where it went. Yarn should be dropped quickly from sight from tester's hand without arm movement.
7. Pass if child picks up raisin with any part of thumb and a finger.
8. Pass if child picks up raisin with the ends of thumb and index finger using an over hand approach.

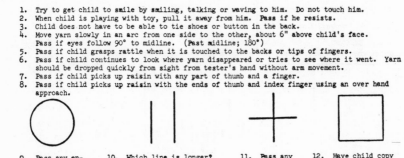

9. Pass any enclosed form. Fail continuous round motions.
10. Which line is longer? (Not bigger.) Turn paper upside down and repeat. (3/3 or 5/6)
11. Pass any crossing lines.
12. Have child copy first. If failed, demonstrate

When giving items 9, 11 and 12, do not name the forms. Do not demonstrate 9 and 11.

13. When scoring, each pair (2 arms, 2 legs, etc.) counts as one part.
14. Point to picture and have child name it. (No credit is given for sounds only.)

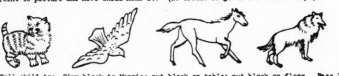

15. Tell child to: Give block to Mommie; put block on table; put block on floor. Pass 2 of 3. (Do not help child by pointing, moving head or eyes.)
16. Ask child: What do you do when you are cold? ..hungry? ..tired? Pass 2 of 3.
17. Tell child to: Put block on table; under table; in front of chair, behind chair. Pass 3 of 4. (Do not help child by pointing, moving head or eyes.)
18. Ask child: If fire is hot, ice is ?; Mother is a woman, Dad is a ?; a horse is big, a mouse is ?. Pass 2 of 3.
19. Ask child: What is a ball? ..lake? ..desk? ..house? ..banana? ..curtain? ..ceiling? ..hedge? ..pavement? Pass if defined in terms of use, shape, what it is made of or general category (such as banana is fruit, not just yellow). Pass 6 of 9.
20. Ask child: What is a spoon made of? ..a shoe made of? ..a door made of? (No other objects may be substituted.) Pass 3 of 3.
21. When placed on stomach, child lifts chest off table with support of forearms and/or hands.
22. When child is on back, grasp his hands and pull him to sitting. Pass if head does not hang back.
23. Child may use wall or rail only, not crawl. May not crawl.
24. Child must throw ball overhand 3 feet to within arm's reach of tester.
25. Child must perform standing broad jump over width of test sheet. (8-1/2 inches)
26. Tell child to walk forward, ⊂⊃⊂⊃⊂⊃⊂⊃→ heel within 1 inch of toe. Tester may demonstrate. Child must walk 4 consecutive steps, 2 out of 3 trials.
27. Bounce ball to child who should stand 3 feet away from tester. Child must catch ball with hands, not arms, 2 out of 3 trials.
28. Tell child to walk backward, ←⊂⊃⊂⊃⊂⊃⊂⊃ toe within 1 inch of heel. Tester may demonstrate. Child must walk 4 consecutive steps, 2 out of 3 trials.

DATE AND BEHAVIORAL OBSERVATIONS (how child feels at time of test, relation to tester, attention span, verbal behavior, self-confidence, etc,):

FIG. 8-10. Denver Developmental Screening Test—directions.

The results of the DDST are of very limited value for the occupational therapist without comments on the clinical or informal observations of the child's behavior as suggested on the bottom of the back of the test form (Figure 8-10). The general observations explain and expand the test report. As noted on the screening test, the behaviors described are those which can be visualized by the observer; for example: he *walks well, kicks the ball forward, buttons up* and *combines two different words.* These describe observable behavior; they do not describe the components or dynamics of the behavior required in order for the child to achieve the finished performance, and they do not permit any qualifying comments. The descriptions give the observable end products of a sequence of developmental events. It is the therapist's responsibility to interpret this material and thus to go beyond the observable behavior seen in the test. Frankenburg and Dodds do not require the examiner to perform this analysis; their objective was to identify children likely to have a developmental problem.

Frankenburg and Dodds have identified the primary reasons for which a child may not complete this test or others: (1) he may not have the basic competencies which are necessary for performance; (2) he may be unwilling to perform for dysfunctional or developmental reasons; (3) from the psychological standpoint of anxiety or annoyance at an interruption in his activity; or (4) from the physical basis of fatigue. The child may not be motivated toward performing all or part of the test. This may, in itself, be an indication of difficulty, since the child may have problems later in the performance of tasks which require internal motivation. All of these behaviors give evidence of emotional problems, which are important to the supplementary evaluations of the child.

The elements of easy administration, scoring, and interpretation have been noted by occupational therapists in their use of the test: it takes ten to twenty minutes to administer; the materials for the test are in a convenient kit, which simplifies the task of taking the test into a child's home or into another part of a clinic or hospital. The materials can be used for the age range of two weeks to 6.4 years. The test can be readily scored and interpreted at different points during the testing or at the end to permit the evaluator to repeat different sections of the test and to observe the demonstrated behavior more thoroughly. The child's developmental profile is compared with that of other children directly on the score sheet.

If the test is used to define the presence of a problem, as suggested by its authors, its value to the occupational therapist is necessarily limited, since most children are brought to the therapist because of a known problem. However, Frankenburg suggests that:

> ...the test has a useful place in the hands of an occupational therapist in terms of screening the overall development of a child. The use of the test in this way then would make it possible to identify areas in which the child may be suspect for being significantly delayed. Having identified these suspect areas the child should be further evaluated.[14]

If, for example, the child demonstrates a lag in fine motor-adaptive behavior, the possibility of perceptual-motor problems may be expected, and perceptual-motor tests might be used to further analyze the child's problem. The authors[13] stress the fact that this is not a diagnostic tool: it is a tool for assisting in the recognition of possible developmental problems which would need further investigation. It should be noted, too, that it is not an intelligence test, but a behavioral maturation evaluation, the purpose of which is to evaluate the strengths and weaknesses within the total behavioral complex at a particular time in the child's development. It is not a prognostic tool.

Some occupational therapists consider the DDST to be useful with multiply handicapped children, particularly if their handicaps are not extreme in the area of motor function. The test permits flexibility in timing; it is adaptable to various situations; and it can show a varied profile. This flexibility is needed because the multiply handicapped child is often not able to adapt his behavior to the highly structured test situation. Many of the evaluation observations of a handicapped child's behavior would be incorporated into the summary of the test results.

The DDST also might be a practical tool for determining the presence of developmental problems in every child admitted to a hospital, clinic, or handicapped children's preschool program. This procedure would not only provide the clinicians with guidelines for further observations of behaviors, but would make them quickly aware of outstanding problems for which the children should receive further diagnostic evaluation and specific treatment.

The description of retardation immediately illustrates the wide range of behavior and dysfunction found in a population of retarded children. There are multiple causes of retardation which result in varying syndromes, which may be apparent in both the child's appearance and his performance. Some children have a behavior profile which is consistently low in all areas. Other children show very erratic profiles. Some retarded children have physical characteristics which are symptomatic of a specific etiology, as in mongolism. In other children, it is difficult to diagnose the primary problem because of the absence of an observable syndrome. For example, the question may be asked: is a child emotionally disturbed because of his retardation or is he developmentally retarded as a result of emotional disturbance.

In spite of the varied diagnoses, evaluation and treatment methods usually remain consistent for retarded children unless contraindications, such as a severe cardiac condition, are apparent. Even then, the child is evaluated and treated within the constraints of the condition.

Problems of Retardation

The biggest problem for the family of the retarded child and the health care services is planning for the immediate and future care of the child. The family is involved emotionally and financially; friends and family may feel stigmatized by the retarded child. As a result, the family may reject the child and try to institutionalize him because they feel he will interfere with the normal routine of their lives.

The second problem area for the family is the financial requirement for medical care and institutionalization, if necessary, which becomes acute as the parents and child grow older. The parents must make arrangements for the child in case of death or inability to care for the child.

From the standpoint of the child and the state, the most desirable practice is to maintain the child in his own home as long as possible, for there he can gain the most developmentally from the family and environmental stimulation. This practice is based on studies done on institutionalized children. Studies done by Skeels, DuPan, and Fischer are a sample of the results commonly found in research on institutionalization.[18] The first conclusion is that children who are institutionalized regress severely when taken from the home environment, probably due to the lack of adult and sensorimotor stimulation. The more a child regresses, the more daily care he will require in areas such as eating, dressing and toileting (cost-benefit analysis would show that staffing an institution to be equivalent to the individual care given in the home would be exhorbitant.)

In addition, it seems reasonable to hypothesize that in comparing the normal child who is institutionalized with the retarded child who is institutionalized, the retarded child would lose his limited learning potential more rapidly than the normal child. The latter probably could make better use of his environment with less adequate stimuli and probably could regain many of his performance skills if placed in a favorable environment.

Treatment planning for the individual child from the results of the DDST is not appropriate, according to Frankenburg and Dodd's specifications for the test. They state that developmental delay or dysfunction cannot be judged accurately on the basis of a single discrepancy in performance, or on such a limited number of test items. This idea supports the need for supplementary observations during the evaluation: if a problem is recognized during the evaluation, the evaluator may expand his formal observations through further standardized testing to support the presence of the problem. For example,

> ...it would be inappropriate to plan a language stimulation program for a child who is delayed in the language sector without first having a complete speech and language and hearing evaluation. This is obvious since the child may have a hearing loss which may cause him to be delayed in language. Treatment for a hearing loss is obviously not confined to language therapy. In a similar way the use of the screening test would also make it possible to pinpoint areas of delayed development.[15]

Such delayed development may not be evident upon cursory informal observation of the child.

DEVELOPMENTAL RETARDATION

Definition

Developmental retardation is the disability area which most often requires the comprehensive developmental evaluation described in this chapter. The term *developmental retardation* refers to delayed development in more than one area of behavior — not just intellectual, motor or speech. It has been categorized into four areas for the President's Panel on Mental Retardation (Figure 8-11).[16] These terms were further defined in the *Massachusetts Plans for its Retarded* as follows:

Mild Retardation. I.Q. of 51-70. Development slow. Children capable of being educated ("educable") within limits. Adults, with training, can work in competitive employment. Able to live independent lives.

Level	Preschool Age 0-5, Maturation and Development	School Age 6-21, Training and Education	Adult 21 and over, Social and Vocational Adequacy
Profound	Gross retardation; minimal capacity for functioning in sensori-motor areas; needs nursing care.	Obvious delays in all areas of development; shows basic emotional responses; may respond to skillful training in use of legs, hands and jaws, needs close supervision.	May walk, need nursing care, have primitive speech; usually benefits from regular physical activity; incapable of self maintenance.
Severe	Marked delay in motor development; little or no communication skill; may respond to training in elementary self-help, e.g., self-feeding.	Usually walks barring specific disability; has some understanding of speech and some response; can profit from systematic habit training.	Can conform to daily routines and repetitive activities; needs continuing direction and supervision in protective environment.
Moderate	Noticeable delays in motor development, especially in speech; responds to training in various self-help activities.	Can learn simple communication, elementary health and safety habits, and simple manual skills; does not progress in functional reading or arithmetic.	Can perform simple tasks under sheltered conditions; participates in simple recreation; travels alone in familiar places; usually incapable of self maintenance.
Mild	Often not noticed as retarded by casual observer, but is slower to walk, feed self and talk than most children.	Can acquire practical skills and useful reading and arithmetic to a 3rd- to 6th-grade level with special education. Can be guided toward social conformity.	Can usually achieve social and vocational skills adequate to self maintenance; may need occasional guidance and support when under unusual social or economic stress.

FIG. 8-11. Retardation defined.

Moderate Retardation. I.Q. 36-50. Backward in their development, but able to learn to care for themselves. Children capable of being trained ("trainable"). Adults need to work and live in sheltered environment.

Severe Retardation. I.Q. of 20-35. Motor development, speech, language are retarded. Not completely dependent. Often, but not always, physically handicapped.

Profound Retardation. I.Q. of less than 20. Need constant care or supervision for survival. Gross impairment in physical coordination and sensory development. Often physically handicapped.[17]

The second conclusion is that children show severe developmental delay if placed in the institution in the early months of infancy, particularly in language and social behavior. Although the studies generally indicate that neuromotor abilities are not as delayed, personal experience suggests that the gross neuromotor behaviors of posture and lower extremity function follow this pattern, but that the refined neuromotor behavior of the upper extremity may be delayed. I question the effect of delay of the latter on auditory and visual-perceptual-motor behaviors, upon which much cognitive and language development depend. Increased developmental delay would decrease the child's immediate learning potential and, therefore, his potential for employment and productivity in adult years.

The third conclusion is that children can make marked gains in institutional settings with appropriate stimuli. Skeels substantiates this conclusion by showing that young children who were cared for by older retarded girls progressed developmentally; and DuPan found a similar result when the children were placed in small living units in which they received individual attention.

This information leads one to conclude that the best institutional setting would be that which most closely approximates the home: small units for small groups of children with a limited number of consistent adults; a routine program suited to meet the developmental needs of each child; experience with the community outside the institution; and training which would lead to productivity.

Occupational Therapy Evaluation

The therapist's evaluation of the child is developmental and emphasizes different areas of behavior, depending upon the division of professional responsibilities, the problems of a particular child, and the type of program in which the child is functioning on a daily basis. Generally, the developmental evaluation is done by the therapist with the routine follow-up treatment performed by the parents of the child, educators, COTA's or institution aides. However, special training of complex behaviors is usually performed by the therapist after the evaluation. The main objective of the evaluation is to determine the developmental profile of the child and, from that, to plan a highly specific training program which will extend and solidify the child's living experience.

Occupational Therapy Treatment

The therapist cannot treat every retarded child whom he tests because of the large number of these children — both in and out of institutions. In making the decision about which child to treat, questions such as the following may serve as guidelines: (1) How much will treatment benefit the child, both today and tomorrow, according to the cost-benefit analysis? (2) Who needs the help, the parents, the child or both? (3) Under what circumstances can the child learn best — a social group, work group, classroom, or an individual treatment session? (4) What person is best equipped to work with the particular problems of the child? (5) Does the child need only a maintenance program because he is progressing very slowly, or does he need a stimulating developmental program because he is making gradual gains?

A single statement cannot be made about the treatment responsibilities of the therapist, simply because the needs of each child vary. However, it seems appropriate for the therapist to (1) serve as consultant to families and institution staff on the children's developmental needs, (2) provide sensori-perceptual-motor experiences and (3) provide prevocational experiences. The first of these areas is self-explanatory, since it is based on the information presented in the previous chapters.

The second area is the stimulation of perceptual-motor behaviors — with emphasis on the development of motor proficiency. As noted in Figure 8-11, the moderate, severe, and profound retardates all have motor problems. Through the repetition of sequenced motor patterns at an increasingly rapid and efficient pace, the child develops motor control, which permits him to function more easily and effectively in his daily routine.

The third area in which the occupational therapist has a function is in the prevocational training of the retarded. This area utilizes all the child's developmental abilities in planned productivity to evaluate his potential for employment. The therapist uses his knowledge of development, behavior, and task requirements in a prevocational or work setting to serve as a link between school or social settings, and a work setting in which the child must meet specific standards for performance.

Kramer discusses three of the primary elements of the realistic work setting in terms of work adjustment, training, and evaluation. Each area has specific characteristics which can be evaluated by the therapist whether the child or adolescent is in an informal or formal work setting. Although he describes the setting for the teenage retardate, with some adaptations and more limited requirements, the setting can be made appropriate for children functioning at a lower developmental level, such as the names of tools for the child would be "paper" and "pencil" instead of "saw" or "hammer."

Basically, work adjustment attempts to develop a configuration in which an individual will learn proper work behavior and proper work attitude on a job working with others. The psychological dynamics for such development are complex but the basic goals should be simple, concrete, and realistic.

1. Learning to sit and work with other people
2. Knowing when to talk and when not to
3. Paying attention to a job
4. Developing familiarity with work situations
5. Achieving the ability to take orders and criticism
6. Learning how to ask for things
7. Developing punctuality
8. Using proper channels for requests

...A number of other benefits accrue during the work adjustment process which are as important to the worker but may not be directly work-related. These intangibles grow with any adjustment process. They include:

1. Increased social maturity
2. Pride in oneself through accomplishment
3. Greater self-sufficiency and independence in the home by being a productive worker
4. A feeling of being equal to or the same as normal siblings
5. Improved favorable relationships between the child and parents

The basic element of this process (training) is to develop in these youngsters the sense that they can be productive if given appropriate work. This is work training at its most basic level.

In achieving this goal, we use tools, our hands and ourselves. Our objectives are to teach:
1. The purpose and use of time cards
2. The names of tools
3. The use of tools, hand and power
4. Safe tools versus dangerous tools
5. Recognition of quality performance
6. Self-reliance in a job
7. Initiative and independence
8. Attention span
9. Proper precautions
10. Clean up and organization of work

The overlap of work training and work adjustment is fairly obvious since all these experiences are interrelated. Work training develops skills that form a pattern to mold the teenager into a worker. Every phase of work adjustment and work training is observed by the foreman and considered in the final evaluation.[19]

Kramer suggests that the written evaluation of the child be kept simple and be validated with specific observations of performance. The evaluation must explicitly describe the child's abilities for the individuals who will work with the child following his prevocational experience. Kramer's evaluation report includes:

1. Learning ability
2. Work habits
3. Work tolerance
4. Work quality
5. Hand use
6. Personality
7. Recreation
8. Summary
9. Impression [20]

Problems for the Therapist Who Works with the Retardate

Working with the retarded child requires patience. Because the child usually progresses very slowly and performs a single task repetitively, the immediate rewards for the therapist are minimal. As a result, the therapist must learn to adjust to the slow pace and develop his own patience.

In attempting to satisfy his own frustrations, the therapist may be inclined to push the child more rapidly than he is able to perform, which often results in failure for the child. If the child experiences chronic failure, emotional problems may become an additional burden to him. To alleviate this, the therapist rewards the child step by step — either with a tangible reward (as used in operant conditioning), or a preplanned success experience. This means that the therapeutic program must start at a very low level and proceed very gradually within the child's rate of ability to accomplish.

The discrepancy between the mental age, the size of the child's body and his drives may be very obvious. It is difficult initially for the adult to accept a child, the chronological size and age of seventeen, who behaves like a four-, seven- or ten-year-old. It can also be disconcerting to the adult when the child who is five feet, seven inches tall shows an affectionate response to him.

It is for these reasons that the therapist must assess the total development of the child. Only with an awareness of the child's profile can the therapist respond to the child at the appropriate developmental level and plan a stimulating developmental treatment program — rather than responding to his physical appearance, size, speech patterns, and so forth.

References

1. Ames, L.B. Personal communication, 1970.
2. Sharpe, B.J. "Developmental Appraisal—Perspectives and Procedures." In Fehr, M.J. (ed.) *Normal Growth and Development with Deviations in the Perceptual-Motor and Emotional Areas* (St. Louis, Mo.: Washington University School of Medicine, 1966), pp. 50-51.
3. Ames, L.B. "Predictive Value of Infant Behavior Examinations." In Hellmuth, J. (ed.) *Exceptional Infant—The Normal Infant: Volume I* (New York: Brunner-Mazel, 1967).
4. Gesell, A.L. and Amatruda, C.S. *Developmental Diagnosis* (New York: Paul B. Hoeber, 1941), pp. 115-116.
5. Ames, L.B., in Hellmuth, J. *Exceptional Infant—The Normal Infant,* p. 11.
6. Ames, L.B., in Hellmuth, J. *Exceptional Infant—The Normal Infant,* pp. 210-211.
7. Ames, L.B. "Individuality of Motor Development." In Fehr, M.J. (ed.) *Normal Growth and Development with Deviations in the Perceptual-Motor and Emotional Areas* (St. Louis, Mo.: Washington University School of Medicine, 1966), p. 45.
8. Ames, Personal communication, 1970.
9. Gesell, A.L. *Studies in Child Development* (New York: Harper and Row, 1948).

10. Gesell, A.L. *The First Five Years of Life* (New York: Harper and Row, 1940). Gesell, A.L. and Amatruda, C.S., 1941.
11. Gesell, A.L. and Amatruda, C.S., pp. 383-384.
12. Frankenburg, W.K. Personal communication, 1970.
13. Frankenburg, W.K. and Dodds, J.B. "The Denver Developmental Screening Test." *Journal of Pediatrics* 71:2 (1967), p. 183.
14. Frankenburg, W.K. Personal communication, 1970.
15. Frankenburg, W.K. Personal communication, 1970.
16. President's Panel on Mental Retardation. *Mental Retardation: A National Plan for a National Problem* (Chart Book) (Washington, D.C.: U.S. Government Printing Office, 1963), p. 15.
17. Massachusetts Mental Retardation Planning Project. *Massachusetts Plans for Its Retarded* (Boston: 1966), pp. 9-10.
18. Skells, H.M. "A Study of the Effects of Differential Stimulation on Mentally Retarded Children: A Followup Report." *American Journal of Mental Deficiency* 46 (1942), pp. 340-350; DuPan, R.M. and Roth, S. "The Psychologic Development of a Group of Children Brought Up in a Hospital Type Residential Nursery." *Journal of Pediatrics* 47 (1955), pp. 124-129; Fischer, L.K. "Hospitalism in Six-Month-Old Infants." *American Journal of Ortho-psychiatry* 22 (1952), pp. 522-533.
19. Kramer, J. "Work Adjustment, Training, and Evaluation for Teenage Retardates." In West, W.L. (ed.) *Occupational Therapy for the Multiply Handicapped Child* (Chicago: University of Illinois College of Medicine, 1965), pp. 258-259.
20. Kramer, J., p. 259.

Bibliography

Ames, L.B. and Ilg, F.L. "Search for Children Showing Academic Promise in a Predominantly Negro School." *Journal of Genetic Psychology* 110 (1967), pp. 217-231.

Currie, Catherine. "Evaluating Function of Mentally Retarded Children Through the Use of Toys and Play Activities." *American Journal of Occupational Therapy* 23 (1969), pp. 35-42.

Fenlason, J.T. "An Occupational Therapy Program for the Developmental Habilitation of Congenital Rubella Children." *American Journal of Occupational Therapy* 22 (1968), pp. 525-529.

Frankenburg, W.K. and Dodds, J.B. "The Denver Developmental Screening Test: Materials." Distributed by Ladoca Project and Publishing Foundation, East 51st Avenue and Lincoln Street, Denver, Colorado 80216.

Gesell, A.L. and Ilg, F.L. *The Child from Five to Ten* (New York:Harper and Row, 1946).

Gesell, A.L. and Ilg, F.L. *The Child from Five to Ten* (New York: Harper and Row, 1946).

434

Knobloch, H. and Pasamanick, B. "An Evaluation of the Consistency and Predictive Value of the 40-Week Gesell Developmental Schedule." In Shagass, C. and Pasamanick, B. (eds.) *Child Development and Child Psychiatry* (Washington, D.C.: American Psychiatric Association, 1960).

Koppitz, E.M. *The Bender Gestalt Test for Young Children* (New York: Grune and Stratton, 1964).

Perlmutter, S.A. "Developmental Appraisal—A Prelude to Treatment." In Fehr, M.J. (ed.) *Normal Growth and Development with Deviations in the Perceptual-Motor and Emotional Areas* (St. Louis, Mo.: Washington University School of Medicine, 1966).

Robinson, H.B. and Robinson, N.M. *The Mentally Retarded Child: A Psychological Approach* (New York: McGraw-Hill, 1965).

Ruess, A.L.; Dally, A.; and Lis, E.F. "The Gesell Developmental Schedules and the Physically Handicapped Child." *American Journal of Occupational Therapy* 13 (1959), pp. 117-124.

Stevens, H.A. and Heber, R. (eds.) *Mental Retardation* (Chicago: University of Chicago Press, 1964).

Terman, L.M. and Merrill, M.A. *Stanford-Binet Intelligence Scale: Manual for the Third Revision, Form L-M* (Boston: Houghton-Mifflin, 1960).

Wechsler, D. *Wechsler Intelligence Scale for Children* (New York: The Psychological Corporation, 1949).

Wright, S.W. and Tarjan, G. "Mental Retardation: A Review for Pediatricians." *American Journal of Diseases of Children* 105 (1963), pp. 511-526.

NOTES

NOTES

Chapter Nine

Illness and Disability:
Implications for the Child

Barbara Sharpe Banus, M.A., O.T.R.

(November 1970)

This chapter surveys the psychological problems which surround *illness or disability, location of treatment* and *people* involved in the treatment of the child. The etiology of psychological problems is seldom distinct because of the child's multiple and interacting responses to this triad. The complex interaction between the child and his environment is again evidenced (see Chapter One); however, the scope of the interaction is now telescoped into the child and the environment in which he finds himself when he is ill. The actual environment may not change for the child, but he may perceive it differently — the child may feel that his bedroom is different when he is sick and confined to bed, as compared to the time when he is well and able to romp around the room. The environment in which the child lives when he is sick or disabled is the environment in which the therapist usually functions and the one in which he encounters the child.

The responsibilities which are attributed to the therapist in this chapter are basic to good health care and are equally applicable to all health-care workers in pediatrics. The term "therapist" is used only for convenience — because the book has been written for occupational therapists.

VARIABLES WHICH COMPOUND
THE CHILD'S PSYCHOLOGICAL
PROBLEMS AND THEIR TREATMENT

The variables of illness, location of treatment, and the people involved in the child's life during his illness may cause psychological problems for any child depending upon (1) his developmental status, and (2) the implications of these variables for him. Most of the variables, such as the type of treatment procedures and the length of illness, are imposed upon the child with little or no possibility of his controlling them. These variables increase the child's dependence upon the adult, and may cause developmental delay or regression. The child cannot make the major decision, for example, about the medical or surgical procedures to be used in his treatment. He may be able to make some of the less critical choices, such as the kind of food he will eat or the room in which he will sleep. Frequently the child has more problems dealing with enforced dependence than the adult. The child often lacks a realistic understanding of what is occurring and the reasons for it. The preschooler, for example, may feel good at the time he is hospitalized for his tonsilectomy and may be unable to associate his past sore throats with the immediate separation from home and the unanticipated physical discomfort. In another situation, such as corrective surgery, there may be no obvious secondary symptoms with which the child can associate the reason for the surgery and the resulting discomfort. In addition, the child who is developing basic self-care behaviors and autonomy, such as the three-year-old who has recently learned to use the toilet, may become anxious if he is not permitted to practice these behaviors. The child who is put back into diapers for his medical condition or to simplify the nurses' work may feel that his parents will disapprove of his not using the toilet. The anxiety results from the conflict created by the hospital's requirements and the child's expectations of his parents' desires.

The complex interrelationships among the triad of variables and the individuality of each child makes it difficult to discriminate among the specific factors which are detrimental to an individual child. If a child is hospitalized, for example, he is probably receiving diagnostic or treatment procedures (or both) from a variety of hospital staff. It may be impossible to determine whether a three-year-old is crying because of the separation from mother and daddy, fear of the diagnostic procedures, possible discomfort caused by the disease, or a combination of all three factors. The possible stimuli which cause psychological upset are multiple, but some are common to most children. It is the effects of the stimuli which are child-specific.

The therapist explores the variables which may affect a specific child prior to making decisions about evaluation and treatment. Although he does not make the final decision about all treatment, he offers recommendations to the child care team which are drawn from his knowledge of therapy, child development, and the care of sick and disabled children. For example, in choosing the best location for the child's treatment, the therapist weighs the value of using the child's home, the neighborhood clinic, and the hospital. He may suggest that the child receive therapy at his home under the supervision of the therapist in the hospital outpatient clinic because (1) the parents can carry out treatment procedures under supervision, and (2) the child is only two years old and will have problems of separation in the hospital which could be psychologically detrimental to him—and, therefore, to the success of treatment.

The child's psychological problems are commonly relegated to treatment sessions with a psychologist, psychiatrist, social worker or, sometimes, an occupational therapist—in conjunction with the parents' group therapy or counseling. This procedure may not resolve the problems for the parents or for the child. Often nurses or other service personnel are in the environment which causes the problem and are therefore in the ideal position to help the child deal with his fears concerning the medical and surgical procedures. Formal therapy sessions may help the child to better cope with his disability, but seldom dispel all of his anxieties and concerns about immediate problems. Psychological problems, such as fears of medical staff, interfere with functional treatment, such as perceptual-motor training. The therapist must be prepared to handle the psychological difficulties of the child before implementing the functional treatment if he wants the therapy session to be successful.

The concept of the occupational therapist who provides a kind of psychotherapy for all patients is somewhat different from the historical perspective of the pediatric occupational therapist whose work was described as *diversional* or *supportive.* The term, *"diversional,"* is contradictory to the goals of occupational therapy; the term, *"supportive,"* is too superficial to describe the benefits derived from occupational therapy.

Diversional therapy, in its most apparent definition, means to avoid the confrontation of a problem by ignoring the existence of the problem, or by redirecting the child's attention toward more pleasant situations to "get his mind off the problem." This procedure is contradictory to *therapy,* which includes the concept of helping the person change behavior in a healthy or positive and permanent direction, through the *resolution* of the problem.

The child must look at his problems directly or indirectly. Direct confrontation of a problem is appropriate when a child storms into the treatment room and throws furniture or tools regardless of the danger to himself, other children, or the therapist. The therapist must intervene and confront the child with his behavior. If the therapist asks questions concerning the reasons for the behaviors, he may not get a direct answer; but the child is given the opportunity to explain and to regain control of his own behavior. If the child can regain control, this approach is more beneficial for him than the response of, "Okay, let's sit down at the table and do our work for today" (diversional procedure). If the child has totally lost control, the behavior is stopped and, at a later time, the therapist explores the cause of the problem with the child in an effort to resolve it. If the etiology is not explored, this behavior may snowball and expand to other areas of the child's environment and the problem will not be solved. Most likely the child is acting out because he needs assistance.

The occupational therapist may need to focus on the problem indirectly, as can be seen in his approach to a child who was scheduled for open heart surgery (see Chapter Five for a description of play therapy). The therapist was asked by the nurse to take David, a restless ten-year-old boy, to occupational therapy "to play with something and get his mind off surgery" for he was obviously anxious about the surgery to be performed that afternoon. In occupational therapy, David was given a choice of several symbolic materials through which it was hoped he would express some of his anxieties about the coming surgery — it was known that the boy would not verbally discuss his fears. David chose a pencil and drawing paper and immediately began drawing a picture which he described as a battle between the Germans and the Americans in World War II. While drawing the picture, David told the therapist about several episodes of injury, some of which he had experienced, such as falling from a fence and getting stitches, and some of which his friends had experienced. Interspersed with these stories were comments about his previous cardiac catheterization and the behaviors displayed by the doctors and nurses—including those of a doctor who became very angry with the nurse. It was pointed out to David that the doctor might have been upset because he wanted the catheterization to proceed perfectly so he would not hurt the boy, one of the few and brief comments made by the therapist, who primarily asked questions to encourage David to talk. About twenty minutes later David said, "I'm finished"—to which the therapist replied, "Who won the battle?" David picked up his paper and pencil, replied, "The Americans"—and walked out of the treatment room. Apparently, through this period David had a chance to work through many of his feelings concerning the coming surgery, and came to some resolution of the problems emotionally, at least to the point of his being able to cope with the immediate situation without anxiously pacing the halls of the ward, as he had done prior to therapy.

This was not diversional therapy. It focused directly on the child's immediate problem, even though the therapist discussed the surgery with David only indirectly through the exploration of his past experiences with doctors. The validation of the need for only this single session with the therapist was illustrated in the sequel to the episode after David's surgery. He never approached or talked with the occupational therapist again, although he acknowledged her once very briefly when she said "hello" to him. It was apparent that he had a very specific need of her assistance in helping him to cope at a critical time. Once this need was met, she was no longer necessary to his rehabilitation.

The term *supportive therapy* can be defined as the superficial prophylactic measures which are used to prevent regressive behavior patterns. It connotes the use of developmentally appropriate objects by the child for the maintenance of his present function. Sick children do need normal developmental experiences, but do not need these experiences provided by the highly trained occupational therapist. The materials for the normal developmental play experiences can be provided by volunteers or "playladies" under the guidance of those who know child development.

In the past it was assumed that the objects were the most important aspect of the treatment and that with only a brief and superficial contact (five to ten minutes daily) from the therapist, the child would interact successfully with the nonhuman object for several hours. Supportive occupational therapy in pediatrics was originally merely taking the cart of toys from bedside to bedside. From this cart the child chose his toy for that day and the therapist briefly gave him directions for its use before going on to the next child. Another aspect of supportive therapy was the supervision of a playroom full of children by the therapist. This was not a planned grouping to meet specific needs of each child, but a place for all children to recreate.

The objective of the occupational therapist is to help the child cope with his illness, not to entertain him momentarily. Within this context I believe that children must have satisfying interpersonal communication before they are able to constructively make use of their environment or of the objects within it. If the therapist talks with and listens to the child's expression of his concerns (his illness or absence from school), and satisfies the child's social and emotional needs, the child then may be able to concentrate on play, through which he can further explore and release his feelings. In addition, the therapist may help the child find ways to meet other concerns, such as using the telephone to call his parents or friends. Without an interpersonal commitment between therapist and child, the child cannot develop a lasting interest in the object, which substitutes for human communication. (A parallel situation is the college student's inability to concentrate on his studies until he has sat down with a friend or roommate, talked about and at least temporarily resolved a pressing problem.)

In other words, this chapter is concerned with *the prevention of psychological problems which children often develop unnecessarily—because of the professional person's ignorance of the psychological effects of the triad of illness, hospitalization and people on the child.* Some of the primary psychological problems with which the handicapped child must cope are described in this chapter, and both general and specific suggestions are given for the amelioration of the problems. Some of the situations which require coping are obviously relevant to the occupational therapist's work with the child; others may not appear to be relevant. However, the therapist must be aware of potential problems and of the most effective and commonly used means of coping with them so that he, the therapist, can work in accord with other members of the child care team to prevent psychological pathology from developing.

THE RELATIONSHIP OF DEVELOPMENT TO ILLNESS

Not all children of the same developmental age are affected to the same intensity by apparently identical stimuli because of the variables of the child's development, the range of his experience and his environment. Two children may have identical illnesses at the same age. But, because of the *extrinsic factors* of different homes and families, different hospital environments, different treatment procedures, different handling by the medical personnel and the *intrinsic factors* of maturation and growth, these children may show very different responses. Thus, the developmental elements which may affect any one child at any one time are a primary variable and are investigated first.

Three concepts concerning illness and development seem to be most significant. First, the child's ability to cope with illness, dysfunction, treatment, and so forth, is a function of his immediate developmental status and ongoing progress — the older the child is, the greater is his capacity to understand the facts and implications of evaluation and treatment. Second, during acute and sometimes chronic illness, a child regresses to those behaviors which are most comforting to him. Third, if the maturation and growth of the behaviors which are in the forefront during a particular phase of development are inhibited, the child may become excessively anxious.

The significance of the first concept, *the child's developmental status,* is primarily associated with his cognitive and language development, which in turn are both affected by his emotional status. The problems of communication become acutely obvious to the adult when the toddler tries to express his needs through jargon and vocabulary which are understood only by his parents. Not only is the toddler unable to express himself adequately, but he cannot understand much of the conversation around him. As the child develops more cognitive and communicative skills, he may understand a few more words, but may not hear or may not understand the total context in which they are used. As a child hears conversation around him, for example, he may hear and understand the word *die* but he may not actually hear the rest of the conversation—or he may emotionally block out the other words. Through fantasy or projection he may think that the people are talking about him, rather than hear that "Tom would *die* laughing if he heard that joke."

Lack of comprehension increases the young child's anxiety, because he does not know when or if his illness or disability will terminate—nor what will happen from moment to moment. The preschool child has negligible concepts of time to give him cues.

He cannot understand that there will be surgery *tomorrow* or a blood test in *thirty minutes*. In response to the preschool child's confusion between reality and his own personal needs and desires, wishful thinking is more prevalent than in school-age children. "My mommy and daddy are coming to live here with me," says the hospitalized four-year-old who wants his mommy and daddy to stay with him.

The second significant concept in the treatment of ill or disabled children is that of *regression*: the younger the child is developmentally, the more rapid is the process of regression. In children of all ages, the habits which have been learned most recently and the social competencies usually diminish first. The child of less than five-years-of-age may show the most rapid regression because he has acquired the basic behaviors — walking, talking, self-dressing — more recently than the school-age child.

Regression in developmental tasks is often the result of forced decreased practice of the skill. The child who is put into a hospital gown and slippers may quickly lose the ability to button the back of a blouse or tie shoes if these skills have been learned recently.

Social competence may regress to the infantile stage, or to the primitive stage of maximum dependence, in which the child seeks food and affection from the parent or parent surrogate. These behaviors may be seen in the eight-year-old boy who wants to be cuddled or the eleven-year-old boy who sobs loudly in pain. These boys would not permit themselves to demonstrate these "babyish" behaviors if they were healthy!

If the illness is temporary and if the child's pre-illness behavior was mature, the regressive behaviors probably will be transitory and serve only as an expression of an immediate need. However, if the child has been immature or insecure prior to the illness, enforced dependency may result in the maintenance of the comfortable immature patterns.[1] As the child regains health, he may whimper when he cannot have his own way in games with peers, he may demand special food or toys, he may cling to mommy and refuse to be separated from her.

The third concept concerns the *focal points* of a developmental stage, and the anxiety which the child develops when he is unable to practice the behaviors which are foremost in his present repertoire. The second concept dealt with the enforced *regressive* patterns which occur from decreased usage; this concept is concerned with the *anxiety* created by the inhibition of growth and maturation.

Both positive and negative developmental and personality characteristics may become reinforced and strengthened during illness. The toddler who already shows negative behavior may become increasingly negative as he becomes more restricted, frustrated, and fearful. This may be his only way of drawing attention to the anxiety he feels — he is indirectly asking for help. The nine-year-old girl who is shy and a "loner" may become very withdrawn, refuse to interact with other children on the hospital ward, or placidly remain in bed. The adolescent girl who is concerned with her physical appearance may spend hours preparing herself for the visit of a boy friend.

If the child is frustrated in his attempt to mature, he may demonstrate a wide range of maladaptive behaviors, some of which may be blatant, others subtle. If the behavior is recognized as an extreme expression of a developmental stage, the child is permitted to maintain the expression (adolescent girl), or is redirected into adaptive patterns (toddler).

Children of identical developmental ages, but of discrepant chronological ages, have different needs. The problems of a child who is developmentally two years old, but who is chronologically four years old, may differ considerably from those of the child who is both chronologically and developmentally two years old. The primary difference between these two children is in their ability to learn, which is critical during an extensive illness or hospitalization. The retarded child, for example, might adapt at a different rate and in a different way from that of the normal child. This implies the need for the therapist to know the developmental ages of all the children with whom he works.

MAXIMIZING THE DEVELOPMENTAL POTENTIAL

The therapist has the responsibility of eliciting the maximum healthy response from the child. To do this he makes specific demands, of the child and of himself. If the chronological and observed developmental behaviors are congruent, the therapist's task is to help the child maintain his present level of performance and to help the child develop further. Treatment objectives for the child and the process of implementing them should be in accord with the values and practice already established in the child's home—if they are healthy and beneficial for the child and his family. The therapist expects the child to perform tasks appropriate to his developmental age — self-dressing, self-feeding and helping in the housekeeping tasks which are similar to those he performs at home — if he is able to do so. The child is encouraged to explore new behaviors — cognitively, socially, motorically and so forth.

To incorporate developmental experiences into all spheres of treatment, the therapist must be aware of the general developmental needs for all children as well as the specific needs of the individual child—for example, the need of all two-year-olds for mastery of the environment, and the accentuated need for mastery of a particular two-year-old who is restricted to bedrest. The number of variables which lead to a child's psychological upset are reduced each time a child's developmental need is met. Sometimes this is a simple procedure. For example, instead of establishing one bedtime for all children on a ward, appropriate bedtime hours can be established for each child according to his past experience, his age and his immediate health and sleep requirements. The children may complain just as they do at home when they feel their siblings are receiving more just regulations. But it is part of the hospital staff's responsibility to decrease the discrepancy between health and illness and home and hospital and they must cope with these normal developmental frustrations.

Frequently, it is impossible to meet all the developmental needs of the child, particularly in the acute stage of his illness when diagnostic procedures and experimental treatments are being given. If a two-year-old, for example, is restrained for an intravenous feeding, he cannot be permitted to walk because he does not understand that he must move slowly. (School-age children sometimes are allowed to push a stand with their intravenous equipment attached to it while they walk around the ward.) Instead of stimulating the motor behavior of the two-year-old, the therapist may provide stimulation for the other developing behaviors, such as language or visual-perceptual-motor patterns. In order for this therapy to be successful, the task must be correlated with the child's needs.

If the child has regressed severely before the therapist begins to work with him, the therapist may need to begin at the primitive stage of emotional-social behavior and gradually wean the child from extreme dependence. In this situation the therapist is initially the therapeutic agent from which the child gains satisfaction. Gradually, objects which are appropriate to the child's usual developmental behavior are inserted into the dyadic relationship. This procedure balances the child's immediate needs for the human relationship with his known or anticipated developmental potential in multibehavioral areas. For example, the therapist might give a twelve-month-old two or three two-inch-block rattles, but he would give a four-year-old (temporarily behaving emotionally as a twelve-month-old child) more complex stimuli, such as a small dump truck and four blocks. The therapist permits the child to use the objects at the performance level of immediate capability, while at the same time he subtly encourages him to regain his potential developmental level. Children often seem to maintain their depressed or regressive behaviors because the adults do not choose the appropriate human or object stimuli, and do not, therefore, motivate the children to respond appropriately. Because the child may be physically or verbally incapable of obtaining his wants — often because he does not know his needs — he remains dependent upon the often unknowledgeable decisions of adults.

Communication is one of the biggest problems for children. Facilitating communication with children is one of the therapist's primary responsibilities. In conversing with the child, verbal explanations are made at the child's level of understanding, as described by Ginot's "childrenese" (see Chapter Five). This is particularly important in communicating with preschool children. In addition to talking casually with the child during therapy, the therapist may need to help the child separate fantasy from reality. For example, a four-year-old says to the therapist, "I'm going home today," because he wants to go home today. To help the child think realistically, the therapist replies, "You are going home but *not* today."

This communication is not treatment of the child's diagnosed disability; but it is psychological treatment, since it clarifies misconceptions which could be psychologically detrimental to the child. This is an expected developmental problem which needs to be corrected immediately and honestly by the adult — it is not the pathological problem of a mentally ill child. This same example also illustrates an explanation which is at the child's level of understanding, and one which is simple enough to prevent his becoming further confused.

Adults discuss *only* that information which they want the child to hear when conversing in the presence of the child, and then they talk directly with him. This care avoids misunderstandings similar to those described in the child's interpretation of the word *die.* The thought, "He won't understand anyway, so we can discuss it here," is misleading. Children recognize individual words, especially if they have heard the words used previously in relation to themselves. They are aware of tones of voices, facial expressions and gestures. And they misinterpret words that sound similar to other words which they recognize. All technical conversations are held out of the child's presence unless he is to be included in the discussion. When it is desirable for the child to be included, he is encouraged to ask questions concerning the words and ideas he does not understand.

Communication also includes the recording of developmental information from the parents, for the edification of all child care workers, in order to ensure their consistent and meaningful communication with the child. His words for specific needs — the *toilet, water, favorite toys* and *I want to get up* — his prebedtime routine, and his food likes and dislikes help the staff respond to the child's needs if he is to be hospitalized. Although a therapist or other personnel may not agree with the parents' means of communication with the child or the handling of the child's routine, they must respect it and conform to it unless the treatment objective is to change the child's language or routine behaviors.

ILLNESS AND DYSFUNCTION

Problems directly related to illness and dysfunction might be categorized into four units: the onset of the illness; the type of illness or dysfunction; the type of diagnostic and treatment procedures; and the prognosis of the illness. A distinction must be made between illness and disability. *Illness* is sickness or unhealthiness which may be temporary or chronic. It may produce a disability, such as spinal meningitis which may produce hemiplegia. It may be physical or emotional. A *disability* is a handicapping condition which does not necessarily affect the health of an individual. For example, a child with an amputated arm is disabled in the use of that arm, but may be physically and mentally healthy.

The Onset of Illness or Disability

The onset of illness or disability may be *traumatic,* (a car accident, for example, in which the child is injured); *gradual and progressive* (muscular dystrophy or arthritis); or *congenital* (cerebral palsy, congenital amputation or mental regardation). The degree of stress experienced by the child is partly dependent upon the child's readiness for the changes which affect him physically and the effect of these changes on his developmental abilities. Illness which occurs traumatically (pneumonia or leukemia), preventing psychological or physical preparation, may create more long-range psychological problems for the child than disability for which the child has been prepared, such as the physical limitations which result after elective surgery. Physical and psychological stress may be extensive if the child has painful exacerbations or constant discomfort during the illness; if the physical discomfort is minimal, the child may be able to function comfortably even though the disease may be progressive.

Each child has different explanations for his illness or disability which are based on his past experience, and on his family's experience and beliefs about illness and disability. However, a common assumption of children is that they are being punished for bad behavior or for disobeying their parents.[2] It is a cause and effect relationship: "I didn't wear my coat so I caught cold"; "I ate too much candy so I have diabetes"; or "I climbed a fence I was told not to climb so I have a bad leg." Children readily make these associations with the assistance of their parents' warnings, "If you don't do this, this and this will happen...." After an illness does occur, in spite of the realistic absence of any correlation with these warnings, both the parents and the child, in their guilt and fear, may respond to the often repeated slogan, "I told you so."

The degree to which the child (1) fantasizes about the etiology of his handicap, (2) understands the implications of his disability, and (3) accepts the handicap, affects his ability to deal with it constructively. For example, a child can see and feel his broken arm and understand that he must be careful of it; but the child is less able to understand a disease such as rheumatic fever, which requires bedrest or minimal activity even though he may feel fine physically.

Children with congenital disabilities have some problems which differ from the problems of traumatically handicapped children. Although the child with a congenital disability may have feelings of anger toward the constraints of his handicap, he may realistically understand that "it won't go away." His psychological stress probably would develop from the frustration he experiences in not being able to perform "like the other kids" or from the difficulties he experiences in adapting to his physical limitations. Initially, the congenitally disabled child knows only how he feels and the behaviors he can perform; he does not compare his body image or developmental abilities with other children. The congenital amputee, blind child or cerebral palsied child knows his limits and may live comfortably within the confines of his disability until he begins to compare himself with others, or until he has the desire to perform a specific developmental task and finds that he is unable to do so. Cognitively he may understand the concept of feeding himself, but due to a neuromotor handicap he may be physically inept in holding a spoon or cup and in bringing the food to his mouth. The child's problems of self-acceptance begin during the early social contacts of the preschool years, as he watches normal children of his size and sees their accomplishments. At this time it may become difficult for the handicapped child to develop social relationships, particularly if he has problems in communication or motor function.

The Type of Illness or Disability

Each type of illness or disability has specific characteristics which psychologically affect children in some identifiable ways.

Anna Freud, Langford, Blom and Prugh, among others, have ennumerated some of these disabilities.[3] Some of the characteristics are experienced only by the child, others are evident to the casual observer. Frequently, it is the characteristics which are evident which create the most problems for the child both socially and emotionally. For example, the child with residual affects from rheumatic fever may be required to limit his physical activity. This handicap is not readily observable to other children, however, and therefore is not as susceptible to ridicule as a disability such as cerebral palsy.

Disfigurement

The degree of disfigurement is prominent in the child's acceptance of himself and in others' acceptance of him. Richardson describes a unit of research which he and his colleagues performed in order to determine how handicapped and nonhandicapped children perceive other handicapped and nonhandicapped children, and to determine whether children really have the values about disability which adults assume they have.[4] To determine the normal child's perception of handicapped children, a sample of individual children were given six pictures of the same child (for the boys the picture was a boy, and for the girls it was a girl), each of which illustrated a different handicap. The child named or pointed to the picture of the child which he liked the best in response to the question, "Which boy (girl) do you like the best?" Each time the child pointed to a picture, that one was removed, and the child was given the same choice with the remaining pictures until there were none left. The results of the experiment showed that the nonhandicapped child was best liked and most frequently chosen first. The remaining order of preference for the children was (2) the child with braces and crutches, (3) the child in a wheelchair, (4) the child with an amputation at the elbow, (5) the child with minimal facial disfigurement, and (6) the obese child. It is interesting to note that obesity — which is relatively common — is least liked by children, although it is not generally described as a disease.

It should be noted that this study contained only static pictures of children instead of real children who might have demonstrated some of the weird motor patterns of severe neuromotor dysfunctions. If the grouping was changed to more severely distorted children, the results might be very different. However, the implications of this study are very relevant to the therapist's planning of individual and group treatment for children with visible handicaps.

Another aspect of the problem of disfigurement is the reaction of the child whose total body image changes as a result of traumatic injury. It is very difficult for this child to accept the radical change in his body from that which was healthy and active to that which is crippled — people now stare at him, which constantly reminds him of the disfigurement. The main problem resulting from extreme disfigurement is the psychological affect on the child and the family. This requires more extensive rehabilitation for parents, child and possibly siblings than the surgical-medical repair itself.[5]

One of the greatest problems for the disabled person is society's reaction to him. Although the kind and degree of disfigurement varies with each disability and with each child, even the most subtle may be observable. An example of this is the child with a heart defect (blue baby), who as a child must rest periodically and who does so in a squatting position. Although this is subtle, other children do notice the odd behavior and may respond negatively to his "always sitting down" and "the funny color of his lips and fingers."

Wright has discussed several of the possible reactions to disabled children and adults.[6] Among these are pity, teasing, curiosity and embarrassment. *Pity,* as Wright defines it, causes a status-conscious relationship in which the nonhandicapped person looks down upon the handicapped person and automatically assumes that the handicapped person is incapable or incompetent in one or more areas of behavior. The reaction of the pitying person may be over-helpfulness toward the disabled child—both attitudinally: "Oh, you poor thing!" and functionally: "Let me carry you," or "Let me feed you." These comments frequently are spoken as though the child were an infant or toddler; because the child cannot walk as fast as another eight-year-old, it is automatically assumed that he cannot think on the level of an eight-year-old. The pitying behaviors of the adult conflict with the child's primary goal of developmental independence. If physical assistance is needed, the adult's behavior is useful; if not, it increases the child's feelings of inadequacy through demanding his dependence.

Teasing or *taunting* is most frequently directed at children who are "different," and therefore not easily understood. It is an earthy and unsophisticated response used by the children who are themselves insecure; it makes the taunter feel superior to the child who does not have the strength to fight back. This behavior can be emotionally and socially destructive to the disabled child who is teasingly assaulted by a group of children without a means of coping with it.

Both adults and children stare at and ask questions of disfigured children to satisfy their _curiosity._ Children may do this (to both adults and other children) without realizing that the other person may be very sensitive to his disfigurement. On the other hand, children can be sensitive to and supportive of the handicapped child when they become aware of his feelings. As with most new experiences, the young child needs some guidance in handling his reactions. If this guidance is positive, he can be an asset to the handicapped child's emotional and social development.

The adults and children who do not perceive the person behind the handicap as a person with the same needs as all people, usually focus on the handicap and may show _embarrassment_ in the presence of a handicapped person. This limitation is primarily true of adults, but can be true of adolescents who are very concerned about the group's reaction to themselves and their friends. Thus in the early years, when values and opinions are malleable, it is beneficial for all children to have some contact with handicapped children.

The handicapped child may cope with the hurtful behaviors in any of several ways — some of which may be constructive, others destructive. The success of his dealings with other people depends upon his acceptance of the disability: if he has a good self-image and feels worthwhile, he can deal with the negative behaviors of others. However, if he perceives himself as being unworthy, ugly or bad, the negative reactions of others may reinforce his thinking and he may not be able to deal constructively with them.

Nonconstructive ways of coping, which include increased dependency on family and withdrawal from other children, are taken on by the young child who does not know how to respond effectively. Older children and adolescents may ignore their disability as though to say, "There's nothing wrong with me; treat me like the rest of the kids." Or they may joke about it to make themselves and others feel at ease; or they may express their anger directly or covertly through sarcasm. If the child or adolescent is forced into a conversation about himself, he may change the subject abruptly or answer curtly and briefly. Meaningful discussions about the problems of disfigurement are not legitimately expected among casual acquaintances, but are expected within the child's family or with understanding friends.

It can be expected that all children and adolescents use one or more of these ineffective coping devices at some time during the process of learning to cope effectively with society. They may be described as _ineffective_ because these coping devices do not help the hurt feelings of the disabled; nor do they resolve the constant problem of communication between the nondisabled and handicapped populations.

Coping with Disfigurement

There are many ways to assist the disabled child in coping with his handicap and the society around him. Let it be assumed that no one outside the child's immediate family and his medical team knows how to interact appropriately with the child. And, because one therapist cannot teach all of the society how to assist the child, one must teach the child how to handle people. Parents and friends will not be available throughout the child's life to cushion all his bad experiences.

First, the therapist is a model adult in demonstrating his healthy concern for and understanding of the child. The child must trust the therapist before he will begin to learn the desirable attitudes and behaviors from him. Before the child learns specific behaviors, he must learn that his attitude toward the people with whom he is interacting can alienate or befriend them. If he asks the right question, but states it in an angry or sullen manner, he may not receive the desired response; the expression of his attitude, therefore, directly reflects his own feelings of self-value. By providing the child with practical ways for dealing with the public before he is unexpectedly confronted, the child's behavior automatically will improve because he will be prepared to handle people.

The therapist gives the child ways to describe his dysfunction or disfigurement to other children and to adults. These descriptions should be developmentally appropriate to the child's understanding, so that he knows what he is saying and is not parroting the adult's definition. The five-year-old with an upper extremity amputation might be encouraged to reply simply that he has a "different hand" called a "prosthesis"—with which "I can write, play games, ride a bicycle, and do other things."

Help the child learn to recognize the times when he realistically needs to seek help and when he can function independently. Explain to him that it is alright for him to say, "No, thank you" in a matter-of-fact but sincere way to the person who offers unnecessary assistance. He may also need support in understanding that it is acceptable for him to perform tasks more slowly than other children — that he should ask for or accept additional time when it is provided for him, such as when eating meals at school. He needs to learn which tasks, tools or physical facilities must be adapted for him — he may need a different size or type of chair to use at the table with the other children, and he may need his paper taped to the table.

Encourage the child to do all the activities which are within his developmental and functional range of behaviors. These include eating, dressing, studying, playing, and working. Inability to participate is based only on the realistic limits in his performance, not on the expectations of other children: "He can't play ball; he has only one leg." If potential performance is unknown, it should be tried experimentally unless contraindicated medically.

Wright suggests that a child should not be exposed to taunting or ridicule in the early years because the child is too young to handle it; because the child is vulnerable and unsure of himself, doubts about himself are easily learned and reinforced.[7] The limited child is inclined to agree with the taunter (bully) that he is stupid or ugly.

To give the child opportunities to practice important social behaviors, he may be taken on excursions during which he will have contact with unknown adults and children while still being supported by the therapist. Appropriate places might include a children's playground, supermarket, park or recreational area, and the library. Because the therapist and child have explored possible negative situations which the child might encounter on the excursions before the actual trip, the therapist tries to let the child handle new situations with people. The therapist intervenes in conversations or situations only if the child has difficulty in coping with the other people. Then he must support the child and later talk with the child and explore healthier ways for handling the uncomfortable situation.

The most effective way for a child to learn to cope with the reactions of other children is for him to participate in a group. Ideally, this group participation begins in the preschool years—as it does for any child (in the case of handicapped children, some consideration is given to the developmental age in addition to the chronological age). This is important because handicapped children often are more dependent on their parents than are healthy children. Handicapped children often have less opportunity for social interaction with children, other than their siblings, than do nonhandicapped children.

If disfigurement and dysfunction are minimal, the child can be directly introduced into a normal preschool group. However, if the child has moderate to severe involvement, preschool programs for children with handicapping conditions are preferable. Once the child has the preschool experience, he is sent to the most appropriate school program, which might be one of several alternatives: kindergarten, special education classes in a public school, a school for handicapped children, or day care centers. The preschool might be described as a long-term evaluation center in which the child learns the basic self-care skills and has the opportunity to develop his potential in a stimulating, planned environment. Preferably before going from a handicapped children's preschool program into a regular school program, the child will participate in a preschool with nonhandicapped children, so that he will have the opportunity to learn when he can or cannot interact in their activities successfully, and to experience their attitudes toward him while still in the protected environment.

A procedure for integrating the handicapped child into a group of children is described as follows. Ideally, a staff member who works with the children visits the child in his own home to evaluate the child's assets and liabilities, and to introduce himself to the child. After this introduction (or in place of it), the child and mother visit the classroom when the children are not present so that he can become acquainted with the facility. This visit is recommended to prevent the child's being overwhelmed by the group of active children and developing a fear of the new environment. At the same time the child discovers the materials which he enjoys, and those to which he can retreat if the classroom does become too active for him.

If the children in the class cognitively function at about an age of five years or more, they are told about the new handicapped child before he joins them. In this way they are prepared for him and probably will be more sensitive to his needs than if they are not prepared. The parent preferably (or the therapist or teacher who knows him best) describes his own child. The description includes the name, a brief description of the handicap and the identification of things the child can do (this procedure illustrates how the child is like them, so that they can identify with him and interact in these areas), and the things he cannot do (which shows the children his limits so that they do not make unreasonable demands of him). Knowing these facts, both the teacher and children can make some reasonable adaptations in the classroom activity to make participation possible for the handicapped child. Realistically, the whole class is not expected to change its routine just to meet the handicapped child's needs — this would not be useful to the child, because he must learn to function in a society which cannot change totally for his benefit.

Some members of the group may reject the disabled child because of their feelings of discomfort and may show one of the behaviors described previously. If the handicapped child is being ignored, the therapist or teacher can choose a respected member of the group (often the leader) and encourage him to assist and interact with the disabled child. The leader may need some suggestions on how to do this, but probably has the initiative and openness to interact easily once he begins. Once the interaction is initiated, other children may imitate the leader and play with the handicapped child.

The Type of Diagnostic and Treatment Procedures

Some diagnostic and treatment procedures may produce the secondary effects of pain, isolation, restraint, or restriction. Each of these characteristics has different meanings for each child, based on the degree of their imposition, the length of time they are required, and the development of the child.

Pain

Some diagnostic and treatment procedures elicit pain which cannot be alleviated; the child must, therefore, have assistance in coping with them. One question arises concerning the etiology of the child's response to pain: how much of the response is physiological and how much is psychological? Research on the effects of surgery suggests that the psychological effect of pain on the child—or the child's reaction to it—is in direct positive correlation to the extent of the surgical procedure.[8] Thus, it can be anticipated that the child with extensive surgery on a critical part of the body (heart or lungs) would have a greater psychological response to pain and discomfort postsurgically than the child with a minor operation (tonsilectomy). The comparison also must recognize that more fears are usually built into the child preceeding major surgery than minor surgery through the extensive diagnostic procedures and, possibly, through previous illness. In addition, as a greater area of the body is affected, it is expected that more pain receptors will be affected.

In Anna Freud's discussion of pain it was suggested that the primary factor which increases or decreases the child's pain tolerance is the anxiety created by the child's interpretation of the cause of pain.[9] Children may perceive pain as punishment, retribution, maltreatment, or persecution; and they may respond to it in the form of anger or submissiveness, according to their individual interpretation of the pain eliciting stimuli. If the fantasy about the cause of the pain is stronger than the child's reality reaction, he will proportionately feel more pain and, at a later time, will remember it as being extreme. The anxious child may even respond to nonpainful stimuli as though he were in pain. The child who factually understands and accepts the cause of pain and has minimum fantasies will have greater tolerance for pain and will respond in less extreme ways.

The responses may be developmentally appropriate and are not necessarily pathological. Anxiety concerning operations has been reported by Prugh in children six years of age and younger, and particularly in those of four years and younger.[10] These findings may in part substantiate Anna Freud's theory. At about the age of four years, children are very concerned with their bodily functions, and have difficulty separating fantasy from reality. As they develop more cognitive skills, these fantasies usually decrease and reality becomes prominent in their lives.

Children physically respond to pain from infancy, but it is not known at what age it begins to have psychological significance for the child. Anna Freud discussed the nondiscriminating pain and anxiety reactions of two- and three-year-olds to painful and nonpainful stimuli. Both age groups showed almost the same symptoms of distress to the two kinds of stimuli: the first stimulus was an injection which was painful and anxiety provoking; the second was a sunlight treatment which was only anxiety provoking. This also implies that the child cannot distinguish between the apparent cause of pain and the real cause of pain. As a result, the child's anxiety may be aroused by an apparent cause of pain during treatment because it is the only visible reason for the pain and fear. In turn, the child may attribute the cause of pain to the person(s) who inflict the treatment and not the treatment method (injection) itself. It is no wonder that young children cry at the sight of medical personnel!

Isolation, Restriction and Restraint

The degree of isolation, restriction or restraint required of the child formulates a different problem for the child than that of pain, even though the symptoms may appear similar — crying, withdrawal, whimpering, anger. _Isolation_ is detrimental because of the decreased sensory stimulation and consequent regression or delay in development.[11] Isolation extends from the child's complete segregation in a private room into which only masked and gowned adults are admitted, to the separation from others in the same room by an oxygen tent. Isolation may last from a few days to several months. I have observed that when isolated children are given toys for their own self-entertainment, children younger than five years old have almost no ability to use them without the help of adults, and even adolescents have limited tolerance for the bleak environment. The young child in particular has problems dealing with the apparent rejection of the staff and other children. Even the people who do enter the isolation room often avoid getting any closer to the child than is absolutely necessary.

Motor restrictions and *restraint* create difficulty for several reasons. First, motor behavior is the child's means of mobility within his environment and his only means of learning about the environment in the early years. Older children, on the other hand, can ask questions about the hospital, the room, the illness, and so forth. Second, motor behavior is a means through which the toddler expresses the feelings which he cannot describe verbally. Because the restrictions do limit the child's emotional expression of internal tensions, anger and hyperactivity are commonly observed. The anger may appear overtly or covertly while the child is restricted; the hyperactivity may appear when he receives his freedom. Although the child may appear to accept or put up with restraint or restriction, he is likely to show his anger by a negative response which is out of proportion to minor incidents which elicit it, such as a change in the location of his bed from one side of the children's ward to the other.

Coping with Diagnostic and Treatment Procedures

Helping the child cope with the diagnostic and treatment procedures refers to helping the child tolerate a necessary, but often uncomfortable, procedure. This help does not decrease the actual pain, shorten the period of isolation, or remove the restraints. The therapist may help reduce the child's anxiety and fears by helping him understand the realities of the situation (at his own level); by acting as a caring parent surrogate himself; and by providing materials with which the child can express his needs and anxieties and maintain his ongoing development.

There are occasions when medical personnel must inflict pain on the child. Nothing can be done to reduce the pain. The therapist can only stay with the child, talk to him, and physically comfort him as much as possible. Even with this psychological support, the child may protest and cry. The therapist neither ignores the child's pain nor avoids it—even though it may be difficult for him to watch a child being "hurt."

The therapist must be aware of his own behavior when working with the child who is in pain. It is tempting to say, "Oh, that doesn't really hurt. Let's exercise it some more," or, "Okay, it does hurt, but let's do it once more." The actual comments may be true (according to Anna Freud's analysis) but the "therapeutic" behavior which accompanies them may not help the child. The child perceives that his feelings are not important to the therapist and that the therapist neither trusts nor believes him — the child may refuse to cooperate. The therapist's tactics are unfair to the child. A child who is not in pain usually does not cry in anxiety once he becomes acquainted with the therapist and the tasks expected of him (except, perhaps the infant of less than seven or eight months of age). The child usually does his best to perform as desired. The child in real pain does cry, which should limit the therapist's present work with him, unless he knows that the therapy will decrease the pain. The child in pain can usually be distinguished from the fussy child, who is generally irritable and whose behavior cannot be differentiated between the time when he is left alone and the time when he is being treated. In this case, it is doubtful that the pain is physical or that the therapist is hurting him.

Schad has described some of the ways in which a child's motion may be restricted and also suggests some treatment goals for this problem.[12] Restriction may be in terms of confinement to the bed, wheelchair or oxygen tent; restrictions from bandages, casts or intravenous equipment; restrictive disabilities, such as amputations or cerebral palsy; or environmental restrictions caused by limited space in the home or hospital. The obvious objectives are to help the child function within the confines of the restrictions—or to reduce the restrictions. In the former, the goal is to help the child continue his development and to tolerate the restrictions while permanently or temporarily confined to bed—or to help him stay within the boundaries of the restrictions if, for example, they are broadened to his room. The reduction of restrictions is a treatment goal for any restricting disability, such as cerebral palsy or blindness, in which the child is learning to cope with his environment.

Restraints are usually precautionary measures which are imposed to prevent the child from injuring himself by scratching himself, removing bandages, disturbing surgical corrections, falling out of bed, or otherwise harming himself.[13] For example, the child who is a postoperative eye patient may not be allowed to move or to be moved during the early phase of recuperation in order to prevent injury to the delicate surgical treatment. This is a problem for most children!

Children in restraint who have a disease or illness which is repulsive to others need the opportunity to develop a close interpersonal relationship in order to counteract the rejecting elements of the disease process. These children include those with severe burns or eczema or some unpleasant dermatological conditions. They are frequently ignored by other children and by the medical personnel because of the horrible odor of the disease.

Children in restraint need satisfying sensory experiences to promote the release of tensions and to prevent sensory deprivation. Infants and young children may respond rapidly and negatively to the restraints which result essentially in isolation and restriction, because they are unable to stimulate themselves. The result can be marasmus.

Isolation also may include restriction or restraint. The child who is in an isolation ward may have very limited restraints or restrictions within that one area. On the other hand, the child who is isolated within an oxygen tent is very restricted—although he may not be restrained unless he is undergoing a treatment procedure such as intravenous feeding. Isolation in these circumstances obviously is a sensory depriving experience for the child; he may hear only muffled sounds and may see only distorted objects and people through the oxygen tent. Isolation of a child is used to prevent the infecting of the nonisolated children or to prevent the child in isolation from becoming infected (sometimes this procedure is called *reverse isolation*). Isolation unintentionally results from enclosure in the oxygen tent which is a barrier between the child and others.

Helping the child cope with these procedures is a problem because of the need to correlate (1) the child's developmental needs with (2) his illness or dysfunction and with (3) the limitations resulting from secondary effects of the illness or dysfunction. It is not requisite for the therapist to actually decrease the problems of restriction, restraint, and isolation. It *is* requisite that he be aware of their effect on the child and be able to make suggestions that will alleviate the development of additional problems. It is most difficult for the preschool child who is developing social interaction to handle these complexities of illness, particularly isolation which prevents direct interaction with other children.

A resolution to this problem (from which there are multiple possible adaptations for other situations) is illustrated in the case of four-year-old Wanda, who was both isolated and, in a sense, restricted because of a recurrent dermatological infection. Each time that Wanda was readmitted to the hospital with this condition, she was isolated to prevent her from infecting the other children; and each time she withdrew from interpersonal communication and refused to talk with anyone—except two permanent staff nurses whom she knew well and the occupational therapist who treated her on each hospitalization. During one hospitalization in her fourth year, Wanda became very withdrawn and would not talk with anyone. The staff became very concerned about the detrimental effects of isolation on her development.

After the occupational therapist had again established rapport with Wanda, so that she would make an occasional comment and would respond nonverbally, group play was initiated for Wanda and three preschoolers between three and one half years and five years of age. Since isolation continued to be in effect, the children met Wanda by standing outside her doorway while the therapist and Wanda stayed several feet inside the room. Wanda had been told of this plan prior to the actual introduction of the children and told that, since the children could not be in her room, there would have to be a "river" separating them which no one but the therapist was big enough to cross (this appealed to the four-year-old imagination).

The materials chosen for the group were based on the developmental needs of the children and Wanda's known performance. The quiet, creative activity of clay and sticks (tongue depressors) was chosen to encourage verbalization between Wanda and the other children. The clay also elicited exploratory and imaginative play, which was ideal for all the preschool children, who were at various levels in the manipulative stage of learning about the materials. The therapist gave Wanda her clay at her small table, and the three youngsters their materials at a small table just outside the door (the table provided automatic limitations of movement and thus assisted in maintaining isolation).

Wanda and the children gradually began talking back and forth with each other and the therapist, who continuously mentioned each of the children's names (to help them identify each other rapidly). They talked about what each one was doing and explored all the possible means of using clay. As the days passed, the activities changed and the conversation increased. Communication with the other children was facilitated by the communication of the children in the play group, since they had the freedom to move about the ward outside Wanda's door. Because of the difficulties created by the children wanting to go into Wanda's room and her wanting to go out, a physical barrier in the form of a "fence" was placed at the door. This limited only the mobility, not the verbal interaction. Wanda ceased to withdraw from the activity on the ward; instead, she would stand at the door and call the other children and ask them to talk with her, to find the nurse so she could use the potty, to get the OT, and so forth.

Once she was out of isolation, Wanda was not a stranger to the ward, but immediately began to interact with the other children and they with her, instead of having to begin the get-acquainted process and to regain developmental abilities lost through regression. In other words, a micronursery school had been arranged for the stimulation of emotional, social, and cognitive developmental needs and the maintenance of all other developmental behaviors.

The Prognosis

The prognosis of the illness or disability is usually reported first (and often, only) to the parents. Consequently, it is their emotional response to this information to which the child responds, not the actual prognosis, which the child does not know. The parents may show anxiety and mourning responses toward the child who is dying and toward the child who is critically ill. Senn and Solnit describe these responses as

anticipatory mourning reactions, which represent their preparation for the inevitable loss to themselves and their family. Mourning is the repetitive and intense review in feelings and thoughts of past and present relationships to the child, accompanied by bitter and resentful emotional reactions to the tragedy of a child dying before his life has unfolded. Such reactions refer not only to the loss of the child, but to the impact of this loss on family relationships and atmosphere. For many parents the death of the child represents a permanent severing of one line to immortality.[14]

This is quite a different set of behaviors from that which is seen in the atmosphere around the child who is temporarily, but not severely, ill — the parents talk about the healthy aspects of the child's life, his going back to school, playing outdoors with friends, visiting grandma, and so forth. This behavior again differs from the reaction: to the child who is chronically ill but who does not have acute exacerbations, or the child who is handicapped. There is a mixture of pleasure and happiness for the child, with sadness for his disability, but there is not an overwhelming fear of loss.

Death

It is generally accepted that children are anxious about death from their early years until the time of adulthood or until they have resolved their own feelings about it. Mitchell has concluded from her study that children today are very anxious about death of both the individual (from cancer, cigarette smoking, automobile accidents) and the masses (from a nuclear explosion).[15] Accepting the hypothesis that children who have had only minimal experience with death still wonder about and fantasize about it, one can imagine the concern of the child who has experienced death within his own family or among close friends. Add to this the child's own illness and his lack of understanding concerning it, plus many of the other unknowns about death, and one would anticipate extreme anxiety in all acutely ill children.

The child who is dying elicits many conflicts and anxieties in the health care worker who is generally poorly prepared to help the child or the parents. Adults prefer to avoid the issue of death because there are no absolute answers to give a child. The answers are based on religious beliefs or on the individual's sociological background. In addition to having no concrete answers, many adults have not resolved their own fears of death and thus feel incapable of discussing it with a child. Mitchell states that of all the deprivations a person may experience, death may be the major one. There is no recourse and there are no substitutes for the individual who dies.

Seldom does the occupational therapist have the direct responsibility for informing the parents or child of the prognosis. Usually the therapist works with children who are expected to live and to function in society. However, it is possible that a child's prognosis might change, and that the therapist would continue to work with the child until the child no longer responds to therapy.

The biggest fear of most health care workers is the need to respond to the child who confronts them with, "Am I going to die? The response may be easy to give if the child is incorrectly identifying his disease with that of a friend whose disease is fatal. However, if the true answer is "yes," the answer is not simple. There is no single best answer to this question.

In choosing the best answer for a specific child, whether or not the question is asked directly, the therapist must know the policy of the hospital, the child's physician, and the parents. He must give an answer which is congruent with answers which have been given by others. He must know the child's understanding of the term *death*.

A combination of cues may add up to creating much anxiety for the child: his parents' over-solicitousness and grief and his own physical discomfort and pain. Although the child knows something is seriously wrong, he may not ask questions because (1) he does not want his fears confirmed, or (2) he is not supposed to know his diagnosis. The preschool child has no concept of the real meaning of death, and may release his anxiety through physical activity. He may have put words together and devised an explanation of death, but he remains unaware of the permanence of the deprivation or of its effect on him. His anxiety can be alleviated best through the reduction of pain as much as possible and by the presence of his parents.[16]

Children in the school years may ask questions about death or about their illnesses, but generally they do not directly ask about their own anticipated deaths. The early school age child may ask about the illness and when he will get better. (Some acting out may occur as seen in preschool years.) Only as he develops the ability to conceptualize, and thus understand, the irrevocability of death, can he become fully aware of his position. Senn and Solnit suggest that, in addition to the anxiety and sadness which accompanies death in all children, the later school-age child and the adolescent feel a kind of helplessness. This is based on their developing independence and individuality, through which they have gained success and satisfaction in social and intellectual pursuits, and which they themselves can recognize.

The question remains: how much does one discuss the child's illness and coming death with the child himself? And who is the appropriate person to discuss it with him? There is negligible research or information on this topic. Richmond and Waisman reported observations of forty-eight children with leukemia.[17] Generally the children showed "an air of passive acceptance and resignation" toward their malignancy, which they had not been told would lead to death. The children, including the adolescents, rarely showed overt concern about death. The authors felt that the absence of behavioral manifestations was an attempt to repress anxiety about death. When the child asked about his illness, he was given a description of it without the diagnostic title. In other words, the child was never told directly that he had leukemia—or that he was dying.

Vernick and Karon have directly confronted the issue of how to talk with the dying child.[18] Fifty-one children, ages nine to twenty years, who were hospitalized for acute leukemia, were interviewed individually and in groups in activity settings. From their reported observations, the usual practices of avoiding the topic of a child's coming death can be challenged.

First, a hospital ward grapevine is very efficient. Children know when a child dies because he disappears from the ward. In conjunction with this, a child usually recognizes symptoms of his own disease in the other child and often discusses them with his friend. Once the other child dies (even though the patients are not told the facts) the obvious question arises: "He had what I have and he died. When will I die?" This probably would increase the child's anxiety, temporarily at least. Vernick states that the adults usually must initiate talk about a child's death—adults have more emotional strength. I believe that, by bringing up a topic which is usually taboo, the child feels he is given permission to talk. Otherwise, the child may feel that he should not talk about death—that it is horrible and too frightening.

The authors also observed increased tension between parents and child during the time that each attempted to hide his knowledge of the disease from the other. Instead of openly being able to support their child, their energy was expended in avoiding the real issue. Once the child was told the truth, both parents and child relaxed considerably and began meaningful communication. Some of the behavior problems decreased with the child's real knowledge of his prognosis. The child no longer needed to resent the medical care he was receiving for a purpose which he could not acknowledge and did not want to know. He became part of the team working toward his health, instead of fighting the treatment. Telling the child the truth about one part of his illness also demands that he be told of each aspect of treatment before it occurs. Vernick clearly identified the unfairness of seeking permission to operate on a child from the parents and not from the child on whom the operation will be performed, if the child is old enough to understand the implications of surgery. Although legally the child is not responsible, it is *his body*, and he is the one who must live with the results of the treatment.

In telling the child about his disease, the parents and physician are eliminating the child's being crudely informed of his status by a playmate, unthinking neighbor, or sibling when the child is at home. One can imagine two siblings arguing over a toy and the healthy child saying angrily to his leukemic brother, "Keep your old bicycle. You're going to be dead soon anyway, then I'll get it!

By preparing the child's siblings for the child's death and acknowledging that the dying child knows of it, the siblings begin to understand why mom and dad are so unhappy—and why they spend a disproportionate amount of time with their brother or sister. Although the siblings may feel somewhat neglected, the children usually will offer much support to their parents. Instead of being angry that mother won't be home from the hospital in time to make their dinner, for example, the children may offer to make dinner because they are sensitive to their mother's exhaustion.

The occupational therapist may be able to offer assistance to the dying child and his family. The therapist can provide the child with an opportunity to act out his feelings about death constructively in play, or he can encourage the child to talk about his concerns (which may be only distantly related to himself and death). He can communicate the child's concerns to other health care staff. In all cases, the therapist must look at his own personal feelings toward death, for these will give him cues as to how he is responding to the child. No matter what his own feelings are concerning the informing of a child about coming death, the therapist can only present his feelings on this topic to the staff. He cannot contradict the practice of the staff because of the possibility of creating real and unfair confusion for the child, who may be too anxious to clarify the conflicts with his parents and physician.

HOSPITALIZATION AND INSTITUTIONALIZATION

Hospitalization and institutionalization connote different objectives in the treatment of the child. The former usually refers to a relatively short-term experience of weeks or a few months for the medical or surgical treatment of an acute condition. Children with chronic conditions, on the other hand, such as extreme emotional disturbance or mental retardation, may be institutionalized for extensive treatment or for permanent care. This procedure is appropriate when families are not equipped to care for their child at home until the child shows some positive developmental changes in his behavior. If the child is severely disabled, as in the case of the profoundly retarded child, these positive changes may be negligible, and the child may receive custodial institutional care for the remainder of his life.

Chronic, convalescent hospitals or institutions can create problems for children over a period of time. External stimulation from the real world and a variety of people is limited or nonexistent (except through television, magazines, and so forth), and the child's development may be impeded (see Chapter Eight). Once the child is discharged from the institution he must deal with community problems which, he either had never experienced, or had not experienced recently (transportation, people who look at or comment to him about his appearance or disfigurement, the use of money, and the routine of a public school, for example).

There can be healthy effects from hospitalization; there has been little research in this area, however. Fourteen-year old Terry, who came from a very deprived environment, recognized the benefits of the hospital; he periodically had asthma attacks and admitted himself to the hospital for treatment. As the social worker found out (through Terry's own admission), he inevitably had an asthma attack when he wanted to sleep in a bed with sheets and blankets, when he was hungry and wanted good meals, and when he wanted to talk with someone who would be interested in him. Essentially the boy was telling his social worker that the hospital was much more comfortable than his home: "I would prefer to live here." The problem for the hospital staff and community was to make life outside the institution desirable enough so that Terry would maintain his health, since he knew that by doing so under the present circumstances, he would eliminate a "home" and contact which was vital to him.

Although treatment objectives may differ within an institution and hospital, the child's social-emotional responses to both may be similar. Institutionalized children show the same reactions qualitatively as the hospitalized child, but quantitatively they may be more extreme. Thus, the following discussion in which the term *hospitalization* is used refers to both situations.

Three factors which may cause emotional disturbance in children during or after hospitalization or institutionalization are (1) the age of the child, (2) the personality and living experience of the child, and (3) the actual type and quantity of diagnostic and treatment procedures.[19]

Some research has been done on the effects of the child's age. Several studies have documented the fact that children four years of age and under show the most detrimental emotional effects. Schaffer and Callender have demonstrated that the baseline division for reactions to separation is seven months.[20] Infants under this age show a minimum reaction; children older than this show extreme reactions to separation, which may lead to Robertson's description of the stages of a process of settling in or adapting to hospitalization: protest, despair, and denial (see Chapter Five). Prugh found that children between two and four years of age show the most disturbed behavior during hospitalization — particularly those who are restricted to bed — and most often show the long-term posthospital effects. Children of more than four years are affected if hospitalization is their first experience with separation.[21]

The second area which may lead to emotional disturbance is the personality and living experience of the child. The child who had personality problems or problems with his parents prior to hospitalization, adjusts more poorly than the child from a healthy environment.[22] This is an expected correlation because the child who is insecure in his relationship with his parents may fear abandonment when his parents leave him in the hospital. Comments by parents, such as, "If you don't behave and stop crying, I'm going to leave you here in the hospital," seem very real to the child who has little understanding of the purpose of hospitalization. This is particularly true for the child who has never been separated from his family and has not experienced their leaving him and returning to him. On the other hand, children who have a variety of living experiences, such as trips to other communities, visits to grandparents and overnights at the homes of peers, understand the process of leaving and returning home. Correlated with this is the fact that the older a child is, the more opportunities he has had for separation.

The effects of multiple, varied diagnostic and treatment procedures have previously been described. Reactions to these procedures, in combination with hospitalization, multiply the problems of the child.

Elements of the hospital environment which influence the child's response are multiple and have been described by Prugh, Robertson, and others. Among the elements already mentioned are the physical characteristics which differ considerably from the characteristics of a home. The hospital room in which the child lives is generally bleak in comparison with his bedroom at home. It may contain only a bed, a chest, or closet for his clothing and perhaps his toys and a chair. There may or may not be curtains on the windows and pictures on the walls; there may or may not be a playroom available in which the child can play, and there may or may not be any play toys or materials on the ward. On the ward there are rooms, such as the medical treatment room, which are off limits for the children. The kitchen, if on the ward, may be on or off limits.

The routine of the hospital also differs from that in the home. It may encourage the children to get out of bed and dress in their own clothes for breakfast, straighten up their rooms, and, possibly, make their own beds, go to school, recreation, and so forth. All of these routine activities are interspersed with regular mealtimes in a dining room, treatments, medications and doctors' rounds. On the other hand, the child may have none of these normal routine experiences to neutralize the negative effects of the hospital procedure, because of the child's particular illness or the particular hospital into which he is admitted.

The routine of a convalescent hospital or institution for chronically ill children usually emphasizes the healthy aspects of a child's environment—with variations added to meet the child's need for treatment. The child may be in and out of the schoolroom or playroom for therapy, but have an otherwise dependable schedule. A regular schedule is most desirable for the child and helps him maintain a feeling of the outside world (into which he must return) while he is dealing with the problems of illness.

Coping with Hospitalization

The occupational therapist is concerned with the child's reactions to hospitalization and usually has a part in planning a healthy hospital milieu (see Chapter Five). This is primarily an administrative problem, but, because it can affect the child's response to therapy, the therapist must use his knowledge to create necessary changes to provide a healthy environment.

Helping the child cope with hospitalization begins before the child enters the hospital. The process of preparation as suggested by Senn and Solnit begins one or two days prior to admission.[23] This gives the child some time to prepare himself for the experience and separation, but prevents the development of excessive anxiety. Each of the following suggestions is individualized for the child and his situation.

The value of the child's being prepared for hospitalization is most relevant for the child of three years and older, with an increase in detail with the added years. Though it does not seem to make as much difference in the child's behavior during hospitalization, it seems to decrease the after-effects in posthospitalization when the child returns home and must readjust. In other words, by his being prepared honestly for each event as it occurs, beginning with prehospital preparation and ending with his return home, the child knows what to anticipate—and believes his parents when they give him information. He will trust them when they say, "The needle will hurt," and, "The doctor's stethoscope won't hurt." When the child returns home and his parents say, "You are not going back to the hospital," or, "You are not going back for a long long time." the child can believe them and settle into the process of readjusting to home life.

Preparation may include children's books which are written for the purpose of preparing the child, a visit to the hospital to see where it is located in relation to home, or a tour of the hospital ward and a room comparable to the one he will stay in when hospitalized, and an introduction to some of the hospital personnel. If a child tends to be very anxious about new experiences and has limited conceptual abilities, a visit to the hospital ward may be detrimental to him because he probably will see children who have obvious defects, bandages, and so forth. As a result of this, the child may fantasize that he, too, will be the recipient of such bandages. Once the child is in the hospital, his concerns about the other children and his becoming like them may decrease as he becomes acquainted with them as children who are like himself in many ways.

The child also is encouraged to participate in the process of packing for the trip to the hospital. This includes his choosing the favorite toy with which he associates home, and which gives him comfort in the absence of his parents.[24] (Some hospitals discourage children from bringing favorite objects from home because of their being carriers of disease and the possibility of their being lost or getting broken. I strongly disagree with this policy.) The child also may fix his room in readiness for his return home, which signifies and reaffirms the fact that he will come home. He may choose the clothing which his parents are to bring the day he is to come home.

If the child is going to a convalescent hospital for an extensive period, adjustments must be made in preparing him for the return home. Otherwise, if he has limited conceptual abilities, he may assume that the return will be immediate and he will respond negatively to the extended absence from home. Adjustments also must be made according to the age of the child, since the very young child will not understand the verbal description and preparation. He will, however, associate the presence of a known object — *not* new toys — with home, family and comfort.

Once the child is in the hospital, the detrimental factors can be decreased in several ways. In some hospitals, arrangements are made for the mother (or father) to live-in with the child who is less than four years old and to assist in his care. Anna Freud suggests that there is a considerable decrease in the child's problems when the mother is present—even if she does nothing—her physical presence and support are the reassuring elements for the child.[25] Living-in is recommended particularly during the child's first two and one-half years, when he has very limited use of language, both receptively and expressively. As the child reaches the school-age years, the need for the parents' living-in decreases (he can communicate his needs and comprehend his parents' absence). In addition to the parents relieving the nursing staff of some of their routine tasks (if they are emotionally and physically able to assist in the care of their child), the parent's presence makes it easier for the therapist to communicate with parent and child together, and to teach the mother the therapeutic procedure prior to the child's discharge. This is ideal, for the therapist then does not have the problems of "catching" the parents when they happen to visit.

It is generally thought that children need both the facts about their illness, treatment and hospitalization, and the opportunity to express their feelings about them during hospitalization. It has been hypothesized that the benefit of verbal and nonverbal expression of feelings is that the children learn to deal with their problems at the time of their occurrence and thus reduce immediate anxiety and long-range negative personality changes. In one pilot study, Rie et al. tried to determine whether the learning of facts through lectures (with no opportunity for the discussion of feelings) or the expression of feelings through ventilation sessions (with no learning of the facts of the illness) was the most effective means of reducing the children's anxiety.[26] Although Rie and his associates emphasized the tentative nature of the results because of the small sample, their results suggest some clues as to the relative values of obtaining facts versus ventilation from the child's point of view. Learning the facts took place in both groups of children; however, the group which was tutored in the facts of the illness showed a decrease in the anxiety level. (Perhaps this is comparable to the results of Vernick and Karon, who found decreased anxiety in telling the dying child about his prognosis.) [27]

Rie hypothesizes the reasons for the unexpected results, one of the most plausible of which is that the physicians who were directly responsible for the care of the children were the tutors; while the leader of the ventilation group was a consulting psychiatrist who had no responsibilities for the children's physical health. One might speculate about the value of ancillary health care personnel in helping the child deal with problems of illness and hospitalization, if upon further research these results are substantiated.

Prugh et al. did a study in which the experimental group was placed in an optimal hospital environment and compared with the control group, which received the routine hospital care.[28] Results demonstrated that children over four years of age protested more overtly (Manifested their distress during their hospitalization, both in crying when treatments were given and when their parents left) than the children in the control group who were hospitalized in a rigid emotional and physical environment (essentially a "don't cry" and "don't express yourself" environmental attitude). There was a decrease over a period of time in the frantic crying of children whose parents visited in the experimental group. The overt reactions which make adults feel uncomfortable—such as the crying, whimpering, hyperactivity, and noisiness—are the reactions that frequently discourage hospital personnel from permitting expression of feelings; they don't always know how to deal with the behaviors or don't want to be "bothered" because it interferes with their "care" of the children. (More often than not, *care* refers to the physical care and not the psychological care.)

The environmental factors, most of which have been described, distinguish the rigid from the expressive atmosphere. As the hospital practices become less rigid, the child is better able to use his environment constructively and to benefit from it. In other words, hospitalization can provide healthy experiences through which the child can continue his development. It can provide appropriate developmental stimulation for the child. This stimulation avoids gross regression in the child's development, unless the illness is overwhelming (as in acute stages, when the child has energy enough only to deal with his illness).

One way to help the child maintain his developmental level and begin understanding his own problems is to involve him in becoming a *doer* (described by Petrillo [29]) within his environment, rather than making him the passive object to which everything is done. The child becomes an active participant in the process of his own habilitation or rehabilitation. He can participate by taking his own pills and by preparing his own snack, or it can be symbolized by having him perform surgery or nursing care on a doll. Among other real tasks, he can also assist the physician or nurse with his treatment — by holding some of the tools, by helping to watch the level of the intravenous bottle and reporting to the nurse the level of its contents.

Blom describes essentially the same idea as the child's transfer of his positive feelings from his parents to the hospital staff.[30] As the child identifies with the staff, he cooperates with them and helps them, perhaps in a manner comparable to that of his cooperation with his parents.

It becomes evident that the attitudes and behaviors of the people who care for the child are primary in determining the child's ability to tolerate his illness and separation from home. The best physical facilities are valuable only with a staff which is knowledgable about and empathetic toward children.

PEOPLE

The Parents

Parents and family are the most important people to the child. The parents prepare the child for his hospitalization or the treatment of his illness; they support the child emotionally and help him tolerate the disease during the acute phase of illness and during hospitalization; ultimately, the parents have the total responsibility for the care of the child. During this process there are many factors which affect the parents' relationship with the child (some of which have been mentioned in Chapters Two and Three).

The objective for any health care professional working with the parents is to understand the parents' attitudes and behaviors toward the child, for they will be reflected in the child's behavior, his reaction to the illness, to hospitalization, and to the people around him. This is not to say that the therapist analyzes every parent. It does mean that the therapist is aware of parents' possible feelings and tries to identify those of a particular parent, so that he, the therapist, can respond to the needs of both the child and the parent.

The Parents' Anxieties about Their Sick Child

The parents' perceptions of illness and hospitalization evolve from their socioeconomic background, religious beliefs, and their personal experiences with illness and disability. When their child becomes sick, the parents may perceive that they are being punished. Sometimes parents use the threat of illness loosely and flippantly to gain their child's cooperation: "You behave—or else you will get sick." At other times religious beliefs are used as the threat: "Be good or God will punish you." The belief that illness or disability is punishment from the parents may occur when the parents are responsible for (or inappropriately feel responsible for) the child's illness or injury. For example, a parent may feel that he should have been present to prevent his child from running into the street and being hit by a car, or the parent may feel guilty because his child pulled a chair up to the stove, spilled a pot of boiling water on himself, and was severely burned. In the case of a child's illness, the parents may know intellectually that they are not responsible and that they could not prevent the illness, even while emotionally blaming themselves: "If we had done thus and so, maybe he wouldn't be sick now." Parents of children who have congenital disabilities may blame themselves or each other—even though they could have done little or nothing to prevent the disability.

Parents' behavior toward their child and health care workers (such as the doctors and nurses who have done only preventive medicine to this point) may change when their child becomes ill.[31] The reactions toward both may be variable and ambivalent. Because the parents may have positive and negative attitudes toward their child, they may have problems interacting with him during the illness. The mother may feel that her mothering responsibilities are being usurped by the hospital personnel, particularly if the child responds better to the staff than to the parents. This is often seen when the child accepts medication easily and without complaint in the absence of his mother, but rebels, cries, and pleads with mommy to stop the nurse from making him take the pills when mommy is present. Mother may feel inappropriately guilty because she has difficulty in quieting the child, and she may withdraw from contacts with either the staff or her child. Other parents demand a great deal of both from the child and the staff because they want their child to recover. The mother may force-feed the child at mealtimes and snacktimes "to give him energy so he will get better fast," and enforce rest during the scheduled rest hour and at other times during the day so that he "doesn't get over-tired and sick again." Even though some of these behaviors may not be beneficial to the child's health, the parent may know of no other way to cope with the child and his own feelings about the disability.

Many parents are handicapped in interacting with their child on the constant intimate basis which evolves with the child's illness. In the home the child is given his toys and a place to play while mother and dad do their work. The parent-child interaction is sporadic as the child asks for brief assistance with a task, shows the parent something he has made, or tells the parent about his activity while the parent continues to iron, wash, cook supper, or mow the lawn. In other words, the child plays parallel to the parents instead of interacting with them as he does with his peers. Parents' inability to play with their child and their consequent discomfort in *playing* with him for hours on end is often observed in the hospital. Yet the parents may feel that they *should* play with their child when they visit him rather than talk with other parents, knit or read.

All parents are expected to have some problems accepting and interacting with their handicapped child. The effort parents are willing to expend in learning to deal with their child separates those parents who accept the child as their own in spite of his problems from those who reject their child because he is imperfect. The anxiety which the parents experience in interacting with their child during the acute illness—or at the inception of the disability—may be symptomatic of the problems they will have in accepting the child's handicap and in dealing with it. In one family, the father of a mongoloid infant requested that the child be institutionalized immediately because he felt that a retarded child would affect his image as a corporation man and hinder his professional progress. The mother's attitude was ambivalent; she loved her husband and their way of life, but she also loved her baby and did not want to give the child up.

One problem with which parents must cope when they keep the child at home is the projection of their own feelings about the disability onto the child. The child incorporates these feelings into his own self-perceptions and, from these, develops his own self-image and body-image. This process is observed to some extent in all families. The child is teased about his freckles, his big ears, his chubbiness or skinniness (just as father is teased about his "pot belly" and mother about her graying hair), or he is commended on his beautiful curly hair, long eyelashes, or happy disposition. Eventually the child becomes very conscious of his body with its assets and liabilities. Not only does the handicapped child recognize the effect of the disability on himself, but he sees that it interferes with family life. A child knows that father has to work at a second job to get money for therapy; he knows the parents may have to take time to travel long distances for his therapy; he knows that his siblings may feel embarrassed about bringing friends home. All these elements are well recognized by the child whose cognitive development is intact — he sees his position in the family and his imposition on the family and their routine.

In their concern for the child and his future, parents may be extreme in demanding the child's dependence or independence. Some parents need to make their child overdependent upon the family. This reaction may be based on guilt about the child and a fear that the child will not be able to care for himself as he grows up. On the other hand, there are parents who push their child to become independent, and who may try to force the child's development before he is ready. Extremes in demanding dependence and independence are usually unrealistic for the child's actual capabilities; the child would either perform too well independently, or not well enough.

Helping Parents Cope with their Sick or Disabled Child

The therapist and other members of the health care team are therapists for the parents as well as for the child. The therapist may help the parents to interact with their child and show them realistically what the child can do—or should be expected to do considering his development and physical status. This is particularly important for parents who emphasize the imperfections of the child and ignore the potential. In other words, the therapist helps the parents to see the assets of the child and to see how they can assist him in coping with liabilities. For example, a four-year-old boy with ulcerative colitis was very "tight" in his physical behavior and emotional expression, and excessively concerned with cleanliness and tidiness. He withdrew from other children who were active because he was afraid of them and their boisterousness. It became apparent that the mother was one of the child's basic problems. Her expectations of his behavior and play were appropriate for a reserved, inactive, intellectually motivated woman. The interaction between mother and child was observed on her visit to the hospital, at which time the boy sat on his mother's lap in the playroom while together they looked at the newspaper and identified words and letters. Meanwhile the other four-year-olds romped around the playroom. With the mother's consent the therapist planned and carried out finger painting as a group activity for all the pre-schoolers—including the boy—while the mother was present. At first, the boy tentatively touched the paints, but then used them only with the aid of a stick, which served as an extension of his fingers. Within a week the child progressed to active involvement and was relaxed and free in his use of the materials. He also progressed to moderate interaction with the other children at various times during the day in both the mother's presence and absence.

Parent-ch-Ther. Inter-action.

Several objectives were accomplished through the therapy: the mother was present and saw the total procedure, instead of hearing about it second-hand from her child and the therapist. Her presence (in spite of the objections she presented to the therapist) showed an initial willingness to learn more about the needs of four-year-olds and her son. Because the task was in conflict with the mother's requirements for the child, it was felt that her presence — which gave the child both verbal and nonverbal permission to participate — would facilitate the therapeutic process; the child would not be pulled between wanting to participate and wondering what his mother would think. For practical purposes, the mother learned how children can participate in play and cleanup and still maintain some cleanliness: a coverall apron, a table and floor which could not be harmed by paint, and a child-size sponge and mop for the children to use in cleaning up the table, chairs, and floor.

Too frequently therapy is carried out only with the child, in the absence of the parents — a practice which does not help the parents learn about their child's developmental and psychological progress. Nor does it help them learn new behavior. In child psychiatry particularly, the child's problem is a symptom of the entire family's problem. Without the participation of the parents, the effectiveness of therapy is questionable for the parents do have some responsibility during both the illness and the rehabilitation of their child.

In addition to the parent-therapist interaction, or the parent-child-therapist interaction, there are parent discussion groups for the parents of children with handicaps. These may be community discussion groups for parents whose children have similar problems within a particular community. They may be formal groups derived from a specific handicapped children's preschool, special education class, outpatient treatment group or day-care program. These groups may be requested and organized by the parents, or they may be initiated by the professional staff for the parents. The group may include only one or two of the health-care professionals who can lead the discussion, or it may include all the professionals involved in the care of the children around whom the group was formulated.

The objectives for parents' groups are multiple. Parents learn that they are not alone with their problems; that other people have similar problems; and that they have learned how to cope with them. Parents and staff help each other learn new ways in which they can help the child cope with his disability as he grows. Through this learning, parents may begin to feel more adequate and secure as the parents of a handicapped child. As a result, they may project a more positive image of the child onto him than they had previously done.

The comments of parents about these groups are varied, but generally show an increased sensitivity to themselves, to others, and to their own children: "I really don't feel so badly any more; after all, look at Mrs. Harrison's problems with her child and she doesn't even have a husband who will help her." "I really learned a lot from Mr. Johnson — he certainly has clever ideas for helping his child." "I found out that my son may have more problems than a lot of kids, but he has a lot less than others. Is our family ever lucky!" The parents are responding with relief because they have finally discovered other parents with similar problems and with whom they can share their concerns. This meaningful communication is often impossible for a family unless there are other families with handicapped children in the same neighborhood.

Through communication with the others, it is hoped that the parents begin to understand the basis for their feelings and thus will be able to readjust their thinking and feel less guilty toward their handicapped child — either because they learn the limits of what they can do to help him, or learn how they can help him most constructively.

As the parents begin to accept their child, they begin to recognize and understand that he is a child first, and *then* a child with a handicap. In spite of the handicap, the child has many of the same developmental needs as any other child. If the child is physically handicapped, he still has the emotional and social needs of other children who are his developmental equivalent; if he is emotionally handicapped, he still needs the neuromotor experiences to help him develop physically.

An occupational therapist is involved in the parents' group in different situations. The therapist may participate only occasionally, when the group wants the different professionals to discuss their work with and plans for the children. On the other hand, the therapist may participate regularly in the parent group if he is working with the total group of children, or if the treatment team works with the parents as a unit. For example, all the personnel in a handicapped children's preschool may be involved on a regular or periodic basis. This helps the parents become acquainted with the personnel, and therefore more comfortable in asking questions and in seeking their assistance.

The Therapist and Other Health Care Personnel

The primary objective of all health care personnel is to provide an atmosphere in which the child can become himself. The therapist shows attitudes and behaviors which encourage the child to develop his own attitudes and behaviors. Axline has described the attitude of the therapist in terms of the atmosphere he provides for the child in the playroom. Although Axline's description refers to the treatment of psychological problems, the idea is pertinent to all therapy—with some variations. A therapist working toward specific objectives in the treatment of a visual-perceptual motor deficit, for example, usually provides both direction and specific tasks for the child to perform. However, the therapist still does not nag or goad or pry or criticize, even though he directs the child's activity. It immediately becomes clear in Axline's description that a positive atmosphere complements the therapeutic relationship and leads to successful treatment.

The play-therapy room is good growing ground. In the security of this room where the *child* is the most important person, where he is in command of the situation and of himself, where no one tells him what to do, no one criticizes what he does, no one nags, or suggests, or goads him on, or pries into his private world, he suddenly feels that *here* he can unfold his wings; he can look squarely at himself, for he is accepted completely; he can test out his ideas; he can express himself fully; for this is *his* world, and he no longer has to compete with such other forces as adult authority...He is an individual in his own right. He is treated with dignity and respect. He can say anything that he feels like saying—and he is accepted completely. He can play with the toys in any way he likes to—and he is accepted completely.[32]

Although Axline describes the play therapy room as "good growing ground," it seems that the attitude and the behavior of the therapist make the room good growing ground. If this is true, the growth can occur anywhere in the presence of a therapist. Although the child's expression of his attitudes and behavior may have to be tempered in the less private setting, most children do not expect or need complete freedom to express themselves.

Adults who work with children also have different needs. They show varying attitudes and behaviors toward children, which are based on their experiences with children, their feelings about children, their own abilities to interact with children, and their knowledge of children learned from other people and from academic study. Although each adult generally shows an individualized approach to and attitude toward children, these attitudes and approaches may vary slightly — or even extensively — under some circumstances. The adult's perception of his own behavior in the adult-child relationship may be very different from the perceptions of the child and other adults. For example, the behavior which the adult considers "good" may not be perceived as "good" by the child. "Good" to one adult may mean quiet, sitting still — "yes, m'am"; "no, sir"; no talking except in response to a direct question; and doing what the adult wants when the adult wants it. "Good" to another adult may mean letting the child act like the child of his developmental age — encouraging his questions, physical activity, curiosity and occasionally being a nuisance. Children's growing can inconvenience adults!

All adults are inconvenienced by children at some time during their interaction. In response, the adult may show rigid behavior and attitudes. Rigidity may occur when the therapist feels pressured to complete a specific evaluation or treatment within a specific period of time. The therapist's conflict is in choosing between the child's immediate psychological needs and his treatment needs, which are costly in terms of time and money.

The development of rigid behavior and attitudes is also understandable in terms of the adult's reaction to the society in which he was raised as a child—in comparison with the society in which children are presently being raised. As a child, he learned the prevailing adult attitudes and incorporated some of these into his own behavior. As an adult, he may have difficulty accepting the changes in society. Although he must be open to the changes and accept them as a natural process, he can still maintain his own value system and let the child know this without becoming rigid in response to threatened change. It is the adult's responsibility to help the child discriminate between the "useful" and "detrimental" changes in society — the healthy versus the unhealthy — the use of drugs for pleasurable feelings versus the therapeutic use of drugs, for instance. The therapist discriminates between the beneficial situations and behaviors for the child and his own personal adult desires; the child needs and wants gross motor activity in therapy but the therapist is "too tired to play." On the other hand, the therapist may limit the length of the gross motor play to prevent the development of fatigue or excessive hyperactivity. Children need mature and knowledgable guidance in making these decisions.

As the child grows, the conflicts between his desires and the standards of rigid adult behavior increase. The child becomes capable of functioning and thinking independently of the adult, and he may no longer accept the rigidity of the adult's thinking. Consequently, he may attempt to break away from it. The adult's response may be (1) to increase the restraints and limits on the child, or (2) to relinquish responsibility for the child's action and let the child go his own way. Tommy exemplified the conflicts which are often presented to the therapist and which gradually increase his rigidity. Tommy, age eleven years, needed successful experiences for which he was initially given a very simple gimp project. Once he completed this project he requested another, and another, and another. In the therapist's enthusiasm for developing Tommy's skills beyond this level of learning, he demanded that Tommy progress to a more difficult task. Tommy refused and continued to beg the therapist for more gimp. The therapist refused Tommy's request until another therapist pointed out that the issue was, who was to be in control, Tommy or the therapist? The therapist forced himself to relax his rigid behavior with "Okay, Tommy, I was wrong — there is no real reason why you shouldn't make more gimp projects," and permitted Tommy to make as many as he desired. Tommy quickly lost interest in the activity, did not complete the new one and requested that he and the therapist "do something else."

The therapist must answer one question for himself: is my rigid behavior really necessary? Is there a real reason for setting the limits I am setting? What harm would be done if I relaxed my behavior? If the therapist answers himself honestly (or finds that another more objective therapist answers these questions honestly) and the answers are negative, the therapist must rethink his demands.

Rigidity in handling children often varies with the therapist's success in handling them. Even therapists who enjoy children have some difficulties in understanding how to cope with them and their problems. The fluctuation between successful (sometimes planned and sometimes lucky) and unsuccessful coping with children raises ambivalent feelings in the therapist: he likes the child but becomes angry with the child, or with himself, when the child responds negatively or refuses to perform. A five-year-old boy with cerebral palsy, for example, yelled loudly, "No! I don't want to do that exercise!" and proceeded to have a temper tantrum in the middle of the occupational therapy department as the therapist tried to coax him into exercising. Needless to say, the therapist was angry with himself and terribly embarrassed. Instead of rigidly demanding a specific schedule at each treatment session, the therapist uses his knowledge of the child and varies the order of treatment, or he goes for a short walk while the child prepares himself for therapy, or he notes the child's distress verbally for the child and inquires as to the cause of the problem. The therapist's rigid requirements for specific behaviors at a specific time seldom gain anything and probably decrease the possibility of successful experiences at the next treatment session.

It is evident that the emotional-social behavior, not the intellectual, motor, and other behavior, is primary to successful adult-child interaction. Some of these emotional and social behaviors, or the "certain somethings," are identified by Sheimo:

> ...it takes a certain 'something' to carry on a satisfactory relationship with normal children and adults. That 'something' can perhaps be called ability to give and take, responsiveness, frankness, honesty — all of which often implies some degree of guts and fortitude...it takes only considerably more of the same thing in dealing with emotionally disturbed or handicapped children...[33]

The therapeutic relationship which results from "give and take, responsiveness, frankness, honesty..." is a primary factor in effecting the outcome of treatment. This relationship may be defined as the interaction between the therapist and child which affects the child's ability to cope with his environment and his problems in the rehabilitation process. The therapeutic relationship can be negative or positive. If it is a poor or negative relationship from the child's point of view, the resulting treatment may be ineffectual or incomplete; the child may go through the treatment superficially, but may then retreat to earlier behavior—or he may refuse to continue treatment. If the relationship is positive, the child wants to perform, partly because he desires to please the therapist. A therapist may have a great deal of knowledge, but if he cannot use himself to stimulate the child's performance, the knowledge is wasted. The child must *like* the adult to attempt change, particularly if the process is painful. (This is not true once the child is internally motivated to improve. In this situation, the child may improve in spite of the therapeutic agent.)

The characteristics which I believe encourage a child's respect and liking for the adult therapist can be categorized in three areas. The first is the therapist's expression of adult behavior through the use of his knowledge and experience to guide the child. The second is the honest display of positive feelings toward the child; and the third is the honest display of negative feelings toward the child.

Honesty is the element which is common to all these characteristics — it is the foundation for mutual communication. Children expect congruence between the actions and words of the adult. This, in turn, implies the honest expression of both positive and negative feelings in the therapist's response and behavior. Often when an individual attempts to hide his negative feelings, his manifested behavior is conflicting; the words are nice but the muscular and vocal tension of the body language appear to be angry. As a result, the child must choose to respond to the verbal or nonverbal behavior. Realistically he could never respond correctly to the therapist's mixed message, for his response would always be partly wrong.

Shirley describes the values of congruent negative behaviors of the therapist. There is a place for them, but not for the mixed messages of incongruence in therapy.

> The therapist must be constantly aware of his own feelings toward the child and the child's reactions and responses if he is to prevent negative feelings from interfering with the therapeutic process...It would be only human for him to feel frustrated, impatient, or irritated if the child's resistances remain high or progress seems slow. It is difficult, also, not to experience feelings of anger if a child behaves in a particularly hostile way...the therapist cannot convincingly pretend and...there is value in the child's experiencing of the therapists' feelings and reactions. There is a certain realism in this view, but there are dangers too; and in any case, the therapist must continually keep under surveillance on his own needs as well as those of the child if he is to maintain his maximum therapeutic effectiveness.[34]

Therapists frequently give mixed messages when they are giving therapy which they know is essential, but which does not quite agree with their own personal values or ideas. The therapist who is naturally neat and tidy, for example, may react with slight tension and negativism when a group of preschoolers mess up the playroom during their therapy; the therapist who does not like the whining of a child may be inclined to shy away from the child while still trying to ignore the behavior. Admission of the therapist's own feeling to the child is the most honest approach because it shows the child specifically what is aggravating to the therapist instead of letting the child imagine a variety of unrelated factors. "I'm upset because the playroom is messy and I have never liked messiness — but that's my problem, not yours (the children's). Please try to put up with me and my grumpiness."

The expression of honesty affects the development of a consistent and trusting relationship of the therapist by the child. The therapist says, "No, your mommy is not coming to visit today," and then helps the child accept this idea—even though some time may be taken from the primary treatment. He does not say, "Oh, yes she'll come," hoping the child will add the "today" silently and then be cooperative and perform as the therapist desires. Sooner or later the child will realize that the therapist tells him only half-truths.

Being the Adult in the Dyadic Relationship

There are two ways in which the therapist demonstrates his adultness in the dyadic relationships with the child. One is the implicit demonstration of behavior—in which the therapist is the model of the correct behavior. His own behavior models the kind of behavior which he desires the child to learn, without directly demonstrating that behavior for the child. As a model of behavior, the therapist inserts those behaviors which he desires the child to learn; but he does not demand that the child learn them. For example, he eats with a spoon instead of his fingers; he says "thank you" to the child who does something thoughtful for him, and he talks about other people in a pleasant way instead of using a supercritical or condemning manner.

The other is the explicit demonstration of the desirable behavior. The therapist guides the child in the correct behavior by initiating an action for the explicit purpose of teaching the child. For example, the therapist may demonstrate how to tie a shoe, how to hold a paint brush, or how to kick a ball. Implicit and explicit behavioral demonstrations occur concurrently, although one may dominate the therapist's action more than another at any one time.

As another adult behavior model for the child the therapist inadvertantly demonstrates the adult behaviors which a child likes and dislikes, and which he will assimilate or reject. A child, for example, may test the therapist, in order to determine his pliability before accepting his word as law. He may be superficially angered when the therapist has the strength and firmness to set the needed limits on the child — to say "No!." But, internally, if the therapist has proven himself honest and reasonable, the child will accept the limits and perhaps be relieved of the responsibility for making the wrong decision, or for making the decision which he felt was wrong.

In all circumstances — happy and sad — the therapist takes the leadership in maintaining the dyadic relationship. If, for example, the child becomes angry at the therapist for not being willing to change the treatment hour, says he will not come to therapy any more, the therapist does not comply with the child's verbalized threat and goes to get him for the next therapy session anyway. The therapist will not permit the child to regret his behavior, and will not let him dominate therapy when his choices are detrimental to rehabilitation.

The therapist, as an adult teacher and model, limits, guides and redirects the child's behavior. He respects the child's feelings and opinions. When the child is angry and rejects the therapist, the adult understands the child's need to express anger through rejection. However, he does not permit the child to express these feelings or opinions inappropriately through hitting, breaking furniture, injuring himself, or other children in play.

The therapist demonstrates his concern for the child through his assistance to the child. "Assistance" may refer to his physical presence, verbal encouragement, or actual help. The therapist chooses a task within the appropriate level of the child's development, and then lets the child perform independently as much as possible. The therapist does not *baby* the child, but encourages his independence and individuality within the boundaries of his development. It is the therapist's responsibility to assess the necessary limits, to define the child's abilities and make only realistic demands on him.

The therapist presents the child with alternatives in problem solving. Frequently the child's living experience has been limited so that he cannot anticipate all possible choices when he is attempting to make a decision. The adult can lead a child toward behavioral change directly or indirectly, by guiding him in the decision-making process, which includes an explanation or demonstration of the consequences of his choices. A child who is aggressive toward other children may not recognize what triggers his behavior. As he becomes aware of the problem and stops blaming the other children for his behavior, the therapist can suggest alternative ways of interacting with the other children, and can support the child as he initiates them.

The therapist must constantly examine his own attitudes, behaviors, and feelings toward the child so that he does not react blindly to the child's behavior. He is aware of his personal likes and dislikes. He recognizes the differences in dealing with different age groups, for example, and accepts the fact that he prefers to work with adolescents, "who talk," as compared with infants, "who don't do anything." He may work better with groups of children than with individuals, or with males than females, or with children with one kind of a personality instead of another kind of personality. Working with the children whom he prefers is ideal, but learning to deal with the children who do not meet his ideal standards is usually necessary.

The therapist separates his personal standards from those of the culture or society in which the child lives. He works with the child toward changing the child's behavior in the direction which will be most beneficial to him in the environment in which that child must live and function. For example, the culture of the therapist may emphasize that only hard work deserves reward; whereas another culture may teach the children to work as little as possible and enjoy life as much as possible. The therapist may have learned the "manners" of his culture which include "please" and "thank you", holding doors open for adults, and standing when an adult enters the room. None of these behaviors may be reinforced in another culture.

The adult therapist who is married and a parent must examine the feelings and behaviors which he displays to his own children and to the children whom he treats. Sometimes it is easier to be a therapist than a parent; the working day is self-limiting for the therapist. He can "get away" from his patients and relax. However, parents have twenty-four-hour-a-day responsibility, even though the children may be asleep. Parents and children may have different personalities, just as therapists and patients have different personalities. However, it is easier to maintain limits and objectivity when working with patients than when dealing with one's own children, who can exert continuous pressure through the constant daily demands to which parents may "give in." The therapist-parent must remember that it is acceptable to respond differently to his own children than to his patients.

In summary, each adult is as different as each child. Each adult expresses similar feelings and reactions to different children, but expresses them differently from any other adult. Although each adult displays different attitudes and works differently with children, each may be equally as effective. There is no one way to work and behave with children; the basic principles for the adult-child interaction are valid for each therapist, but the individual implementation is unique.

References

1. Langford, W.S. "Physical Illness and Convalescence: Their Meaning to the Child." *Journal of Pediatrics* 33 (1948), pp. 242-250.
2. Langford, W.S. "Physical Illness and Convalescence: Their Meaning to the Child."
3. Freud, Anna. "The Role of Bodily Illness in the Mental Life of Children." *Psychoanalytic Study of the Child* 7 (1952), pp. 69-81; Langford, W.S. "Physical Illness and Convalescence: Their Meaning to the Child"; Blom, G.E. "The Reactions of Hospitalized Children to Illness." *Pediatrics* 22(1958), pp. 590-600; Prugh, D.B., Staub, E.M. Sands, H.H., Kirschbaum, R.M. and Lenihan, E.A. "A Study of the Emotional Reactions of Children and Families to Hospitalization and Illness." *American Journal of Orthopsychiatry* 23(1953), pp. 70-106.
4. Richardson, S.A., et al, "Cultural Uniformity in Reaction to Physical Disabilities." *American Sociological Review* 26(1961), pp. 241-247.
5. Wolff, S. *Children Under Stress* (London: The Penguin Press, 1969).
6. Wright, B.A. *Physical Disability: A Psychological Approach* (New York: Harper and Row, 1960).
7. Wright, B.A. *Physical Disability: A Psychological Approach.*
8. Vernon, D.T.A., Foley, J.M., Sipowitz, R.R., and Schulman, J.L. *The Psychological Responses of Children to Hospitalization and Illness* (Springfield, Illinois: Charles C. Thomas, 1965).
9. Freud, Anna. "The Role of Bodily Illness in the Mental Life of Children"; Blom, G.E. "The Reactions of Hospitalized Children to Illness."
10. Prugh et al. "A Study of the Emotional Reactions of Children and Families to Hospitalization and Illness."
11. Robertson, J. *Young Children in Hospitals* (New York: Basic Books, 1958); Schad, C.J. and Dally, A.T. *Occupational Therapy in Pediatrics: A Student Manual* (Dubuque, Iowa: William C. Brown, 1959); Schaffer, H.R., and Callender, W.M. "Psychologic Effects of Hospitalization in Infancy." *Pediatrics* 24(1959), pp. 528-539.
12. Schad, C.J. and Dally, A.T. *Occupational Therapy in Pediatrics: A Student Manual.*
13. Schad, C.J. and Dally, A.T. *Occupational Therapy in Pediatrics: A Student Manual.*
14. Senn, M.J.E. and Solnit, A.J. *Problems in Child Behavior and Development* (Philadelphia: Lea and Febiger, 1968), p. 235.
15. Mitchell, M.E. *The Child's Attitude to Death* (New York: Schocken Books, 1967).
16. Senn, M.J.E. and Solnit, A.J. *Problems in Child Behavior and Development.*
17. Richmond, J.B. and Waisman, H.A. "Psychologic Aspects of Children with Malignant Diseases." *American Journal of Diseases of Children* 89(1955), pp. 42-47.
18. Vernick, J. and Karon, M. "Who's Afraid of Death on a Leukemia Ward?" *American Journal of Diseases of Children* 109(1965), pp. 393-397.

488

19. Wolff, S. *Children Under Stress.*
20. Schaffer, H.R. and Callender, W.M. "Psychologic Effects of Hospitalization in Infancy."
21. Langford, W.S. "Physical Illness and Convalescence: Their Meaning to the Child."
22. Prugh et al. "A Study of the Emotional Reactions of Children and Families to Hospitalization and Illness."
23. Senn, M.J.E. and Solnit, A.J. *Problems in Child Behavior and Development.*
24. Blom, G.E. "The Reactions of Hospitalized Children to Illness."
25. Freud, Anna. "The Role of Bodily Illness in the Mental Life of Children."
26. Rie, H.E., Boverman, H., Ozoa, N., and Grossman, B.J. "Tutoring and Ventilation: A Pilot Study of Reactions of Hospitalized Children." *Clinical Pediatrics* 3(1964), pp. 581-586.
27. Vernick, J. and Karon, M. "Who's Afraid of Death on a Leukemia Ward?"
28. Prugh et al. "A Study of the Emotional Reactions of Children and Families to Hospitalization and Illness."
29. Petrillo, M. "Preventing Hospital Trauma in Pediatric Patients." *American Journal of Nursing* 68(1968), pp. 1468-1473.
30. Blom, G.E. "The Reactions of Hospitalized Children to Illness."
31. Freud, Anna. "The Role of Bodily Illness in the Mental Life of Children."
32. Axline, V.M. *Play Therapy,* Revised edition (New York: Ballantine Books, 1969), p. 16.
33. Sheimo, S.L. "Problems Encountered in Dealing with Handicapped and Emotionally Disturbed Children." *American Journal of Occupational Therapy* 3(1949), p. 303.
34. Shirley, H.F. *Pediatric Psychiatry* (Cambridge, Mass.: Harvard University Press, 1963), p. 771.

Bibliography

Blake, F.G. *The Child, His Parents and the Nurse* (Philadelphia: J.B. Lippincott, 1954).

Bosselman, B.C., Rosenthal, I.M., and Schwarz, M. *Introduction to Developmental Psychiatry* (Springfield, Illinois: Charles C. Thomas, 1965).

Bullard, D.M. "The Response of the Child to Chronic Physical Disability." In Hislop, H.J. and Sanger, J.O. (eds.) *Chest Disorders in Children* (New York: American Physical Therapy Association, 1968).

Calef, V. "Psychological Consequences of Physical Illness in Childhood." *Journal of the American Psycho-Analytic Association* 7(1959), pp. 155-162.

Gillham, H.L. *Helping Children Accept Themselves and Others* (New York: Columbia University Teachers College Bureau of Publications, 1959).

Langford, P.A., Giodesen, A. and Glaser, H.H. "Let's Play Hospital: A Directed Hospital-Play Program for Children with Chronic Pulmonary Disease." In Hislop, H.J. and Sanger, J.O. (eds.) *Chest Disorders in Children* (New York: American Physical Therapy Association, 1968).

Langford, W.S. "The Child in the Pediatric Hospital: Adaptation to Illness and Hospitalization." *American Journal of Orthopsychiatry* 31 (1961), pp. 667-684.

Murphy, L.B. *The Widening World of Childhood* (New York: Basic Books, 1962).

Plank, E.H. *Working With Children in Hospitals* (Cleveland, Ohio: Western Reserve University Press, 1962).

Reed, A.W. "Problems of Impending Death." In Hislop, H.J. and Sanger, J.O. (eds.) *Chest Disorders in Children* (New York: American Physical Therapy Association, 1968).

Richardson, S.A. "The Handicapped Child: Social Obstacles to Growing Up." In *The Social and Emotional Needs of the Handicapped Child* (Waltham, Mass.: The Florence Heller Research Center, Brandeis University, 1965).

Richmond, J.B. "Behavior, Occupation and Treatment." *American Journal of Occupational Therapy* 14 (1960), pp. 183-186.

Spock, B. and Lerrigo, M.O. *Caring for Your Disabled Child* (New York: Fawcett, 1967).

Weston, D.L. and Irwin, R.C. "Preschool Child's Response to Death of Infant Sibling." *American Journal of Diseases of Children* 106(1963), pp. 564-567.

NOTES

Chapter Ten

Health Care for Children

Barbara Sharpe Banus, M. A., O.T.R.

(April 1971)

The first nine chapters of this text explored child development theories and practices in relation to occupational therapy in pediatrics. It is now necessary to explore occupational therapy in relation to other health care practices, for the occupational therapist never functions in isolation.

HEALTH NEEDS OF CHILDREN TODAY

As adults we have the responsibility of providing children with the best health care available. According to Richmond and Weinberger,[1] however, our society is delinquent in meeting this objective. They have described the kinds of changes which need to be made in the society and in health services to help our children develop to their fullest potentials. All of the services reflect the efficacy of prevention which will decrease the need for the treatment of acute and chronic disease and disability.

1. The environments in which children live need to be improved in order to give them the personal opportunity to grow and develop. There are problems in the areas of housing, nutrition, welfare, education and so forth which need to be solved.
2. Children deserve to participate in planned developmental programs or to have informal developmental experiences as infants and young children, particularly those children in low socioeconomic groups.
3. Programs which will lead to the prevention of accidents need to be developed, since accidents are one of the primary causes of death in children.
4. Children need more and better dental care; poor dental care is the health problem most frequently encountered.
5. More attention needs to be focused upon the influence of children's psychological reactions on their learning. Correlated with this is the need for measures to prevent the development of psychological problems and the need for therapeutic resources to decrease and correct problems.

6. Better visual and auditory screening tests need to be made available to all children in the early years, since visual and auditory defects in the school years often lead to problems in learning.

From this brief review, it is evident that both intrinsic and extrinsic factors affect a child's health and, therefore, his development to potential. The dominant question is: how can all these needs be met, considering (1) the dearth of health care and educational personnel, (2) the shortage of available health care facilities and (3) the exhorbitant cost of health care?

TRADITIONAL HEALTH CARE PRACTICES
THAT DO NOT MEET
THE CONTEMPORARY NEEDS OF CHILDREN

When one thinks about today's typical health care, some traditional visual images come to mind. I see pediatricians in their comfortable offices in suburban communities and pediatricians in generally bleak hospital pediatric clinics in rural communities or inner cities. I visualize the treatment or rehabilitation team in the hospital, on the wards or in a specific hospital department, such as the occupational therapist who treats one patient every half hour within the walls of the occupational therapy department. I also visualize some of the finer details, such as the starched white uniforms which many of the hospital staff wear, the bleak faces of the children as they wait to see their families during the restricted visiting hours, and, finally, the team meeting which is presided over by the pediatrician or child psychiatrist.

The team meeting is an institution in itself. All of the appropriate staff are represented at the team meeting, during which each one discusses the problems of the child from his own point of view. From the collective information, the physician makes the final decision about the diagnosis, treatment or disposition of the child. He later communicates the decisions to the parents, at the same time maintaining communication with the staff who are working with the child.

In other words, *team* refers to the people who work together to effect the child's treatment. Traditionally, the pediatrician was head of the team in the pediatric medical setting and the child psychiatrist was the team leader in the child psychiatric setting. Each health care professional reported the findings of his evaluation to the physician and received his orders or prescription from the physician for the treatment of the child. As Beloff and

Willet have noted, the physician was the captain of the team in all decisions and all health care workers were subordinate to him and his decisions.[2]

Traditionally, the pediatrician has multiple responsibilities toward the children in his community. His primary task is to supervise the health of children for the purpose of helping them to reach their full developmental potential. The pediatrician may help to prepare the mother for her newborn child by discussing prenatal and postnatal care with her. Following the infant's birth, he practices preventive medicine through supervisory health examinations of the child from infancy through adolescence. The pediatrician coordinates health care personnel who care for a child with an acute or chronic illness. He serves as a community resource for parents who seek his assistance with problems which may affect the physical, mental or emotional life of their children.[3,4] The variety of these tasks show the range of the pediatrician's responsibilities. One might wonder how any pediatrician can respond to each of these needs for all of his patients.

Problems evolved in the traditional medical model as the evaluation and treatment procedures of each profession became more complex. It became difficult for the physician to prescribe the specific treatment to be performed by the physical therapist, occupational therapist, speech clinician and so forth. The physician has his own time-consuming responsibilities and cannot keep abreast of all the new developments in each profession and, therefore, cannot always prescribe the best procedures.

In addition, the number of physicians, both medical and psychiatric, does not begin to match the number of individuals needing health care services. There were approximately 16.3 pediatricians and 135 general practioners per 100,000 children under fifteen years of age in 1961. This means that only 151 physicians cared for every 100,000 children in 1961.[1] These statistics are even worse than they appear because there was a gradual *decrease* in the overall number of physicians who cared for children during the twenty years before 1960. One can easily project the inadequacy of medical services for children in the 1960-1980 period if this trend continues. In addition, the majority of pediatricians practice in suburban areas, few move to rural communities and many have been leaving the inner city. (One also wonders if the pattern of pediatricians, in terms of changing location of practice, is paralleled by the ancillary health practitioners). *Consequently, the one-fourth of this country's children who live in poverty do not receive even adequate medical services.*[1] If the traditional team approach is maintained, in which the physician must personally supervise all medical services, these children may not receive any health care.

Other problems developed with the traditional team concept in which the pediatrician was "the leader." First, this practice tended to downgrade the potential assets of the other team members. Strong professional identities which have been negatively stereotyped through the years overshadow the newer professional concepts and personal assets which may be beneficial to the team concept. For example, in the traditional setting *only* the pediatrician can head the medical-rehabilitation team; *only* the psychologist can give psychological tests; *only* the psychiatrist can perform psychotherapy; *only* the physical therapist can use neuromuscular facilitation techniques. If the professional health care worker is influenced by these stereotypes, he immediately limits his own development. He does not expand his own abilities (or expect other professionals to expand theirs) in the direction toward which he is best suited or in a direction which could lead to solving the problems of children.

With this stereotyping of professional responsibilities, other problems can arise. Theoretically, only the physician and social worker may be delegated to communicate with parents. Today this is an unrealistic requirement because of the numbers of children who are examined by each physician. On the other hand, if each of the professionals does talk with parents and does communicate his testing results or recommendations to them, problems are created. Grossman suggests that the traditional team approach is "totally antitherapeutic" for the child and his family because a family with a sick or handicapped child needs *one person* with whom it can communicate and through whom it can maintain contact with the other health care services.[5] The physician who, ideally and historically, has held this responsibility seldom has adequate time to be liaison for each of his many clients. Families and children need one person who listens to their needs, who is interested and concerned with them, who helps them obtain the needed services and, most important, who maintains *human* contact. The absence of this sensitive person is often a large part of the family's problem.

Other problems evolve through the traditional treatment of the child in the hospital. As we have discussed in Chapter Nine, the hospital is very unhealthy for a child's emotional life. Many times it is actually physically unhealthy as well, because of the rapid spread of infections. And, finally, most parents cannot afford the cost of hospitalization, treatment in the hospital and individual services over an extended time.

Traditionally, the child from suburbia visits his own pediatrician in the office. The child from the inner city poverty areas, however, attends a pediatric clinic—where he may have to wait as much as five or six hours for his examination by a physician, who may differ with each visit. In either situation this traditional practice is unsatisfactory. The child's doctor has very limited time to talk with families and to help work out ordinary problems with the parent and child. He has even less time to follow up his recommendations for treatment (Is the mother giving the child the correct dosage of medication? Are the parents supervising the child's new diet?). Consequently, health needs are being met only by those children and families who have the money and/or the incentive to seek medical help and those families who then follow that medical advice.

TRENDS INDICATING CHANGE IN
TRADITIONAL HEALTH PRACTICES

Looking at these three traditional units of health care, one can project some of the needed changes. The physician should not automatically be allocated the leadership of the health care team; the team's functions need to be better coordinated in order to provide total services while preventing duplication of services; and treatment should be made available outside of hospital facilities. The objectives for health care services must be reviewed and the means for meeting them must be revised. The objectives are to maintain health, to prevent illness and disability and/or to diagnose and treat disease and disability. Diagnosis and treatment of disease and disability have been the usual and recognized practices of most of the health care professions and need little explanation. Prevention, on the other hand, was the responsibility of departments of public health until recently. With increased emphasis on prevention, however, there will be a decreased need for traditional medical services. Currently, a shift has been initiated from:

...medical to health concern, from problems of treatment to methods of prevention. Although this shift is still incomplete, there are increasing signs of its being a progressive one. Furthermore it appears inevitable if we examine the rationale and forces behind it. We must, for example, recognize that our traditional approach to disease and disability has provided only episodic care for acute-, severe- or emergency-type illness. Though occasional preventive health services such as immunizations and x-rays have been made avilable to some, the great majority of people have no continuing contact with any single medical resource. Thus they represent an unenlightened and indigent population from the medical viewpoint. What is clearly needed, in the preventive versus treatment approach, in the new accent on health versus disease, is comprehensive and quality care in which there is emphasis on maintaining optimum health rather than on intermittent treatment of acute disease and disability.

In order to implement this new focus on health maintenance, then, we are moving into a setting that is relatively new for most of us in the health-related professions. Although the public health physician, the general practitioner and the visiting nurse have traditionally served patients in their homes, in schools or in other community-centered facilities, most of us in the supporting professions have more frequently functioned in the highly structured setting of the hospital. The current shift in the center of gravity from the acute disease hospital to the community health center will necessarily shift our setting from the conventional medical complex to neighborhood service centers in which health activities are a part. In these comprehensive centers, health, education and welfare programs being developed will include units which support each other while maintaining autonomy of action to permit maximum achievement in their respective areas of interest and competence.

Health and medical care in the future, then, will emphasize *human development* (editor's italics) by programs designed to promote better adaptation, rather than by technologically oriented programs offering specific solutions to specific difficulties. The latter will always be seen as a part, although hopefully a diminishingly important part, of a health program...[6]

Richmond and Weinberger[1] have described this same concept of changing health care by stating that the *medical center* will focus on disease and periodic care through diagnostic clinics and research-education hospitals; whereas the *community health centers,* which focus on prevention and continuing comprehensive family care, will provide service through ambulatory health centers and community hospitals. It is recognized that the care of the acute patient is still an important part of treatment. For example, burn patients will continue to need medical care in hospitals and will need rehabilitative services during the acute stages of the disability. However, even the burn patient needs to return to his family sooner and receive more home care.

Prevention begins at or before pregnancy (genetic counseling, for example), at which time the mother receives information on nutrition, infant care, and so forth. Postnatally, the parents are informed of good child health practices which include the need for a good external environment in which to live, good developmental experiences, dental care, prevention of accidents and so forth.

Comprehensive and Coordinated Health Care

Comprehensive and coordinated health care is one of the suggested means for meeting these health needs. *Coordinated health care* refers to the central administration of a program from which the planning, evaluation and treatment services are disseminated.[7] It means that the team makes the plan for the coordination of the health care services and collaboratively executes the needed health care. A coordinated health care unit, for example, might be located in a community service agency in the inner city. The administrators and community workers, such as social workers, occupational therapists, nurses and physical therapists, would have offices at this central location where they would coordinate the planning and communication with the community and from which they would disperse into the community. Or, the center for coordination might be in a local hospital, outpatient clinic or other public health facility.

Comprehensive is the complement to coordinated health care and is the most vital unit of the combination. Comprehensive health care adds a new dimension to health services because it requires that *all* necessary services be made available to people who need them. This is ideal. More often than not, however, it is not implemented because there is not adequate financial backing to support all the prime personnel. In addition, the area within the designated boundaries, such as the inner city, may not be a popular place in which to work. Although comprehensive health care is ideal, it is usually very limited in the inner city or rural community. Instead, the community may have only physicians, social workers and public health nurses. Either the family or the health care workers may have to travel long distances to receive or provide extensive or specialized health care. If the community is fortunate, it may have a regular clinic, such as a monthly pediatric clinic for children. Specialists, such as physical therapists and orthopedists, may attend the clinic periodically and provide diagnostic evaluations and follow-up treatment. However, the sporadic nature of the clinic can never meet all the daily needs.

Roth[7] describes one approach to comprehensive, coordinated health care — coordinated and comprehensive home care. (The program serves families in Erie County in New York State.) Roth discusses the interdisciplinary team approach which may be coordinated by a central agency, but recognizes that although it is coordinated, it is often not comprehensive in the services which it offers. In this case, health personnel either have to substitute services or omit them. The value of overlapping knowledge and skills quickly becomes apparent. This demonstrates the need for pediatric health care personnel to have some knowledge about all facets of development, prevention, evaluation and treatment; to have consulting services available as resources; and to have the opportunity for continuing education in the needed areas. For example, the physical therapist may need additional training in nutrition so he can provide basic information on nutrition; the occupational therapist may have to serve the dual function of therapist and social worker for which he has to gain additional training in counseling; or the nurse may need to learn some of the physical therapist's skills.

If the comprehensive and coordinated health services programs followed the traditional model, the physician would have the responsibility for the planning, execution and coordination of all the services. However, in the model suggested by Roth, the coordinator differs for each family. This suggests a more realistic use of all available personnel. If for no other reason, the quantities of families requiring services make it impossible for one individual (the physician) or a small group of individuals to coordinate the overall planning for the program and the individual family care.

The Coordinator

The person who has the primary responsibility for coordinating all of the health care services for a specific child might be described as *coordinator of health care services* or *coordinator of therapies.* His qualifications should be based on his personal and professional skills in working with families or people, not on his professional title. The coordinator might vary for each family, since different families may trust one professional more than another and vice versa — there *must* be mutual trust. The coordinator would be responsible for the child and his family within the realm of health care. He would make the contacts with the other services and take the family and child to meet the people within these services; he would prepare the family for the experiences they would encounter in the world of health care, in much the same way that the family and health care personnel prepare the child for medical procedures (see Chapter Nine). He would also prepare the providers of service, such as the therapists and physicians, for the child. This procedure would have the additional benefit of eliminating the repetitious taking of case histories. Grossman [5] describes this approach to health care as a much more "humanizing experience" for both parents and child.

The team function varies somewhat as a result of the coordinator's function. The physician is no longer automatically the captain of the team; the person who is now responsible for the overall care of the child is the captain of that child's team. The team functions in order to *communicate* information concerning the child, rather than to pass the child through a series of individuals who will automatically evaluate and treat him — it is the coordinator's responsibility to decrease excessive manipulation of the child. The coordinator serves as the liaison between the family and the other team members who provide services for the child.

The value of this kind of coordinator was illustrated with a family who was very dissatisfied with the visual-perceptual-motor training their child was receiving because treatment frequency was only once a week. Instead of "bothering" their physician, who was "too busy," they contacted and were accepted at another hospital clinic in a nearby community where their child could be treated daily. Meanwhile, the child continued his weekly treatment at the original clinic. If the coordinator of the child's team had been someone other than the overworked physician and someone whom the parents trusted, the parents probably would have felt comfortable in saying to the coordinator "Our child needs more visual-perceptual-motor training. What can we do?" Then an assessment of the real needs, both the parents' and the child's, could have been made and changes implemented, if necessary, which would have been more appropriate in terms of time and money for both the family and the therapists.

There is another coordinator position which differs in responsibilities from the position of coordinator of health care services for the child. This is the person or administrator who is responsible for the coordination of the total program for many children. The responsibilities of this coordinator vary (depending upon the institution for which he works), but continue to focus primarily on communication. The communication may be with state representatives and senators in order to obtain favorable legislation for the program. It may be with people or agencies who will support the program financially. Or, it may be with other members of the team as they need help in communicating with one another. One system of coordination has been worked out at the Handicapped Children's Preschool (described later in the chapter). The Project Director, who is nominally the head of the preschool, defines her major responsibilities in the areas of working for legislative support of preschools for handicapped children, financial support and education of the public. Two other professionals are responsible for the day-to-day function of the preschool. The Educational Director is responsible for planning and coordinating everything that happens within the context of the preschool classroom. The Program Coordinator/Evaluator is responsible for all parts of the program which are not directly related to the classroom. Together the Educational Director and Program Coordinator/Evaluator work to resolve mutual problems and serve as feedback systems for each other, but are then independently responsible for coordinating their own units of responsibility.

A SUGGESTED HEALTH CARE MODEL

Having suggested that (1) coordinated and comprehensive health care is necessary to provide adequate services for children and that (2) the coordinator of the team should be chosen according to the needs of the specific family, we must now consider the ways in which the health care team can function as a unit to provide services most effectively and efficiently.

Johnson [8] suggested a working model for the interaction among health care professions which she described as *complementary* or *synergistic*. She designed a model of sequential educational experiences and information sharing for undergraduate students in the health professions to give them a more common background and understanding of their own roles as well as those of others. She suggests that this synergistic model is more effective than a model which combines all of the "fragmented" professions (occupational therapy, physical therapy, speech therapy and so forth) into a single specialty or a model in which all students have a common core curriculum at the university level from which they develop the same or very similar professional knowledges. Although this model was developed for students, it suggests a framework for the development of a working relationship among the practicing health care workers.

Johnson describes the synergistic relationship as the "complementary relationship of organisms in which one supports the others in mutual action toward a common goal, thereby producing a result greater than any organism could attain alone.'

In other words, each developmental therapist who works with children has a common baseline of knowledge and skill, but has a specialty area of knowledge which complements the specialty knowledge of others. The development of the synergistic relationship among staff members is one of the goals of the Handicapped Children's Preschool in Roxbury, Massachusetts. Within the classroom structure there are approximately twenty-five physically handicapped children between three and seven years of age, one educational director, two teachers, three assistant teachers, one physical therapist, one occupational therapist and one speech therapist. All teachers and therapists work together with the children in the classroom. The basic routine for the preschool day is organized to meet the general developmental needs of preschoolers through developmental stimulation. Therapy for each child is inserted into this routine as needed by a particular child.

Each developmental therapist (teachers and therapists) comes to the preschool with a specific knowledge base, the practice of which he transmits to the other staff. As a result, the staff members complement and supplement each other in their work with the children. This approach to education and therapy is thought to be vital to the preschool's success and to the children's and staff's development. For example, because there is only one physical therapist, it is impossible for her to perform all the physical therapy daily for each child who needs it. It is also doubtful that the physical therapist is the only one capable of performing this function, provided that she supervises the other preschool staff in the therapeutic techniques. The physical therapist has the knowledge base from which she assesses the child's needs and plans the treatment. She then teaches the other developmental therapists how to incorporate healthy neuromotor patterns into their work with the children and how to perform some of the specific therapeutic techniques. The speech clinician performs a similar function in her work with the children. She evaluates and works with the children who show speech pathology while, at the same time, she teaches the other staff how to stimulate healthy speech patterns. In other words, each specialist is a technologist in his developmental specialty, but is a technician in the application of therapy/education of the other specialty areas.

In this setting, the synergistic relationships need not evolve entirely from the formal educational backgrounds of the preschool staff. As the staff's interests change and develop, they are encouraged to explore new areas and to transmit their newly acquired knowledge to the others. One staff member, for example, may become intrigued with the cognitive theory of Jean Piaget and none of the staff may be familiar with this theory. The individual who studies the theory (formally, through a university course, or informally) then describes it and suggests the implications for its use to the other staff and helps them incorporate Piaget's ideas into their own practices.

Only through the synergistic relationship can the preschool program function within the developmental framework, for therapy is incorporated into the classroom activity as much as possible and is made available to the child when he is ready for it. If each child was scheduled for treatment at a specific half hour each day, the time at which he would receive the therapy would not necessarily be his optimum performance time. Developmental therapy in the area of communication might be very successfully handled by a particular child during rest hour when he is ready to be physically quiet, but mentally and verbally active. Neuromotor developmental therapy for the lower extremities might be received best when the child is tired of sitting still — this cannot always be scheduled! Development of self-care behaviors is most successful when the child is motivated to perform a task — when he needs to use the toilet, when he arrives at school and must take off his coat, when he is eating lunch, and so forth. Because of the variables in each child's daily needs and the number of children that have the same needs at the same time, no one therapist can exclusively handle therapy/education in his particular domain. He must share his knowledge and experience with the other staff.

Other possible synergistic combinations of developmental therapists are multiple and are based upon the needs of the population to be served and the availability of personnel. The latter is exemplified by the team of the pediatrician and nurse-practitioner which has evolved from the need to provide more children with more efficient medical care. Pediatric office nurses who take on the role of nurse-practitioner are providing patient-centered services. These require patient care decisions, primarily in the area of preventive pediatrics, instead of clerical, technical and administrative tasks which are traditional for office nurses. The service functions include taking the child's history, examining children routinely as part of preventive pediatrics, responding to parents' telephone inquiries, and contacting the community agencies which can provide a family with needed services. When the child becomes ill, the nurse-practitioner visits the child at his home or the hospital and assists in the management of his illness after the physician has made the diagnosis and has prescribed treatment.[3,10] In other words, the pediatrician and nurse-practioner work as a team in which the nurse-practitioner, under the pediatrician's supervision, assumes increasing responsibility for prevention and health education. This relieves the pediatrician of some of his less exacting and more routine responsibilities.

Beloff and Willet [2] described an innovative team approach which took into consideration the needs of both the inner city population to be served and the lack of health care manpower. The goal of the team was to serve more people more effectively and efficiently by using the manpower of third- and fourth-year medical students, public health nurses, neighborhood health aides and available consultants such as social workers, psychiatrists and nutritionists. It is interesting to note that the public health nurses were the only traditional members of the medical team. The medical students provided needed medical services while at the same time benefiting from a real and, therefore, meaningful learning experience. The neighborhood health aides (sometimes called community workers or something similar) provided the team with knowledge of the community which was vital to the acceptance and, therefore, the function of the program. In this project the health aides were responsible for many of the project details, such as transportation arrangements for the patients and follow-up appointments for families seeking new housing.

Although in title this formed a team, Beloff and Willet found that the group was composed of individuals who had problems overcoming the stereotyped barriers and dividing task assignments. The problems that arose were primarily the result of traditional role concepts. These conflicts were resolved gradually through the collaboration of the team. As each member began to understand and accept the contributions of the others and to understand his own contributions, true teamwork evolved. This clearly demonstrates the traditional hangups which adversely affect innovative health care.

Health care teams may use a physician only as a consultant to the team, particularly in the area of health education and prevention. For example, as part of prevention, a team of an early childhood educator, occupational therapist, physical therapist and speech clinician could compile their individual knowledges about child development into a screening test to identify developmental delay and dysfunction in preschool children. As a part of health education and prevention, a public health team might consist of a nurse, social worker and nutritionist. Their responsibilities might include visiting new mothers in their homes to help them care for themselves and their infants. Each of the team members would learn enough of the other members' skills to be able to recommend treatment or to refer the families to other health services.

When all developmental therapists have a broad knowledge of child development and health, as implied in the above examples, a single evaluation can be performed by a variety of health care workers. Once the general evaluation is completed, the developmental therapist who has the most knowledge concerning the child's problem in the particular area can do more in-depth testing and follow-up treatment. For example, a developmental team of a pediatric nurse, occupational therapist, physical therapist and special educator could each acquaint themselves with a specific formal or informal evaluation. Instead of each one evaluating the same four children within the area of his specialty, each could evaluate one of the children totally and make referrals for more in-depth evaluation to the others.

Because the synergistic team combination differs from the traditional model of the medical team, the head of which is the physician, the change from the traditional medical model is natural. With the change from a group of individuals who work subordinately to the physician, to a group who work parallel and cooperatively with him and each other, the potential for the "captain of the team" changes. No one professional dominates the others because none is all-knowledgable about the needs of children. In addition, with more of the health care services being performed outside of the hospital clinics and wards, the physician is less conspicuous and less involved in the child's daily program. Therefore, it is not realistic for him to remain captain of the treatment team. On the other hand, if the child has an acute exacerbation of his illness, the physician does become the dominant member of the health care team during the acute stages of the disease.

Within the context of the synergistic relationship, the team member with primary care responsibilities for the child is the coordinator of the child's team. The responsibility might rotate as the primary provider of care changes. For example, during the acute stages of illness, the physician would have primary responsibility; during rehabilitation, the therapist who has most contact with the child and is most comfortable with the child and parents might have primary responsibility. The coordinator of care responsibilities could conceivably shift between these two people if the health and treatment of the child fluctuates.

THE OCCUPATIONAL THERAPIST AS A MEMBER OF THE HEALTH CARE TEAM

The Professional Responsibilities

The content of the occupational therapist's knowledge and his experience primarily determine the occupational therapist's job responsibilities. However, the *way* in which he uses his knowledge and experience is significant because of the limited number of practicing occupational therapists. Occupational therapists must work to potential and not become encumbered with tasks that other personnel who have less training can do as effectively, or with tasks that other professionals who have equal or more training can do better. West [11] suggests four significant functions for the occupational therapist of tomorrow in community health care with a diversified patient population. These include evaluator, consultant, supervisor and researcher.

Many new graduates initially respond to the responsibilities described in those titles with "But I want to work with the child!" The role of the evaluator directly implies this function and, as a matter of fact, none of the titles negates the possibility of direct child-therapist interaction. I believe that the therapist who holds any of these four positions should maintain at least periodic contact with the people whom he is serving. Otherwise, he may become less aware of the real needs of the people for whom he is planning. He also may become less understanding of and less sympathetic toward the real problems which his staff is experiencing.

The task of *evaluator* is not new to the reader of this text. This is an assumed requirement for each developmental therapist. An evaluator may use any of the assessment procedures suggested in Chapter Two — informal, formal, standardized, group or individual. Evaluation may be his only task or it may be combined with treatment. West's statement about the role of evaluation summarizes the functions which have been described at different points throughout the text:

> ...it is in this role (evaluator) that some of the current developments promise so much for our future. I refer particularly to the increasing number of instances in which occupational therapists join physicians and other members of the health team in appraising the nature of disability and determining the range and level of functioning abilities. In addition, they share the responsibility for making recommendations regarding future plans. In these kinds of roles, members of our profession are gaining new respect and recognition for contributions they can make to diagnosis and to programming as well as to the treatment process itself. [12]

West's statement reinforces the concept of comprehensive and coordinated team function to which each developmental therapist adds his particular skills. Diagnosis, programming and planning for the future are the professional elements within the therapeutic process. The actual treatment procedure can be performed by a semiprofessional person under the guidance of the qualified person.

Evaluation of a total program is as essential as the evaluation of the child for, unless the overall program is functioning effectively, the parts of it — child evaluation and treatment — probably will not meet the desired standards or objectives. For example, if the evaluation tools or treatment materials are not adequate, it is doubtful that the child will receive adequate evaluation or treatment. If the physical facility in which treatment is performed is poorly arranged or overcrowded, it may interfere with the child's treatment. Or, if there is poor communication among the staff, the child's evaluation and treatment may not be maximized because it is not well coordinated. All these factors must be evaluated regularly.

"Accountability," which is the current word to describe the responsibility of a program to the funding agency, also is one of the reasons for evaluation. The usefulness and value of the program must be objectively evaluated whether it is a rehabilitation clinic, preschool, well-baby clinic or other facility. This procedure for evaluation is similar to that which was described in Chapter Three, but is expanded to cover the overall program.

West's concept of the *consultant* is similar to some of the functions of the developmental therapist which have already been described. This position includes consultation among occupational therapists within their own professions and consultation with members of the other professions or with other developmental therapists. The reasons for this are ". . . intimately related to our appalling paucity of numbers and to our failure, generically, to multiply, but it is even more closely tied in with the public health aspect of twentieth century medicine." [13] West further describes the multiple settings in which professional health care workers are found and the reasons for their developing good communications among themselves:

> They are serving in diagnostic and evaluation clinics, in schools or neighborhood facilities of various kinds. They travel with mobile units to rural areas and smaller urban communities that do not have the resources of the big city. They go individually into patients' homes and help parents and families carry out prescribed routines. They staff university-affiliated centers where patients are seen by specialists in every branch of medicine and the health-related professions.

But regardless of the specific locale in which they work, they are involved with increasingly complex kinds of disabilities — emotional as well as physical — and they are incorporating more of the supporting professions into their multidisciplinary teams. Each of them is advising, counseling, supervising and in other ways serving as a consultant to his professional colleagues, to teachers, to assistants, aides and attendants, to lay people, and to families who carry out the actual patient treatment or training.

The concept of the occupational therapy consultant has received increasing attention since 1967 and today is an essential part of the responsibilities of the occupational therapist. All developmental therapists must be consultants for each other, for no one developmental therapist knows everything about a child's behavior and it is unfair to the child to divide him into segments for treatment.

The role of *supervisor* is a natural outgrowth of learning and experience. Some therapists dislike the position because the administrative and teaching requirements, which usually accompany it, may eliminate patient contact. Work with patients is "second hand" if the supervising therapist teaches or directs students and staff only through verbal communication with no patient contact. On the other hand, a demonstration (or series of demonstrations) in which the therapist interacts with the child is the most effective supervision. For many therapists, this interaction is also the most gratifying part of supervision.

The supervisor also has the primary responsibility of analyzing and critiquing the program which he administers, according to West:

A profession exists not only to provide a service but to look at where that service fails or could be improved, to find new ways to do its work better, and to reduce selected elements to a technical level for accomplishment by less highly trained personnel.

If we (occupational therapists) are to evidence the integrity of the true professional, we must give every job to be done to the least trained person who can adequately perform it, even if this means that some functions traditionally reserved for highly trained (and often over-trained) persons will now be done by someone with less training. Freeing highly trained persons from trivia will permit them to assume appropriate consultative and supervisory functions and maximize the effective use of their experience and expertise.[14]

Although developmental therapists should, and frequently do, function as supervisors, they are not usually described in this way. Whenever a therapist teaches parents, staff or students how to treat a child, he is technically a supervisor. One of the objectives for health care personnel is to teach parents how to care for their own child. This is important financially for the family, developmentally for the child, and psychologically for the parent. In the role of supervisor, the therapist performs the functions of a technologist and problem-definer, while the parent is the direct provider of services.

Research is a fairly recent and very important addition to the responsibilities of the occupational therapist. It is gaining importance as therapists begin to recognize discrepancies in behavior between their observations in practice and reports in the literature. Some developmental therapists are doing research to substantiate theory; others are doing research to validate their observations.

Experimental research enables the developmental therapist to test ideas. This research need not be formidable. A small patient group may be used to validate a hypothesis. If the results are significant, a pilot study or formal research project may be initiated. For example, it might be useful to determine how many health care workers actually contact children upon their admission to a hospital; or to determine which health care workers are most trusted by parents; or to determine what procedures are performed by whom in a community or outpatient clinic and how many of these procedures are repetitive. Through the collection of data, changes which are advantageous to the children can be suggested — and respected because of the concrete evidence which supports the idea.

There is also library research through which inventories of the available research can be made, evaluated, applied to practice and re-evaluated. Too often good data lie dormant in the libraries because "There isn't *time* to go to the library." If the therapist is attempting to update his knowledge and skills, this statement is not valid. Robert Coles [15] (Albee, 1968) suggests that most of what needs to be known about the fears and anxieties caused by life itself is already known in terms of the causes and resulting psychodynamics of mental illness, but that it is rediscovered annually. Instead of moving forward and applying known principles to the care of the mentally ill, people remain at a standstill while further experimentation is continued. There is some relationship between this occurrence in psychiatry and pediatrics. Much is known about the prevention of children's disease and disability, but in many communities nothing is being done about it. Library research helps resolve the questions of the needs and often suggests means of prevention and treatment. Many recent health journals are emphasizing the health needs of American communities, the ways in which health care teams might be used in specific communities and the problems generated by the use of the team. Information is available to the developmental therapist who is committed to improving his services.

The developmental therapist must make a choice. Do I treat many children according to information on development, evaluation and treatment which I learned in the past and which may be out of date? Do I explore new information which is coming out in recent updated journals, compare it with past knowledge and apply it to my practice? Or, do I work with fewer children, collect data on their behavior and then take the necessary time to write up the research results which will update the literature and eventually help more children? The last two challenges are the only acceptable ones in this day of change.

The Places in Which the Occupational Therapist Can Work

Occupational therapists can work with children in many different situations. Goals can range from the traditional tasks of rehabilitation to maintenance, which prevents further disability while stimulating further development, to true prevention. Wiemer [16] described the continuum of health: wellness...latent illness...subclinical illness...clinical illness...and transience. Parallel to this, she proposed a continuum of prevention: promotion...protection...identification...correction...accommodation. Wiemer suggested that too often therapists work with people *after* they become ill (in the areas of correction and accommodation), instead of working to prevent their illnesses and dysfunctions. Accordingly, she suggests that occupational therapists work toward the promotion and protection ends of the continuum.

Typically, the occupational therapist emphasizes correction and accommodation by performing evaluation and treatment for acute and chronically ill patients within the hospital or clinic setting. Because this is the most common treatment setting and the best understood function, it will be pursued only to suggest new uses for pediatric outpatient clinics. *Outpatient pediatric clinics,* which are always resources for the parents of handicapped and nonhandicapped children, can be used more effectively. The therapist has a natural affiliation with the child both at times of his health and illness and thus can maintain continuity in developmental experiences in both circumstances. In the area of prevention, the occupational therapist can evaluate every child's development regularly. They can then maintain a close contact with the children who are hospitalized to receive treatment for acute exacerbations of the illness, surgery and other interventions. This, in turn, prevents the termination of developmental experiences upon hospital or institutional admission (see Chapter Nine).

The pediatric clinic also can provide a setting in which natural play groups can be developed as the children wait for their appointments with the pediatrician. Although the groups constantly change during the clinic day, the child's behavior can be observed in a social situation, even though the clinic is sometimes distracting and stressful. In addition, the parent-child interaction can be observed. This information supplements formal screening tests or other evaluations, even though the behavior is observed in a setting unknown to the child.

Anne Morris, an OTR at Mount Sinai Hospital in New York City, is using the pediatric clinic in another way: to teach mothers how to foster development in their preschool children. Her hypothesis is that parents are the key to a child's preschool education and that the pediatric clinic is a natural place to demonstrate suitable children's toys for them, teach them how to use them and sometimes lend them to the family (this might be described as a toy library). Morris decided to teach the parents about developmental play, instead of the children, because she recognized the parents' desire to help their own children.[17]

In the midposition on the continuum of goals for the occupational therapist is maintenance. This includes stimulating development while preventing further disability. Maintenance functions are found in home treatment programs for handicapped children in which parents are shown the tasks for stimulating development and the techniques for preventing further dysfunction, such as correct positioning to prevent deformity.

Maintenance is also found in preschool programs for handicapped children in which children receive developmental stimulation for their basic needs as children and therapy for their handicapping condition. Maintenance in this sense is a dynamic therapy because it is active intervention to maintain health. It is not just routine physical care which, without stimulating experiences, might lead to regressive behavior. I rank these programs in the midposition because they are no longer hospital-based and because they deal with both prevention and rehabilitation

Preschool programs for healthy children have been available for many years. Now, preschool programs for handicapped children, similar to the Handicapped Children's Preschool in Roxbury, Massachusetts, are evolving to prepare the children for public schools, whenever possible. If not possible, the preschool staff determines the kind of community programs which would be most beneficial to the child's development. These preschools usually define a specific child population. For example, it must be determined which children need experience in a protective emotional and physical environment. A choice must be made as to which place is best for a child, such as the child with hemophilia. He may be most suitably placed in a preschool for healthy, nonhandicapped children because physically handicapped children often lack muscular control and balance which could lead to the unintentional injury of the hemophiliac child.

Preschools for nonhandicapped children might be more willing to accept handicapped children if a support team of therapists and a nurse were available to them. This would be a solution to the placement of handicapped children in preschool programs and would be financially desirable. The support team would serve as a liaison between the child's nursery school teachers and his medical team. The support team might include occupational, physical and speech therapists and a nurse, each of whom could offer the teachers specific information on handling the child and his therapy. The member of the team who could provide the teachers with the most information about a particular child would be the liaison. If the child showed overall developmental delay, the occupational therapist probably would be the teachers' primary resource (other support team members would give the occupational therapist information as he needed it); on the other hand, if the child had primary problems in speech, language and hearing, the speech clinician would be the liaison.

Early treatment in the form of *home care* by the parents, under supervision of the developmental therapist, helps eliminate the incapacitating disability which later appears. For example, the diagnosis and treatment of a visual deficit may decrease the possibility of later perceptual problems. Some correction can be made through therapy after the diagnosis of physical defects is made and before the dysfunction is too well established. Developmental stimulation of the blind or deaf infant will decrease excessive lag in development at a later date. With the recognition of psychological or social behavior problems, suggestions may be made to help parents deal with the behavior. The objective of the therapist's intervention is to prevent the parents from developing a negative attitude toward their infant which could increase as the child grows. With the recognition of environmental deprivation, inexpensive materials and common household items can be recommended for stimulation to compensate for the inadequacies. The values of developmental therapy within the first year cannot be overemphasized. New parents, particularly, need help; some are overanxious while others are unaware of the existing or potential problems.

Perlmutter [18] emphasizes three points in presenting a rationale for early evaluation and treatment. She states that (1) the optimal treatment interventions frequently occur before twelve months of age in cases of birth defects, infant diseases, and so forth; (2) that it is essential for the family to be involved in *designing* and *executing* patient treatment if the treatment is to be successful; and (3) that early treatment offers the pediatric patient the best chance of attaining normal levels of function. In further describing the last point, Perlmutter states that dysfunctional compensatory behaviors have not had time to develop, so treatment time need not be spent on undoing the compensatory behaviors. In addition, the human organism has the unique characteristic of plasticity and potential responsiveness in the first twelve months of age which gradually diminishes with maturation. Successful treatment — which Perlmutter describes as the attainment of a level of functioning that is within normal limits — is also advantageous to the therapist. It is very gratifying to watch an infant develop, especially when the child was originally diagnosed as a poor candidate for life or therapy. It enhances the professional image of the therapist in the eyes of other skeptical health care workers. It provides an opportunity to experiment with and to develop new treatment techniques which can be transmitted to other health care workers.

Richmond and Weinberger's presentation of statistics supports Perlmutter's comments. They suggest that "between 20 and 40 percent of all children suffer from one or more chronic conditions and that the majority could benefit from treatment." [19] They go on to estimate that *through comprehensive care during the first six years of life at least a third of the handicaps would be prevented or corrected and through care during the first eighteen years of life about sixty percent of the handicaps would be prevented or corrected.*

Community-based health facilities are best situated to serve the needs of health education and prevention. Well-baby clinics and day care centers can serve the infant, toddler and preschooler, while school health programs can be developed to meet the health needs of school-age children. Many children's diseases have been conquered and now the majority of health problems occur as a result of the child's interaction with his environment. For example, the main cause of death for children between 1941 and

1961 was accidents.¹ This trend is reversible with more and better health education for children and their parents.

Community health centers offer many valuable services and exciting possibilities for the developmental therapist. With the advent of community health clinics in the low-income and poverty areas, people are more willing to seek health care because they do not have to travel very far and transportation may be more accessible. In addition, the community members have a shorter waiting time in the small community clinic as compared to the time spent waiting in the hospital clinics which serve a much larger population. Within the community clinics, the families become well acquainted with the physicians, nurses and other personnel and become receptive to learning about the prevention of illness and disability. In the long run, this reduces the need for crisis intervention. For example, the pregnant woman learns about nutritional needs of the child which she, in turn, uses in planning meals for the rest of her family; she learns about toxic materials in her home which are dangerous to her young children, such as poison in lead-based paint, aspirin, other common medications and cleaning substances. With this knowledge, the mother can provide a safer environment and better care for her own child. Parents are more willing to bring their child to a convenient well-baby clinic where they know the staff and they are more likely to follow the recommendations for preventive practices made at this clinic than at the large impersonal hospital clinic.

Day care centers may be available for both nonhandicapped and handicapped children. They relieve mother of her child-care responsibilities for a portion of the day so she might work to support her family or to supplement the family income. This may be desirable for parents at any income level. A day care program for nonhandicapped children can be planned which will be therapeutic for the handicapped child. At the same time, the parents can be relieved of some of the intensive 24-hour-a-day care and responsibility which is emotionally draining — sometimes to the point of their being unable to offer much emotionally to their other children.

Caldwell and Smith [20] have briefly described a group day care program for children as young as six months of age. They stress the need for quality day care which again implies the need for highly trained people who have a solid knowledge of child development. They stress planning for the child's developmental age rather than the chronological age, the need for the program to supplement the family unit in preference to substituting for the family and the inclusion of the parents in the program. Because of the work schedules, the latter was difficult to implement and, therefore, the parent program had to be individualized. Observations of the children over a period of time after the initial testing indicated healthy changes and gains in both the cognitive and emotional areas. Since this program's inception in 1964, Caldwell and Smith have concluded that the day care group does serve as an enrichment experience for the infant, toddler and preschooler and have begun to document this information.

Day care centers need developmental therapists to execute or supervise daily developmental therapists to execute or supervise daily developmental stimulation.Experts in early childhood education, occupational therapy, child psychology, special education and other related fields all are potential candidates. Some day care programs emphasize only the routine physical care of the child (balanced diets, toileting, handwashing, naps, and so forth) and have minimal *planned* play experiences based on the children's developmental needs. The most beneficial kind of day care center offers (1) a stimulating environment which suggests play activities to stimulate all areas of development and (2) a staff who know how to use the environment and themselves to stimulate maximum development.

If the handicapped child's dysfunction has been diagnosed early and is not severe, he may adjust readily to a program for nonhandicapped children. However, the staff in the day care program which accepts handicapped children may need psychological support and assistance from the developmental therapists. These therapists can offer specific ideas about self-care and developmental tasks as well as information on the disability and special care needs.

The *public school* also uses the services of the developmental therapists in programs of prevention and corrrection (especially nurses, psychologists, speech therapists and occupational therapists). Traditionally, the occupational therapist evaluated and treated individuals or small groups of children in the occupational therapy room in the school. The occupational therapist, however, may be part of a team of developmental therapists who work with teachers and therapists in the public school to screen children on entrance. As stated by Cowen,[21] who described "Denver's Preventive Health Program for School-Age Children," children should be evaluated and treated for disability and illness long before the school years begin, but since this is not presently feasible, schools must begin to participate in prevention while departments of public health and mental health gradually develop evaluation and treatment programs for the younger age group.

The Falmouth, Massachusetts, school system is another example of ways in which to use developmental therapists. They requested help from the Division of Family Health Services, Massachusetts Department of Public Health, in revising their school health program which was both inadequate and inefficient. As part of the overall plan to provide better health services for the school children, I coordinated an inservice course on developmental evaluation and stimulation for forty Falmouth school staff. Staff included teachers of kindergarten, first grade, transitional first grade, special education, Headstart and physical education; guidance counselors and school nurses. The ostensible objective of the course was to select or develop a screening test for the kindergarten which would pick up developmental delay or dysfunction. However, the secondary goals were equally important: (1) to develop an awareness of and ability to evaluate children's developmental needs (2) to learn ways in which to stimulate children's development and (3) to learn how to use developmental therapists from the community to further evaluate and/or treat children whose problems are greater than the competence of the school teachers.

In addition to screening children for potential disabilities, provisions must be made for the children who are known to be handicapped. Once the child is developmentally ready for kindergarten or elementary school, the parents, child and developmental therapists who have worked with the child choose the school program from which the child will benefit the most. A school without architectural or other barriers, which is located in the community in which the family lives, is most desirable. The teachers and school administrators are even more important for they may have to make adjustments in the curriculum, the classroom environment and their own routines and responsibilities to meet the needs of the handicapped child. Too often the response of school personnel is "We're not insured against an injury to him — he might be knocked down or fall downstairs." Perhaps the educator knows little about the child's handicap and, therefore, legitimately feels inadequate in dealing with him in the classroom. Information gained on disability from inservice training, similar to the Falmouth model, and/or the use of support personnel as described for preschools, probably would help relieve some of these fears.

The occupational therapist has other functions with the school-age child. They may include helping the child shift from the protective environment of the preschool or day care program to the classroom environment in the public school or working with the child in the home classroom. It may involve helping the teacher deal with her fears of the handicapped child. The therapist, for example, may have the child demonstrate his skills for the teacher such as self-care, walking and sitting down on a classroom chair at a desk, and then can explain any restrictions or precautions to the teacher. "Be sure the child holds onto the rail when walking up and down stairs. His climbing is okay, but sometimes unsteady and occasionally, he needs to be reminded to hold onto the rail." (In some situations this education might be the responsibility of the nurse or preschool teacher.) Other useful comments might be: "These are the ways in which we help Sam deal with the laughter or stares of other children..."

The therapist may continue to treat the child directly at his school or may become a consultant to the teacher who will be the provider of the services to the child. Some teachers have responded favorably to a report based on the informal developmental evaluation described in Chapter Eight, which specifically shows the child's progress over a period of time, his immediate goals and recommendations for attaining them. With this information, combined with observation of the child in the preschool or treatment setting, the teacher probably will feel prepared to handle the child and will feel comfortable about referring to the child's developmental therapists for further information.

Not all handicapped children can attend public schools because of the architectural and attitudinal barriers of schools and school personnel or because of the severe multiply handicapping conditions which preclude successful learning. Again, the community health center is the ideal place for dissemination of services to the child. Preferably the child can attend some kind of daily program outside the home, such as a community or prevocational program for severely handicapped children. Otherwise, the developmental therapist may evaluate and treat the child in his home.

The Personnel Choice

Correlating the fact that one-fourth of the children in this country live in poverty with the fact that there are few health services available in poverty areas, occupational therapists and other developmental therapists must reconsider their job aspirations. Therapists must move out of the confines of the hospital and provide services, at least part time, in the inner city and rural areas. According to the multiple reports on contemporary health care needs, children in poverty areas need priority care. Even if the developmental therapist accepts this as his priority, he still has the option of choosing the children whom he will serve.

The question of "With whom will the developmental therapist work?" is difficult for many therapists to answer objectively. There are children whose handicaps are so subtle, they are hardly discernible until the child enters a situation in which his handicap is in the forefront. The environmentally deprived child may function adequately in his neighborhood but have problems in the public school; the perceptually handicapped young child may not realize he has problems until he attends public school. On the other hand, infants with multiple congenital deformities are visibly handicapped from birth and children with syndromes resulting from congenital retardation are soon recognized. There are children with terminal diseases and children with acute but temporary diseases.

It is essential that each developmental therapist work efficiently and effectively as well as working to satisfy his own needs. At the same time, the therapist must provide the child and his family with maximum benefits. Therefore, in selecting the patient population and/or work situation, it may be useful for the occupational therapist to ask himself (and others) some questions. His answers will vary depending upon the community, the needs of the children, the other developmental therapists' availability and his own personal and professional assets and liabilities.

1. Which treatment is essential to the habilitation or rehabilitation of the child considering his immediate and long-range developmental needs?
2. Which therapies can be omitted without being detrimental to the child?
3. With which of the therapists is the child and his family most comfortable?
4. Who helps the child and family communicate with other health care personnel?
5. Is the evaluation and treatment necessary which I plan to do with the child?
6. Are other developmental therapists better qualified to treat the child? Or is someone who is less qualified, but available, able to treat the child under my supervision?

Effective utilization of a professional or nonprofessional person may differ at different points in the individual's career. This may be the result of his own growth within the profession that takes him from the traditional staff therapist position, for example, to student supervisor, and finally to administrator of a department or program. Or, professional development may proceed in an unanticipated direction into another area which is not directly related to the original profession. We should never permit ourselves or others to feel boxed in by a professional title — this can be compared with Piaget who did not want to feel boxed in by a narrow and therefore constricting definition of intelligence and cognition. One person who informally (outside of an academic program) and thoroughly studies and applies new material may become equally or more competent than the person who originally knew the material but ceased to use it or develop it further.

I believe that with the increase in time and experience after the years of formal education, the pureness of professional knowledge and practice decreases. Only in this way does a profession or a person within a profession develop. New ideas always are needed, some of which are discarded as they prove to be irrelevant to work being done or developed; others are incorporated into the theory of the profession. As stated by Zimmerman,[22] the professional titles, content, and divisions of today probably will not be those of tomorrow. For example, much of the content of this text is not pure occupational therapy. Yet, knowledge of this content is important to the successful practice of occupational therapy today, even though tomorrow may see part of it outdated.

Hopefully, the content of this book will help the occupational therapist answer the questions of where, with whom and what to practice. In the final analysis, however, the choice of patient population is a personal one. It may be based on the theory to which the therapist intellectually ascribes. It may reflect the financial considerations of who will financially support the program or from which children will there be the biggest return on the investment of therapy. Or, the choice may be primarily subjective and emotional. Which child do I care about the most or which child rewards me the most by his response to therapy? Or where is there a job opening?

Initially, most therapists are drawn to a particular kind of child. They have varied reasons for working with handicapped children in preference to working with normal children or working with children rather than working with adults. Therapists also choose to "specialize" in one kind of handicapping condition instead of another, such as working with children who are emotionally disturbed as opposed to working with mentally retarded children.

The therapist needs to explore the reasons for his working with one child or group of children instead of another. Does he, the therapist, feel rewarded and gratified by children and their responses to him? Is this based on a fear of working with adults? Is it based on the need to have power and control over handicapped children which appears to be easier than control over active, healthy children? Is it the result of feeling pity for sick children? Or, is it a problem-solving intrigue — a desire to go beyond the normal routine and to explore the problems involved in working with handicapped children? The therapist's reasons for working with the handicapped child should be objective enough to prevent the exaggeration of his own problems or the projection of his own problems onto the child.

Even within the framework of the broad categorization of the treatment group chosen by the therapist, such as children with emotional or physical problems, decisions must be made about which children to treat. Some therapists firmly believe that with the shift to community health care, developmental therapists should emphasize prophylaxis and treatment of the group with minimal problems who can respond to treatment and become contributors to society. Others have more empathy with the multiply handicapped child who already has three strikes against him. There is a place for the treatment of all children with problems of all degrees. The therapist ideally works with the children whom he feels most qualified to help both professionally and personally.

References

1. Richmond, J.B. and Weinberger, H.L. "Session II—Program Implications of New Knowledge Regarding the Physical, Intellectual, and Emotional Growth and Development and the Unmet Needs of Children and Youth." *American Journal of Public Health Supplement* 60(1970), pp. 23-67.
2. Beloff, J.S. and Willet, M. "The Health Care Team." *Journal of the American Medical Association* 205(1968), pp. 663-669.
3. Silverman, I.: Personal communication, 1970.
4. Gellis, S.G. "You as a Pediatrician." In Love, A. and Childers, J.S. *Listen to Leaders in Medicine* (New York: Holt, Rinehart and Winston, 1963).
5. Grossman, F. Personal communication, 1970.
6. West, W.L. "The Occupational Therapist's Changing Responsibility to the Community." *Americal Journal of Occupational Therapy* 21(1967), p. 312.
7. Roth, M.E., Ehinger, R.F. and Mosher, W.E. "The Value of Coordinated and Comprehensive Home Care." *American Journal of Public Health* 57(1967), pp. 1841-1847.
8. Johnson, J.A. *A Systems Analysis of Defined Collaborative Relationships at a College of Allied Health Professions* (Doctoral Dissertation, Boston University School of Education, 1970).
9. Johnson, J.A., p. 40.

522

10. Andrews, P., Yankauer, A. and Connelly, J.P. "Changing the Patterns of Ambulatory Pediatric Caretaking: An Action-Oriented Training Program for Nurses." *American Journal of Public Health* 60(1970), pp. 870-879.
11. West, W.L., pp. 312-316.
12. West, W.L., p. 313.
13. West, W.L., p. 314.
14. West, W.L., p. 315.
15. Albee, G.W. "Models, Myths, and Manpower." *Mental Hygiene* 52(1968), pp. 168-180.
16. Wiemer, R.B. "Prevention: What is Occupational Therapy's Role?" (Paper presented at American Occupational Therapy Association Annual Conference, New York, 1970).
17. Ickeringill, N. "Turning Mother into Teacher." *The New York Times* July 7, 1970.
18. Perlmutter, S.A. Presentation at American Occupational Therapy Association Annual Conference, New York, 1970.
19. Richmond, J.B. and Weinberger, H.L., p. 37.
20. Caldwell, B.M. and Smith, L.E. "Day Care for the Very Young—Prime Opportunity for Primary Prevention." *American Journal of Public Health* 60(1970), pp. 690-697.
21. Cowen, D.L. "Denver's Preventive Health Program for School-Age Children." *Americal Journal of Public Health* 60(1970), pp. 515-518.
22. Zimmerman, T.F. "Laddering and Latticing: Trends in Allied Health." *Americal Journal of Occupational Therapy* 24(1970), pp. 102-105.

Bibliography

Barry, M.C. and Sheps, C.G. "A New Model for Community Health Planning." *American Journal of Public Health* 59(1969), pp. 226-236.

Brown, H.J. "Changes in the Delivery of Health Care." *American Journal of Nursing* 68(1968), pp. 2362-2364.

Cowen, D.L. "Denver's Neighborhood Health Program." *Public Health Reports* 84(1969), pp. 1027-1031.

Ellwood, P.M. "Can We Afford So Many Rehabilitation Professions? *Journal of Rehabilitation* May-June (1968), pp. 21-22.

Fein, R. "The Doctor Shortage: An Economic Diagnosis." *The Brookings Study in Social Economics* (Washington, D.C.: The Brookings Institution, 1967).

Hunter, G.T. "Health Care Through Head Start." *Children* 17(1970), pp. 149-153.

Ishiyama, T. "Staffing Patterns—A Solution to the Manpower Shortage." *Mental Hygiene* 52(1968), pp. 199-203.

Katz, L.G. "Teaching in Preschools: Roles and Goals." *Children* 17(1970), pp. 42-48.

Magraw, R.A. *Ferment in Medicine* (Philadelphia: W.B. Saunders Co., 1966).

Mazer, J.L. "The Occupational Therapist as Consultant." *American Journal of Occupational Therapy* 23(1969), pp. 417-421.

New, P.K. "An Analysis of the Concept of Teamwork." *Community Mental Health Journal* 4(1968), pp. 326-333.

Pochert, L. "Our New Role Challenge: The Occupational Therapy Consultant." *American Journal of Occupational Therapy* 24(1970), pp. 106-110.

Sarason, S.B. et al. *Psychology in Community Settings; Clinical, Educational, Vocational, Social Aspects* (New York: John Wiley, 1966).

Taylor, K.O. "Trends in Hospital Use." *Public Health Reports* 84(1969), pp. 1037-1042.

West, W.L. "1967 Eleanor Clarke Slagle Lecture: Professional Responsibility in Times of Change." *American Journal of Occupational Therapy* 22(1968), pp. 9-15.

West, W.L. "The University-Affiliated Center: History and Philosophy" (Paper presented at the Conference on the Training Function of Occupational Therapy in University-Affiliated Centers, Los Angeles, 1969).

West, W.L. "The Growing Importance of Prevention." *American Journal of Occupational Therapy* 23(1969), pp. 226-231.

West, W.L. and Wiemer, R.B. "Occupational Therapy in Community Health Care." *American Journal of Occupational Therapy* 24(1970), pp. 323-328.

Zigler, E.F. "A National Priority: Raising the Quality of Children's Lives." *Children* 17(1970), pp. 166-170.

NOTES

Index

D

P

Retardation — developmental, 242
Reversibility, 380
Reward (*See* Reinforcement).
Rhythm, 356
Rolling, 137
Rood system, 184, 193
Rooting reflex, 133, 215, 238
Routine, 101, 102

S

Sadistic behavior, 239
Schemes (Piaget), 365, 368
School phobia, 234
Screening tests (DDST), 420
Self-actualizing theory, 11
Self-image.
    self-image, 85, 218
    self-image — evaluation of, 254,
    self-image — failure in development, 242, 243
Semiotic function, 371
Sensorimotor intelligence, 362, 371
Sensory testing, 174
Separation.
    separation-individuation, failure to separate, 244
    separation-individuation, treatment of, 256
Sequencing, 305
Sequential development, 84, 397, 398
Sexuality,
    sex education, 248
    sexual identification, 89
    sexual image defined, 220, 221
Shaping behavior, 262, 263
Sibling rivalry, 235
Signs (Piaget), 369, 371, 373 (*Also see* Symbols)
Sitting, 138 (thought).
Size — discrimination and constancy, 284, 286-289
Sleep disturbances, 232
Smiling response, 215, 225
Social.
    social behavior, 58, 93, 224, 225, 408, 423
    social development, 80, 111, 224
    social behavior in superego development, 225, 226
Sociopathic reactions, 239, 250, 266, 268
Solitary play, 227
Somatotypes, 128
Spastic hemiplegia, 162
Spastic quadriplegia, 160
Spastic paraplegia (diplegia), 161
Speech.
    speech-definition, 344
    speech disorders, 353, 356
Splinter skill, 23, 392
Standardized testing, 32, 34, 45, 58, 50, 302, 406, 420

NOTES